Seventh Edition

BD Chaurasia's

Handbook of General Anatomy

As per the latest NMC Guidelines | Competency Based Medical Education (CBME) Curriculum under Graduate Medical Education Regulation

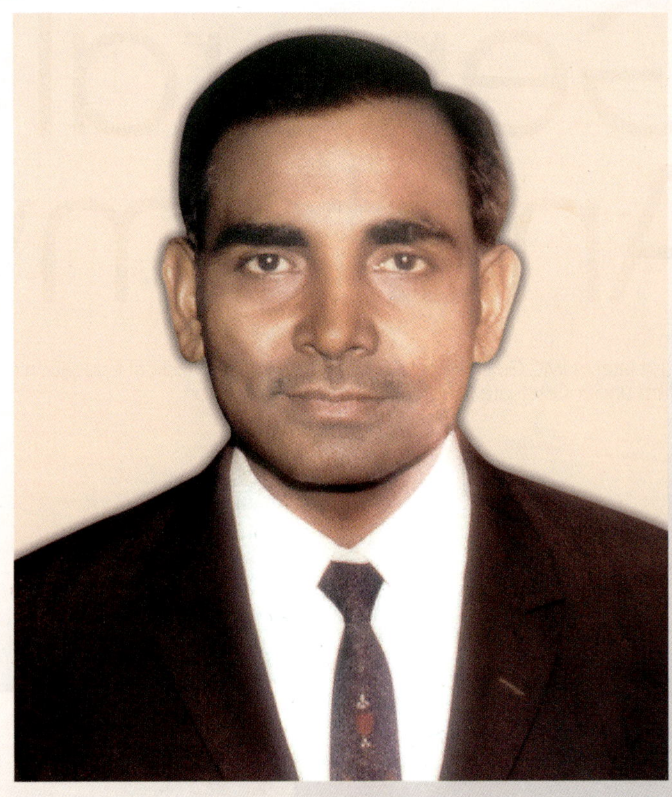

Late Dr BD Chaurasia
(1937–1985)

Seventh Edition

BD Chaurasia's Handbook of General Anatomy

As per the latest NMC Guidelines | Competency Based Medical Education (CBME) Curriculum under Graduate Medical Education Regulation

Late Dr BD Chaurasia

MBBS, MS, PhD, FAMS

Department of Anatomy
GR Medical College
Gwalior, India

Revised and Edited by

Krishna Garg

MBBS, MS, PhD, FIMSA, FIAMS, FAMS,
Chikitsa Ratan and FASI

Ex-Professor and Head, Department of Anatomy
Lady Hardinge Medical College, New Delhi

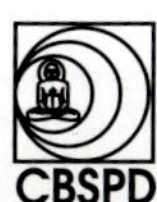

CBS Publishers & Distributors Pvt Ltd

New Delhi • Bengaluru • Chennai • Kochi • Kolkata • Lucknow • Mumbai
Gujarat • Hyderabad • Jharkhand • Nagpur • Patna • Pune • Uttarakhand

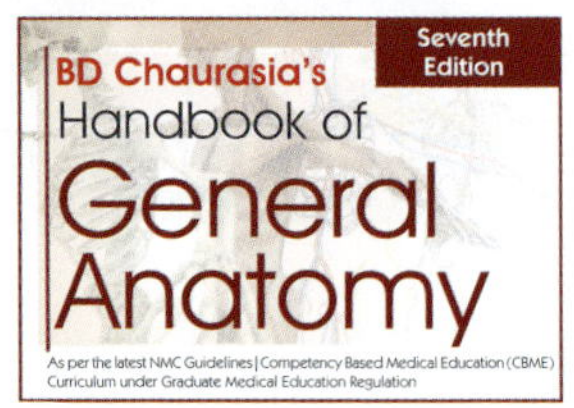

ISBN: 978-93-5466-569-1

Seventh Edition: 2024[1]
Reprint: 2025, **2026**
First Edition: 1978
Reprint: 1980, 1981
Second Edition: 1983
Reprint: 1985, 1987, 1989, 1991, 1992, 1994, 1996
Third Edition: 1996
Reprint: 1998, 1999, 2000, 2001, 2002, 2003, 2004
Fourth Edition: 2009
Reprint: 2010, 2011, 2012, 2013, 2014
Fifth Edition: 2015
Reprint: 2016, 2017, 2018, 2019
Sixth Edition: 2020[3]
Reprint: 2021, 2022, 2023

Disclaimer

Science and technology are constantly changing fields. New research and experience broaden the scope of information and knowledge. The editor has tried her best in giving information available to her while preparing the material for this book. Although all efforts have been made to ensure optimum accuracy of the material, yet it is quite possible some errors might have been left uncorrected. The publisher, the printer and the editor will not be held responsible for any inadvertent errors, omissions or inaccuracies.

Published by Satish Kumar Jain and produced by Varun Jain for

CBS Publishers & Distributors Pvt Ltd
4819/XI Prahlad Street, 24 Ansari Road, Daryaganj, New Delhi 110 002, India
Ph: 011-23266838, 23289259 Website: www.cbspd.com
e-mail: delhi@cbspd.com

Corporate Office: 204 FIE, Industrial Area, Patparganj, Delhi 110 092, India
Ph: 011-4934 4934 Fax: 011-4934 4935 e-mail: publishing@cbspd.com; publicity@cbspd.com

Branches

- **Bengaluru:** Seema House 2975, 17th Cross, KR Road, Banasankari 2nd Stage, Bengaluru 560 070, Karnataka, India
  Ph: +91-80-26771678/79 Fax: +91-80-26771680 e-mail: bangalore@cbspd.com
- **Chennai:** 18/8B, Subbarayan Street, Shenoy Nagar, Chennai 600 030, Tamil Nadu, India
  Ph: +91-44-42032115, 45022115 e-mail: chennai@cbspd.com
- **Kochi:** 42/1325, 1326, Power House Road, Opp KSEB, Power House, Ernakulum Kochi 682 018, Kerala, India
  Ph: +91-484-4059061-65,67 Fax: +91-484-4059065 e-mail: kochi@cbspd.com
- **Kolkata:** 147, Hind Ceramics Compound, 1st Floor, Nilgunj Road, Belghoria, Kolkata 700 056, West Bengal, India
  Ph: +91-33-25633055/56 e-mail: kolkata@cbspd.com
- **Lucknow:** Basement, Khushnuma Complex, 7 Meerabai Marg (behind Jawahar Bhawan), Lucknow 226 001, UP, India
  Ph: +91-522-4000032 e-mail: tiwari.lucknow@cbspd.com
- **Mumbai:** PWD Shed, Gala no 25/26, Ramchandra Bhatt Marg, Next to JJ Hospital Gate no. 2, Opp. Union Bank of India, Noorbaug, Mumbai 400 009, Maharashtra, India
  Ph: +91-22-66661880/89 e-mail: mumbai@cbspd.com

Representatives

- **Gujarat** • **Hyderabad** • **Jharkhand** • **Nagpur** • **Patna** • **Pune** • **Uttarakhand**

For trade terms please contact customercare@cbspd.com
For general enquiries please contact info@cbspd.com

Printed at: Paras Offset Pvt. Ltd, New Delhi, India

Preface to the Seventh Edition

Most popular and student-friendly *BD Chaurasia's Handbook of General Anatomy* for MBBS, BDS, physiotherapy and occupational therapy students has been upgraded by improving the diagrams and revising the text.

However, the highlight of this edition is the addition of chapters of various systems of the body, including their gross and clinical anatomy, thus giving a bird's-eye view of these important areas. These seven newly added chapters are respiratory system, digestive system, sensory organs, endocrine system, urinary system, reproductive system (both male and female) and "Cadaver as our first teacher". This will make the study of gross anatomy and clinical anatomy holistic in nature.

Thus the *Handbook of General Anatomy* now no longer remains the book for general anatomy only but it also includes brief study of all the systems. So it almost becomes a mini textbook for our dear students.

This edition has been designed as per the latest NMC Guidelines | Competency Based Medical Education (CBME) Curriculum under Graduate Medical Education Regulation.

Thanks to Mr Sanjay Chauhan, Mr Sushil Rawat and Mr Prasenjit Paul who have diligently done the graphic designing, formatting and proofreading of the book.

My heartfelt thanks are to Mr SK Jain CMD, Mr Varun Jain Director, Mr YN Arjuna Senior Vice President—Publishing, Editorial and Publicity and Ms Ritu Chawla General Manager (Production) for encouraging and helping me all the time.

Suggestions for rectification and improvement are welcome. These may be sent at dr.krishnagarg@gmail.com

My first and last thanks are to Almighty for directing and guiding the intellect along the right path.

Krishna Garg
Editor

Preface to the First Edition

This *Handbook of General Anatomy* has been written to meet the requirements of students who are newly admitted to medical colleges. It thoroughly introduces the greater part of medical terminology, as well as the various structures which constitute the human body. On account of the late admissions and the shorter time now available for teaching anatomy, the coverage of general anatomy seems to suffer maximum. Since it lays down the foundation of the entire subject of medicine, it was felt necessary to produce a short, simple and comprehensive handbook on this neglected, though important, aspect of the subject. It has been written in a simple language, with the text classified in small parts to make it easier for the students to follow and remember. It is hoped that this will prove quite useful to the medical students.

Gwalior
November 1978

BD CHAURASIA

Index of Competencies

Competency based Undergraduate Curriculum for the Indian Medical Graduate

Contents

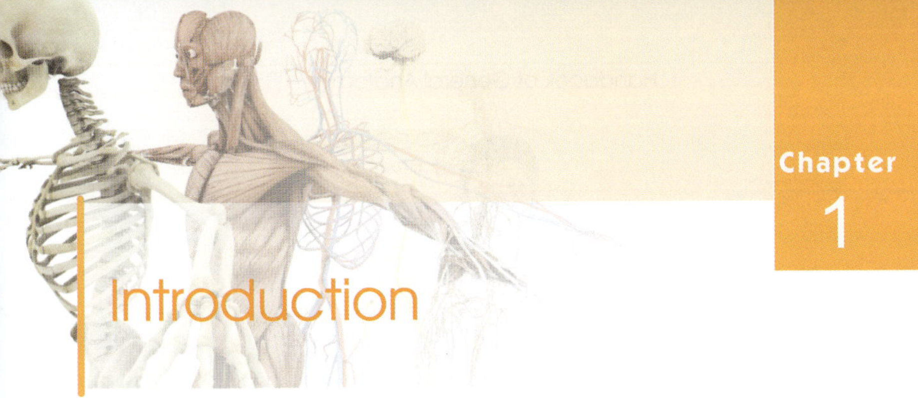

Chapter 1

Introduction

Life is a book with three chapters. Two are already written by God—birth and death. The chapter in the middle is empty; fill it with smile, love and faith.

Human anatomy is the science which deals with the structure of the human body. The term, 'anatomy', is derived from a Greek word, "anatome", meaning cutting up. The term 'dissection' is a Latin equivalent of the Greek *anatome*. However, the two words, anatomy and dissection, are not synonymous. Dissection is a mere technique, whereas anatomy is a wide field of study.

Anatomy forms firm foundation of the whole art of medicine and introduces the student to the greater part of medical terminology. "Anatomy is to physiology as geography is to history, i.e. it describes the theatre in which the action takes place."

SUBDIVISIONS OF ANATOMY

Initially, anatomy was studied mainly by dissection. But the scope of modern anatomy has become very wide because it is now studied by all possible techniques which can enlarge the boundaries of the anatomical knowledge.

The main subdivisions of anatomy are:

1. ***Cadaveric anatomy*** is studied on dead embalmed (preserved) bodies usually with the naked eye (macroscopic or gross anatomy). This can be done by one of the two approaches:
   a. In *regional anatomy* the body is studied in parts, like the upper limb, lower limb, thorax, abdomen, head and neck, and brain (Fig. 1.1).

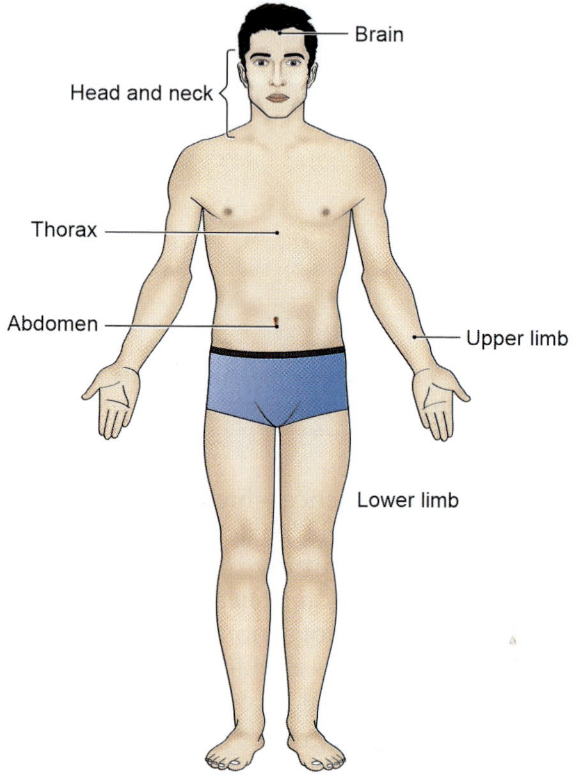

Fig. 1.1: Various regions of the body

b. In *systemic anatomy* the body is studied in systems, like the skeletal system (osteology), muscular system (myology), articulatory system (arthrology or syndesmology), vascular system (angiology), nervous system (neurology), and respiratory, digestive, urogenital and endocrine systems (splanchnology). The locomotor system includes osteology, arthrology and myology. These systems are briefly mentioned close to the end of this chapter.

2. ***Living anatomy*** is studied by inspection (Fig. 1.2a), palpation (Fig. 1.2b), percussion (Fig. 1.2c), auscultation (Fig. 1.2d), endoscopy (bronchoscopy, gastroscopy), radiography, electromyography, etc.

3. ***Embryology (developmental anatomy)*** is the study of the prenatal developmental changes in an individual (Fig. 1.3). The developmental history is called 'ontogeny'. The evolutionary history, on the other hand, is called 'phylogeny'.

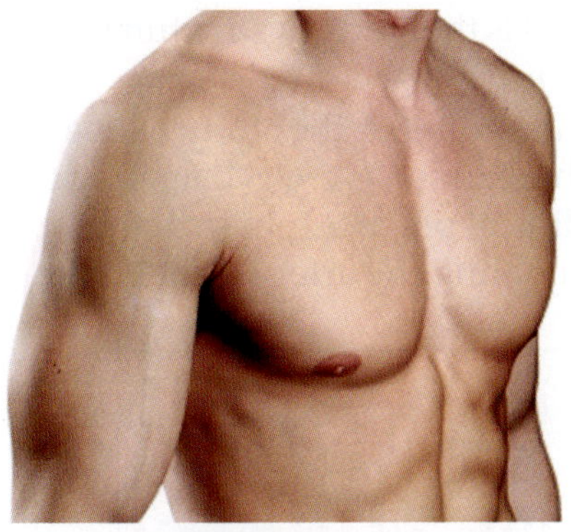
Fig. 1.2a: Inspection of the chest

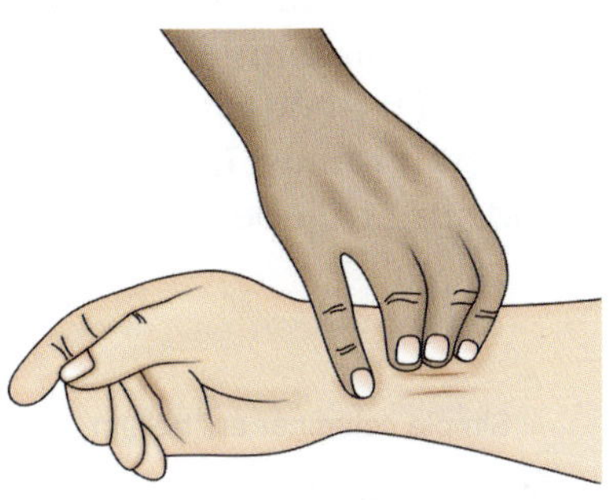
Fig. 1.2b: Palpation

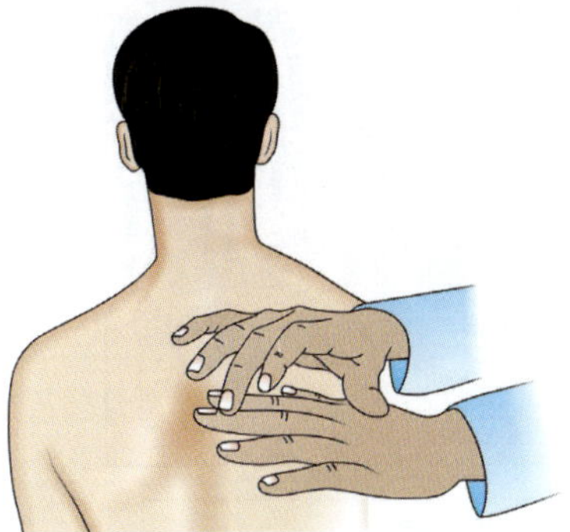
Fig. 1.2c: Percussion

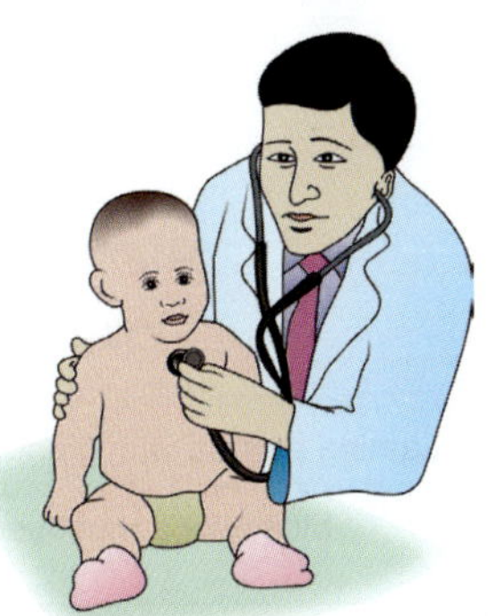
Fig. 1.2d: Auscultation

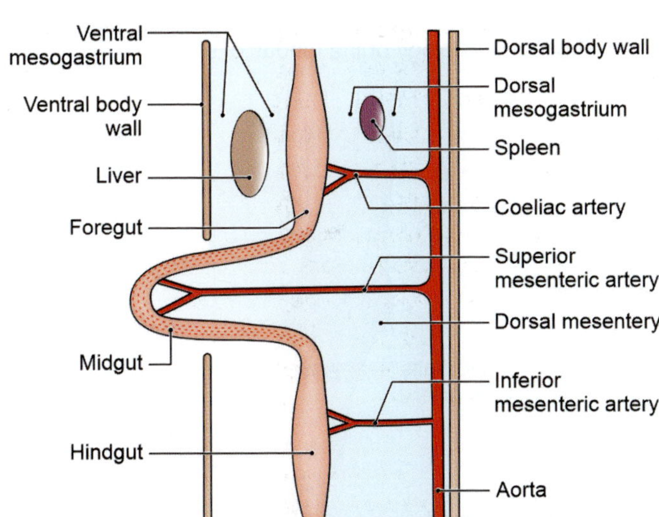

Fig. 1.3: Development of various parts of the gut

4. ***Histology (microscopic anatomy)*** is the study of structures with the aid of a microscope (Fig. 1.4).
5. ***Surface anatomy (topographic anatomy)*** is the study of deeper parts of the body in relation to the skin surface, e.g. palpating the artery. It is most important in clinical practice, physical therapy and surgical operations, e.g. palpating the artery (Fig. 1.5).

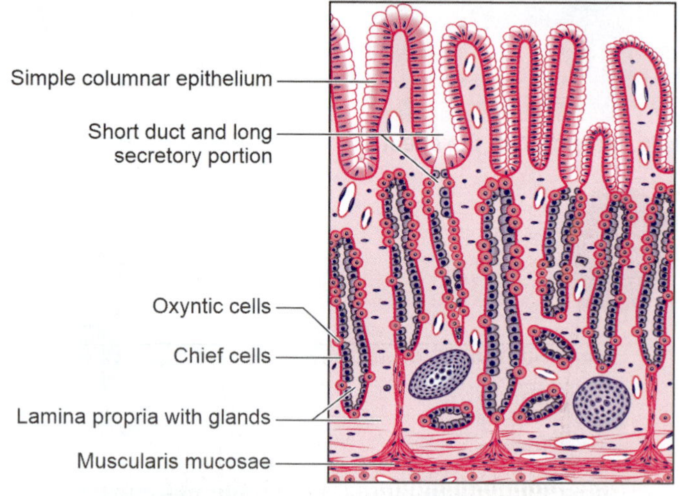

- All epithelial cells are simple columnar in type
- Parietal cells are large and pink, chief cells are small and blue
- Duct is 1/3rd, secretory part is 2/3rd

Fig. 1.4: Histology of the fundus of stomach

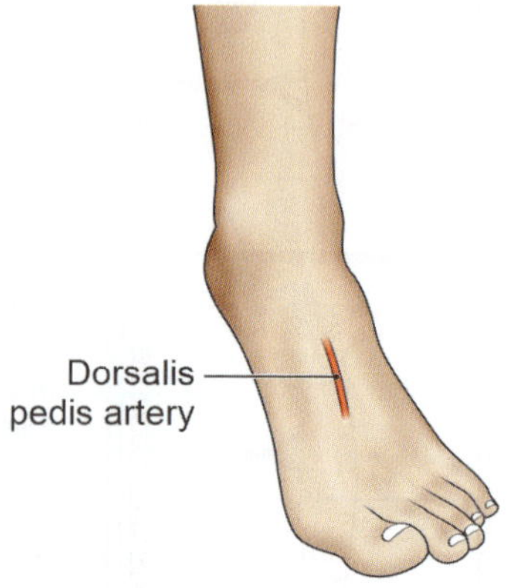

Fig. 1.5: Palpating the dorsalis pedis artery

6. ***Radiographic and imaging anatomy*** is the study of the bones and deeper organs by plain and contrast radiography, by ultrasound and computerised tomographic (CT) scans (Fig. 1.6).
7. ***Comparative anatomy*** is the study of anatomy of the other animals to explain the changes in form, structure and function (morphology) of different parts of the human body.
8. ***Physical anthropology*** deals with the external features and measurements of different races and groups of people, and with the study of the prehistoric remains (Fig. 1.7).
9. ***Applied anatomy (clinical anatomy)*** deals with application of the anatomical knowledge to the medical and surgical practice (Fig. 1.8).

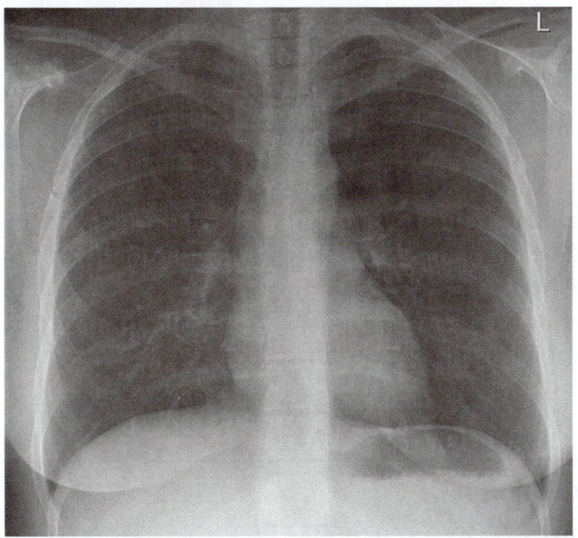

Fig. 1.6: X-ray Chest: Posteroanterior view

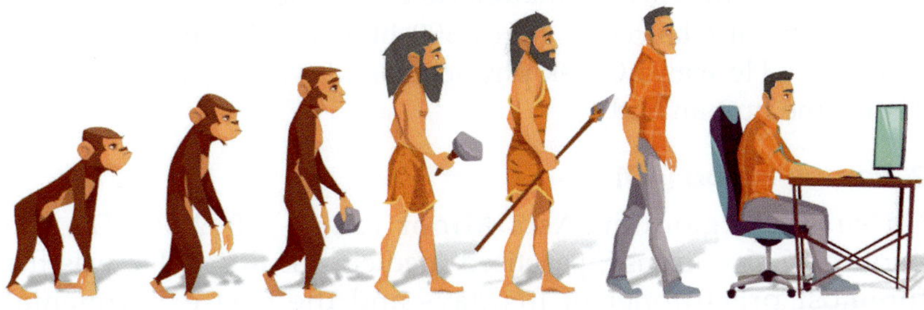

Fig. 1.7: Physical anthropology

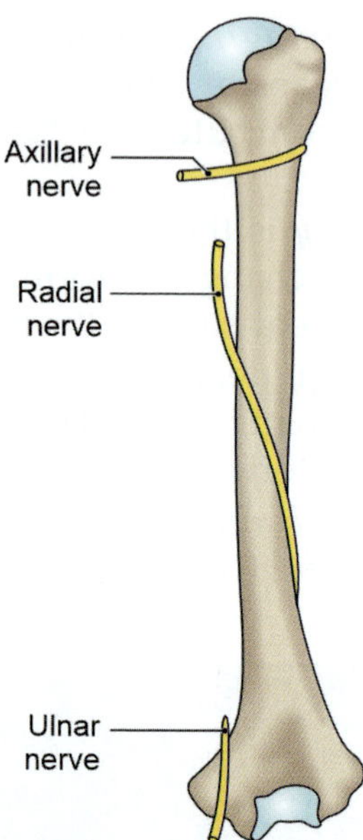

Fig. 1.8: The relation of nerves to the posterior aspect of humerus

10. ***Experimental anatomy*** is the study of the factors which influence and determine the form, structure and function of different parts of the body.
11. ***Genetics*** deals with the study of information present in the chromosomes (*see* Chapter 17).

HISTORY OF ANATOMY

1. Greek Period (BC)

Hippocrates of Cos (circa 400 BC), the 'father of medicine', is regarded as one of the founders of anatomy. Parts of hippocratic collection are the earliest anatomical descriptions.

Herophilus of Chalcedon (circa 300 BC) is called the "father of anatomy". He was a Greek physician, and was one of the first to dissect the human body.

2. Roman Period (AD)

Galen of Pergamum, Asia Minor (circa 130–200 AD), the "prince of physicians", practised medicine at Rome. He was the foremost practitioner of his days and the first experimental physiologist.

3. Fourteenth Century

Mundinus or Mondino d'Luzzi (1276–1326), the 'restorer of anatomy', was an Italian anatomist and professor of anatomy at Bologna.

4. Fifteenth Century

Leonardo da Vinci of Italy (1452–1519), the originator of cross sectional anatomy, was one of the greatest geniuses the world has known. He was the founder of modern anatomy.

5. Sixteenth Century

Vesalius (1514–1564), the 'reformer of anatomy', was German in origin, Belgian (Brussels) by birth, and found an Italian (Padua) university favourable for his work. He was professor of anatomy at Padua.

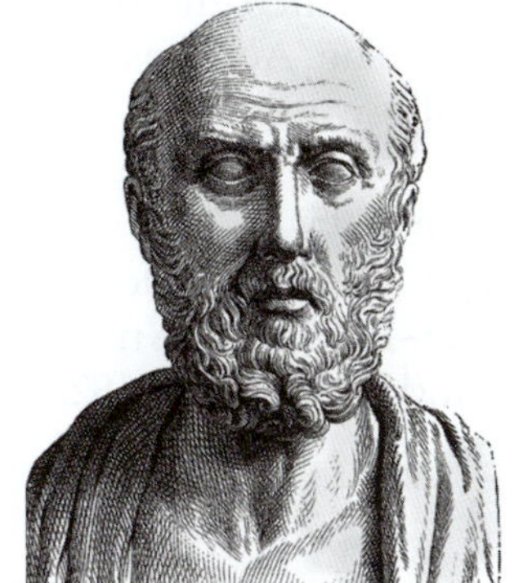

Hippocrates

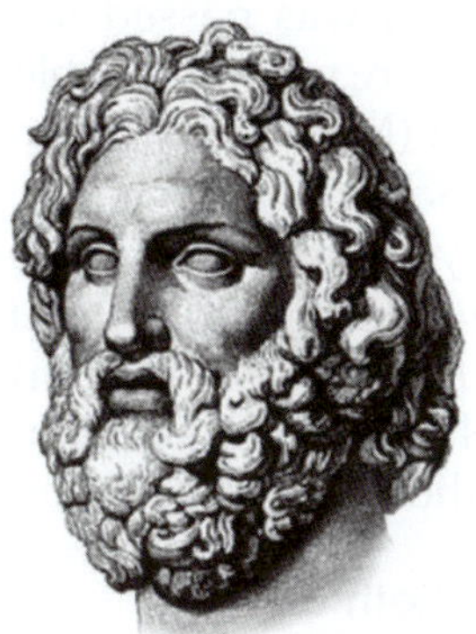

Herophilus

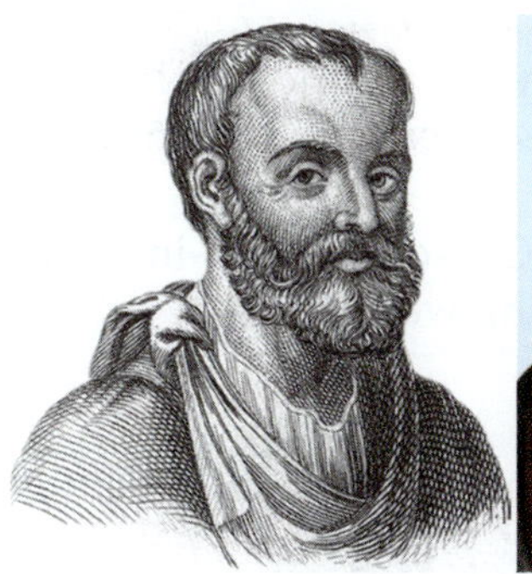

Galen

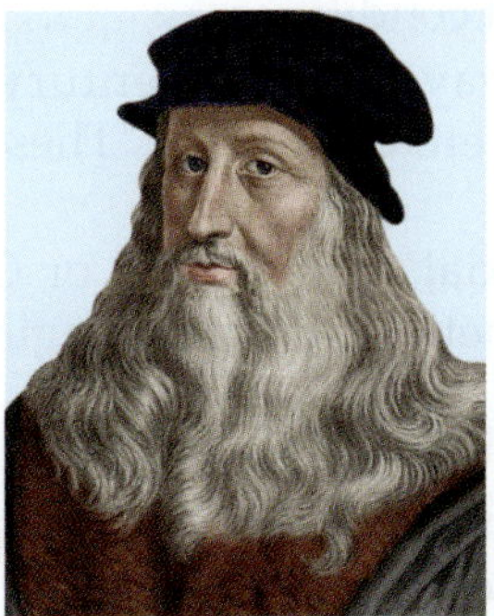

Leonardo da Vinci

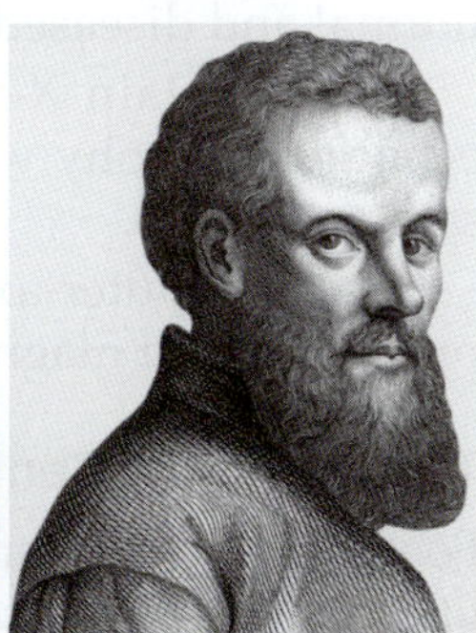

Vesalius

6. Seventeenth Century

William Harvey (1578–1657) was an English physician who discovered the circulation of blood, and published it as *Anatomical Exercise on the Motion of the Heart* and *Blood* in *Animals*. He also published a book on embryology.

7. Eighteenth Century

William Hunter (1718–1783) was a London anatomist and obstetrician. He introduced the present day embalming with the help of Harvey's discovery, and founded with his younger brother (John Hunter) the famous Hunterian museum.

8. Nineteenth Century

Dissection by medical students was made compulsory in Edinburgh (1826) and Maryland (1833). Burke and Hare scandal of 16 murders took place in Edinburgh in 1828. Warburton Anatomy Act (1832) was passed in England under which the unclaimed bodies were made available for dissection. The 'Act' was passed in America (Massachusetts) in 1831. Formalin was used as a fixative in 1890s.

X-rays were discovered by Roentgen in 1895.

The noted anatomists of this century include Ashley Cooper (1768–1841; British surgeon), Cuvier (1769–1832; French naturalist), Meckel (1724–1774; German anatomist), and Henry Gray (1827–1861; the author of Gray's *Anatomy*).

9. Twentieth Century

The electron microscope was invented in 20th century. It was applied in clinical practice, which made startling changes in the study of normal and diseased conditions.

Besides plain X-rays, in this century, ultrasonography and echocardiography were discovered. These were the non-invasive safe procedure.

Also computer-axial tomography or CT scan, a non-invasive procedure and magnetic resonance imaging were devised.

10. Twenty-first Century

Foetal medicine is emerging as a newer subject. Even treatment *in utero* is being practised in some cases.

Human genome has been prepared.

New research in drugs for many diseases, especially AIDS, is being done very enthusiastically. There is also a strong possibility of gene therapy.

Indian Anatomists

Dr Inderjit Dewan worked chiefly on osteology and anthropology.

Dr DS Choudhry did notable work on carotid body.

Dr H Chaterjee and Dr H Verma researched on embryology.

Dr SS Dayal did good work in cancer biology.

Dr Shamer Singh and his team did pioneering work on teratology.

Dr Chaturvedi's and Dr CD Gupta's prominent work was on corrosion cast.

Dr LV Chako, Dr HN Keswani, Dr Veena Bijlani, Dr Gopinath, Dr Shashi Wadhwa of All India Institute of Medical Sciences, New Delhi, researched on neuroanatomy.

Dr Keswani and his team established museum of history of medicine.

Dr AK Susheela of AIIMS, New Delhi, has done profound work on fluorosis.

Dr MC Vaidya and Dr NK Mehra are well known for their work on leprosy, HLA and immunology.

Dr IB Singh of Rohtak did enlightening studies on histology. He has been author of several books in anatomy.

Dr AK Dutta of West Bengal had authored many books on anatomy. Dr Yogesh Sontakke has been writing many books on anatomy.

Pandit Madhusudan Gupta was the first man who dissected a cadaver in 1836 in Calcutta and created a sensation in orthodox Hindu society. He was honored by a 7 cannon salute.

Dr A Halim is a great teacher of many teachers. He retired from KGMC, Lucknow, UP. His book *Surface* and *Radiological Anatomy* is most popular.

Dr Chandrama Anand retired as Director of Lady Hardinge Medical College and associated hospitals. She was Director Professor and Head, Department of Anatomy, a very passionate, all-rounder lovable teacher.

Amongst the medical educationists are Dr Sita Achaya, Dr Ved Prakash, Dr Basu, Dr M Kaul, Dr Chandrama Anand, Dr Indira Bahl, Dr Swarna Bhardwaj, Dr Rewa Choudhary, Dr Smita Kakar, Dr Anita Tuli, Dr Shashi Raheja, Dr Ram Prakash, Dr Veena

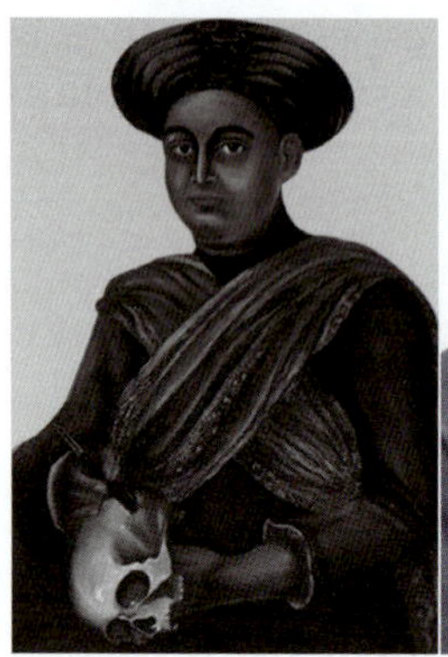
Dr Madhusudan Gupta

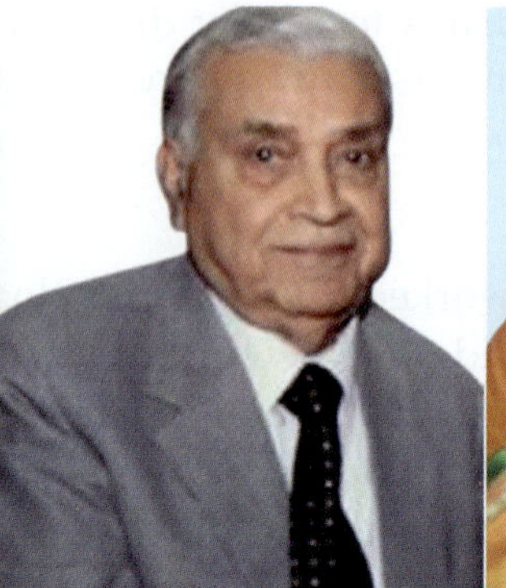
Dr A Halim

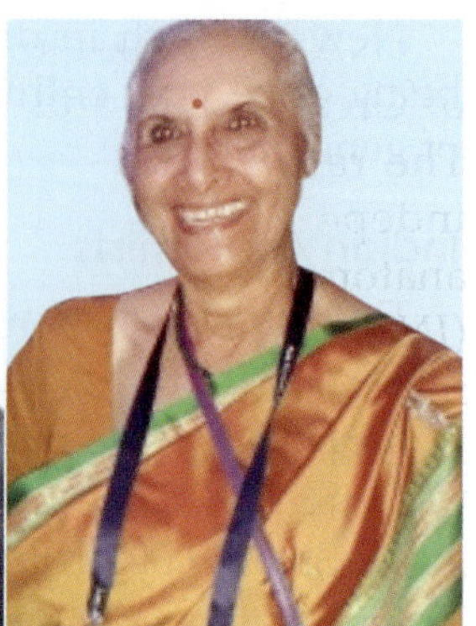
Dr Chandrama Anand

Bharihoke, Dr Madhur Gupta, Dr Neelam Vasudeva, Dr Sabita Mishra, Dr Raj Mehra, Dr Rani Kumar, Dr Satyam Khare, Dr JM Kaul, Dr Shipra Paul, Dr Dharamnarayan, Dr AC Das, Dr A Halim, Dr DR Singh and many others.

Dr Harish Agarwal, an anatomist, worked in jurisprudence for a number of years.

Dr Cooper of Chennai, Dr M Thomas and Dr Kiran Kucheria did commendable work on genetics.

Dr Mehdi Hasan and Dr Nafis Ahmad Faruqi did pioneering research in neuroanatomy.

Dr Balasubramanyam is a computer anatomist.

ANATOMICAL NOMENCLATURE

Galen (2nd century) wrote his book in Greek and Vesalius (16th century) did it in Latin. Most of the anatomical terms, therefore, are either in Greek or Latin. By 19th century about 30,000 anatomical terms were in use in the books and journals. In 1895, the German Anatomical Society held a meeting in Basle, and approved a list of about 5000 terms known as **Basle Nomina Anatomica** (BNA). The following six rules were laid down to be followed strictly: (1) Each part shall have only one name; (2) each term shall be in Latin; (3) each term shall be as short and simple as possible; (4) the terms shall be merely memory signs; (5) the related terms shall be similar, e.g. femoral artery, femoral vein, and femoral nerve; and (6) the adjectives shall be arranged as opposites, e.g. major and minor, superior and inferior.

BNA was revised in 1933 by a committee of the Anatomical Society of Great Britain and Ireland in a meeting held at **Birmingham**. The revised BNA was named Birmingham **Revision** (*BR*). An independent revision of the BNA was also done by German anatomists in 1935, and was known as **Jena Nomina Anatomica** (*JNA* or *INA*). However, the *BR* and *INA* found only local and restricted acceptance.

In 1950, it was agreed at an International Congress of Anatomists held at Oxford that a further attempt should be made to establish a generally acceptable international nomenclature. In the Sixth International Congress of Anatomists held at Paris (1955), a somewhat conservative revision of BNA with many terms from BR and INA was approved. Minor revisions and corrections were made at the International Congresses held in New York (1960), and Wiesbaden, Germany (1965), and the 3rd edition of **Nomina Anatomica** (Ed. GAG Mitchell, 1968) was published by the Excerpta Medica Foundation.

The drafts on *Nomina Histologica* and *Nomina Embryologica* prepared by the subcommittee of the International Anatomical Nomenclature Committee (IANC) were approved in a plenary session of the Eleventh International Congress of Anatomists held in Leningrad in 1970. After a critical revision, the 4th edition of *Nomina Anatomica* (Ed. Roger Warwick, 1977) containing *Nomina Histologica* and *Nomina Embryologica* was published by the same publisher.

> *Competency achievement:* The student should be able to:
> AN 1.1 Demonstrate normal anatomical position, various planes, relation, comparison, laterality and movement in our body

ANATOMICAL TERMINOLOGY

Various positions, planes, terms in relation to various regions and movements are described.

Positions

- ***Anatomical position:*** When a person is standing straight with eyes looking forwards, both arms by the side of body, palms facing forwards, both feet together, the position is anatomical position (Fig. 1.9).

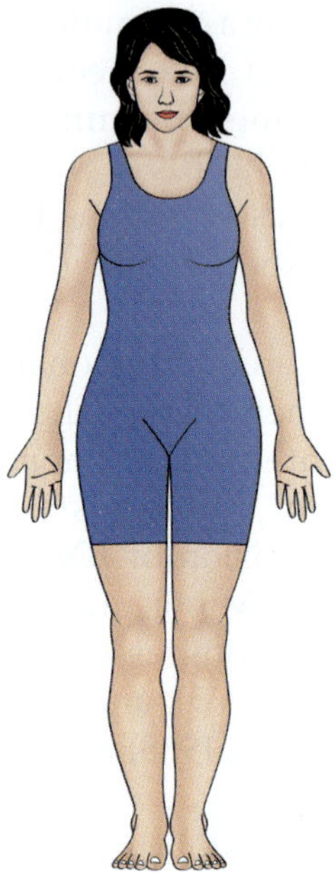

Fig. 1.9: Anatomical position

- ***Supine position:*** When a person is lying on his/her back, arms by the side, palms facing upwards and feet put together, the position is supine position (Fig. 1.10).
- ***Prone position:*** Person lying on his/her face, chest and abdomen is said to be in prone position (Fig. 1.11).
- ***Lithotomy position:*** Person lying on her back with legs up and feet supported in straps. This position is mostly used during delivery of the baby (Fig. 1.12).

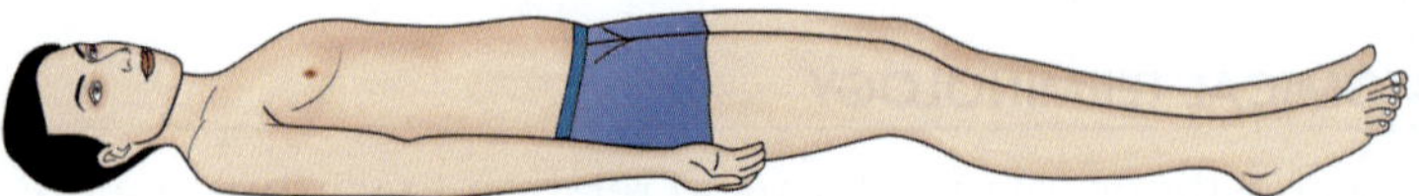

Fig. 1.10: Supine position

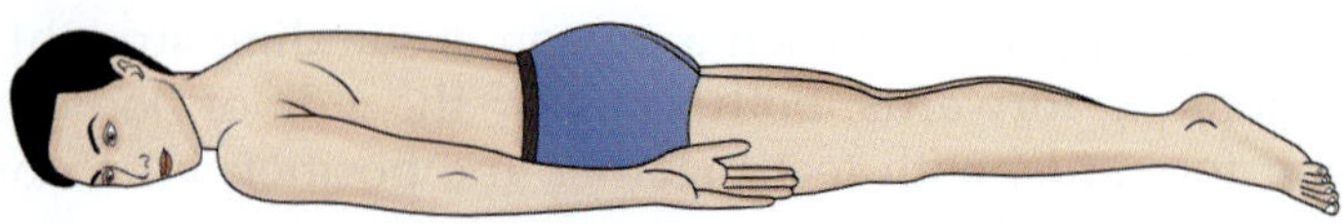

Fig. 1.11: Prone position

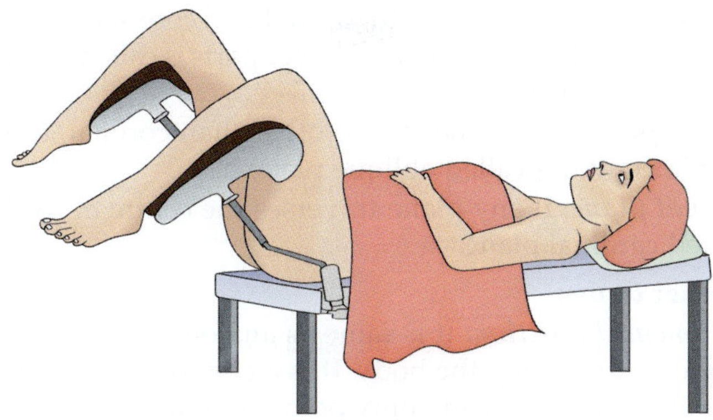

Fig. 1.12: Lithotomy position

Planes

- A plane passing through the centre of the body dividing it into two equal right and left halves, is the median or midsagittal plane (Fig.1.13). Plane parallel to median or midsagittal plane is the sagittal plane.
- A plane at right angles to sagittal or median plane which divides the body into anterior and posterior halves is called a **coronal plane** (Figs 1.14 and 1.15).

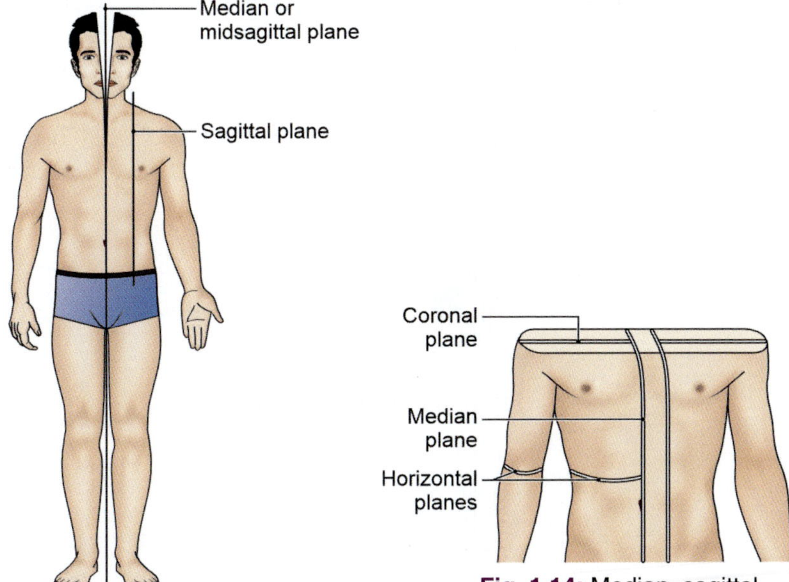

Fig. 1.13: Median and sagittal planes

Fig. 1.14: Median, sagittal, coronal and horizontal planes

- A plane at right angles to both sagittal and coronal planes which divides the body into upper and lower parts is called a **transverse horizontal plane** (Fig. 1.15).
- *Oblique plane:* Any other plane other than coronal, transverse and midsagittal is called oblique plane.
- *Cardinal plane:* If any plane traverses the centre of the body, it is called cardinal plane.

Some other terms:

- *Fundamental position:* It is same as anatomical position except that palms are facing the body. It is a comfortable position and is not important from anatomy point of view.
- *Centre of gravity:* The point where three cardinal planes intersect in the body is called "centre of gravity".

Terms used in Relation to Trunk, Neck and Face

- *Ventral* or *anterior* is the front of trunk, neck and face.
- *Dorsal* or *posterior* is the back of trunk, neck and face (Fig. 1.17).
- *Medial* is a plane close to the median plane (Fig. 1.16).
- *Lateral* is plane away from the median plane.
- *Proximal/cranial/superior* is close to the head end of body.

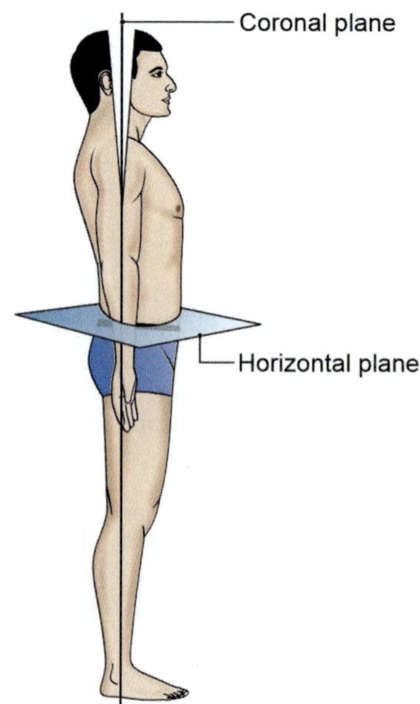

Fig. 1.15: Coronal and horizontal planes

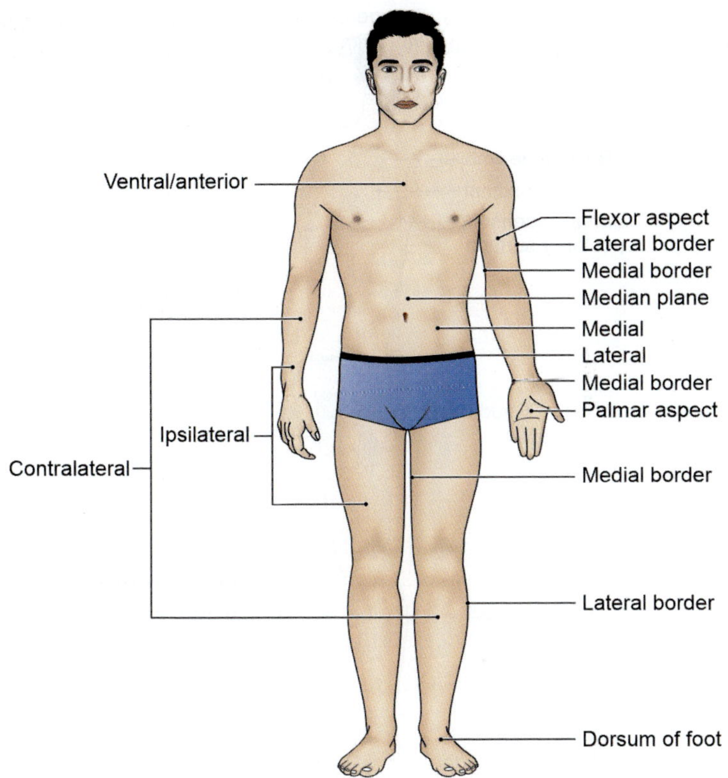

Fig. 1.16: Language of anatomy

- *Distal/caudal/inferior* is close to the lower end of the trunk.
- *Superficial is close to skin/towards* the surface of body (Fig. 1.18).
- *Deep* is away from skin/away from the surface of body.
- *Ipsilateral* is on the same side of the body as another structure.
- *Contralateral* is on opposite side of body from another structure.
- *Invagination* is projection inside.
- *Evagination* is projection outside (Fig. 1.19).

Terms Used in Relation to Upper Limb

- *Ventral* or *anterior* is the front aspect (Fig. 1.17).
- *Dorsal* or *posterior* is the back aspect.
- *Medial border* lies along the little finger, medial border of forearm and arm.
- *Lateral border* follows the thumb, lateral border of forearm and arm (Fig. 1.16).

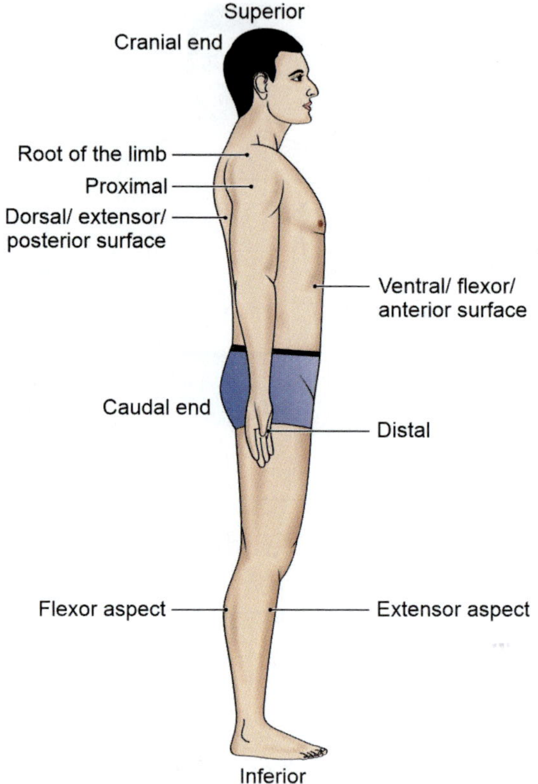

Fig. 1.17: Language of anatomy

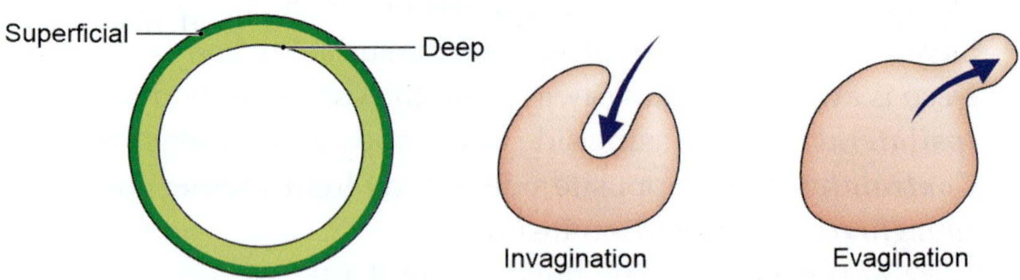

Fig. 1.18: Language of anatomy

Fig. 1.19: Language of anatomy

- ***Proximal*** is close to root of limb, while ***distal*** is away from the root (Fig. 1.17).
- ***Palmar*** aspect is the front of the palm (Fig. 1.16).
- ***Dorsal*** aspect of hand is on the back of palm.
- ***Flexor*** aspect is front of upper limb.
- ***Extensor*** aspect is back of upper limb.

Terms used in Relation to Lower Limb

- *Posterior* aspect is the back of lower limb.
- *Anterior* aspect is front of lower limb.
- *Medial border* lies along the big toe or hallux, medial border of leg and thigh (Fig. 1.16).
- *Lateral border* lies along the little toe, lateral border of leg and thigh.
- *Flexor* aspect is back of lower limb.
- *Extensor* aspect is front of lower limb (Fig. 1.17).
- *Proximal* is close to the root of limb, while *distal* is away from it.

Terms of Relation Commonly used in Embryology and Comparative Anatomy, but Sometimes in Gross Anatomy

a. *Ventral*—towards the belly (like anterior).
b. *Dorsal*—towards the back (like posterior).
c. *Cranial or rostral*—towards the head (like superior) (Fig. 1.17).
d. *Caudal*—towards the tail (Fig. 1.17).

TERMS RELATED TO BODY MOVEMENTS

Movements in general at synovial joints are divided into four main categories.

1. *Gliding movement:* Relatively flat surfaces move back-and-forth and from side-to-side with respect to one another. The angle between articulating bones does not change significantly.
2. *Angular movements:* Angle between articulating bones decreases or increases. In **flexion** there is decrease in angle between articulating bones and in **extension** there is increase in angle between articulating bones (Fig. 1.20). **Lateral flexion** is movement of trunk sideways to the right or left at the waist. **Adduction** is movement of bone toward midline, whereas **abduction** is movement of bone away from midline.
3. *Special movements:* These occur only at certain joints, e.g. pronation, supination at radioulnar joints, protraction and retraction at temporomandibular joint, inversion and eversion at subtalar joint.
4. *Rotation:* A bone revolves around its own longitudinal axis. In **medial rotation** anterior surface of a bone of limb is turned towards the midline. In **lateral rotation** anterior surface of a bone of limb is turned away from midline.

In Upper limb

Shoulder Joint

- ***Abduction of shoulder:*** When limb is taken away from the body (Fig. 1.21).
- ***Adduction of shoulder:*** When limb is brought close to the body.
- ***Flexion of shoulder:*** If arm is taken towards the front of the chest wall.
- ***Extension:*** Arm is taken backwards and laterally (Fig. 1.22).
- ***Circumduction:*** It is movement of distal end of a part of the body in a circle. A combination of extension, abduction, flexion and adduction in a sequence is called circumduction as in bowling.
- ***Medial rotation of shoulder:*** When the arm rotates medially bringing the flexed forearm across the chest (elbow in contact with trunk).

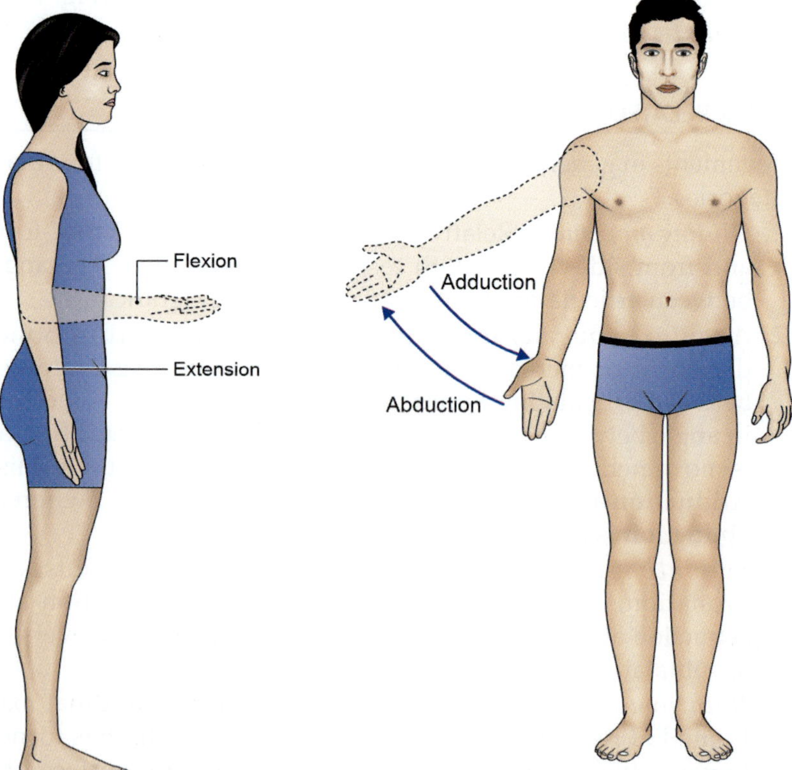

Fig. 1.20: Angular movements

Fig. 1.21: Abduction and adduction of shoulder joint

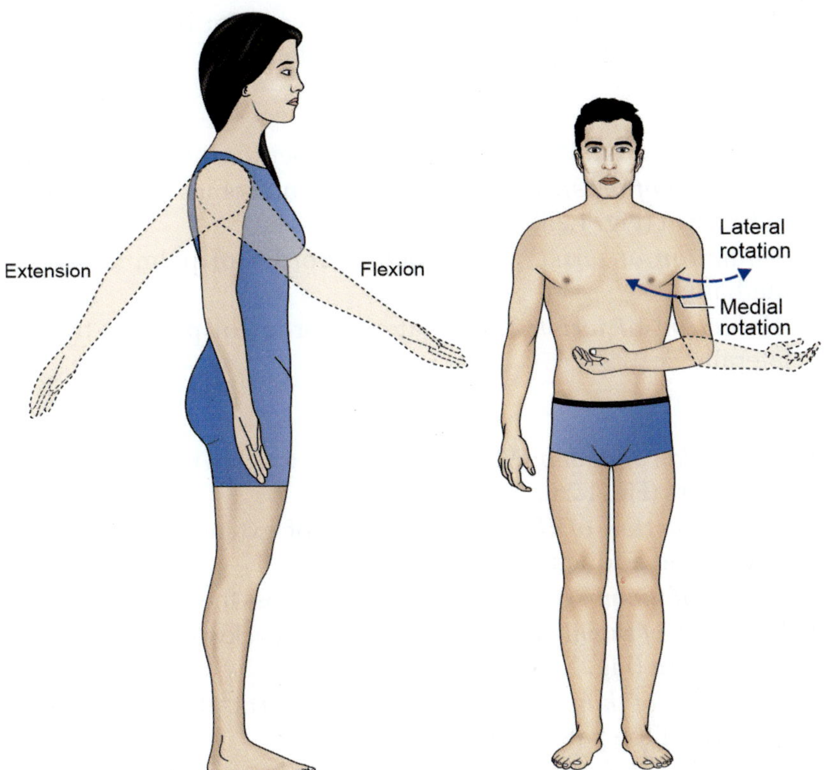

Fig. 1.22: Flexion and extension of shoulder joint

Fig. 1.23: Medial rotation and lateral rotation of shoulder joint

- ***Lateral rotation of shoulder:*** When arm rotates laterally taking the flexed forearm away from the body (Fig. 1.23) (elbow in contact with trunk).

Elbow Joint

- ***Flexion:*** When two flexor surfaces are brought close to each other, e.g. in elbow joint when front of arm and forearm move close to each other (Fig. 1.20).
- ***Extension:*** When extensor or dorsal surfaces are brought in as much approximation as possible, e.g. straighten the forearm at the elbow joint (Fig. 1.20).

Forearm

- ***Supination:*** When the palm is facing forwards or upwards, as in putting food in the mouth (Fig. 1.24).

- ***Pronation:*** When the palm faces backwards or downwards, as in picking food with fingers from the plate.

Wrist Joint

- ***Flexion of wrist:*** When palm comes closer to front of forearm.
- ***Extension of wrist:*** When dorsum of hand comes closer to back of forearm (Fig. 1.25).
- ***Adduction of wrist:*** When medial border of palm is turned medially.
- ***Abduction of wrist:*** When lateral border of palm is turned laterally.

Thumb

- ***Opposition of thumb:*** When tip of thumb touches the tips of any of the fingers (Fig. 1.26).
- ***Circumduction of thumb:*** Movement of extension, abduction, flexion and adduction in sequence.
- ***Flexion of thumb:*** When thumb is taken across the palm (Fig. 1.27).
- ***Extension of thumb:*** When thumb is taken backwards in the plane of the palm (Fig. 1.28).
- ***Abduction of thumb:*** When thumb is put vertically at right angles to plane of the palm (Fig. 1.29).
- ***Adduction of thumb:*** When thumb is in close contact with lateral side of index finger (Fig. 1.30).

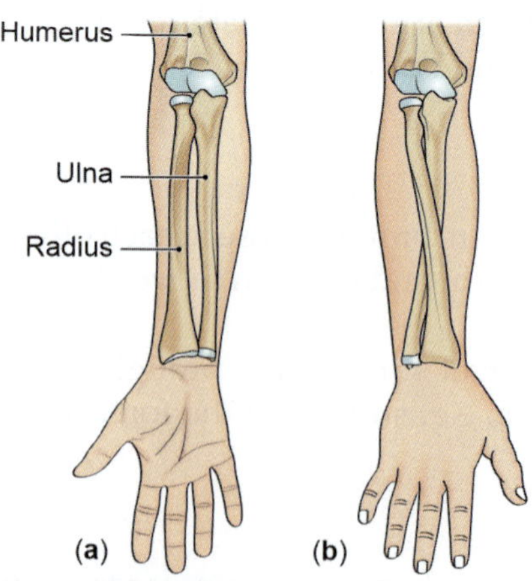

Fig. 1.24: Supinated forearm (a) and pronated forearm (b)

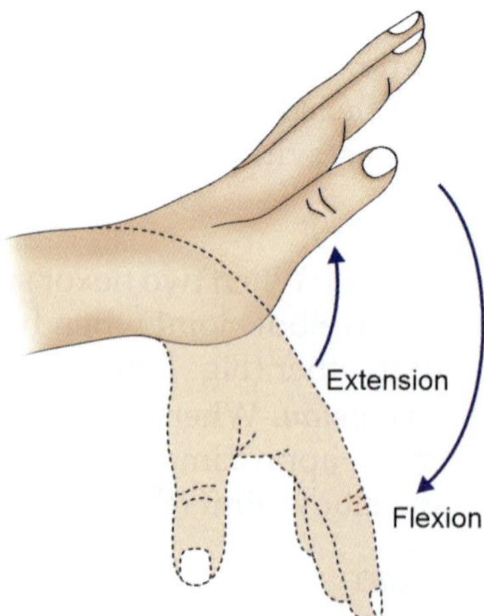

Fig. 1.25: Flexion and extension of wrist joint

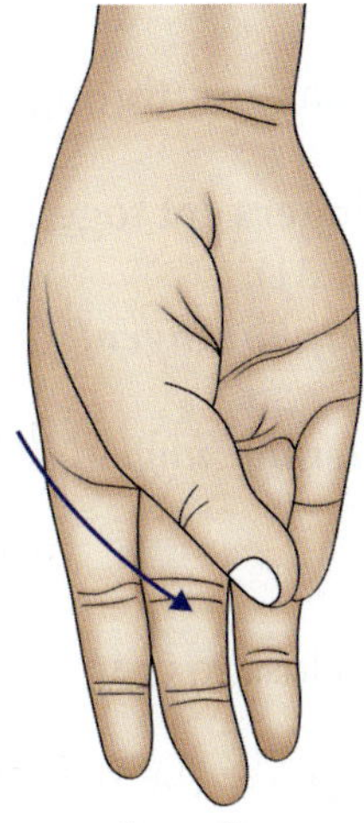

Fig. 1.26: Opposition of thumb

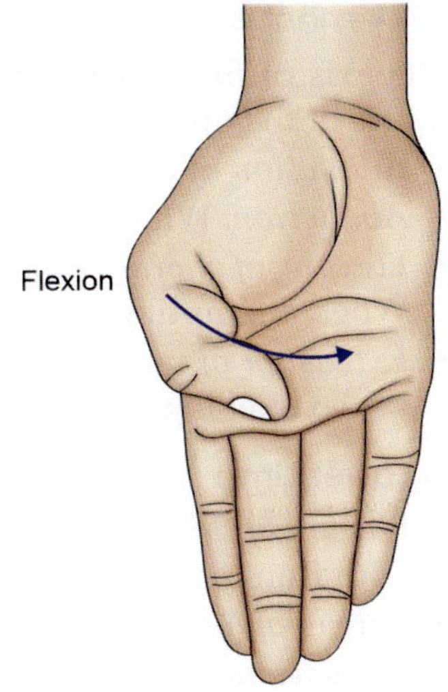

Fig. 1.27: Flexion of thumb

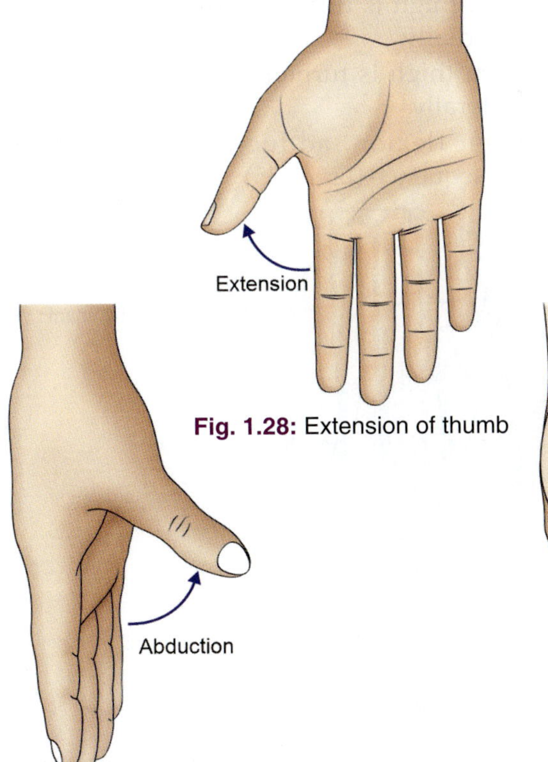

Fig. 1.28: Extension of thumb

Fig. 1.29: Abduction of thumb

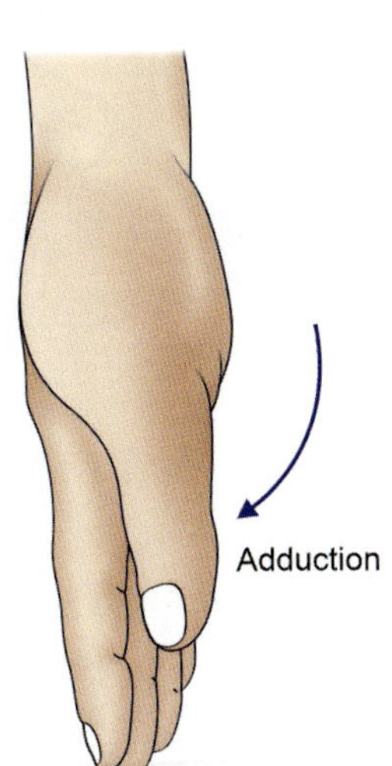

Fig. 1.30: Adduction of thumb

Movement of Fingers

The axis of movement of fingers is the line passing through the centre of the middle finger (Fig. 1.31).

- ***Adduction of digits/fingers:*** When all the fingers get together.
- ***Abduction:*** When all fingers separate (Fig. 1.31).
- ***Flexion of metacarpophalangeal and interphalangeal joints:*** When attempting to make a fist.
- ***Extension of metacarpophalangeal and interphalangeal joints:*** When opening the fist (Fig. 1.32).

In Lower Limb

- ***Flexion of thigh:*** When front of thigh comes close to or in contact with front of abdomen (Fig. 1.33).
- ***Extension of thigh:*** When person stands erect.
- ***Abduction:*** When thigh is taken away from the median plane.
- ***Adduction:*** When thigh is brought close to median plane.
- ***Medial rotation:*** When thigh is turned medially. It is done by pointing the big toe medially.
- ***Lateral rotation:*** When thigh is turned laterally. It is done by pointing the big toe laterally.
- ***Circumduction:*** When flexion, adduction, extension and abduction are done in sequence (Fig. 1.35)

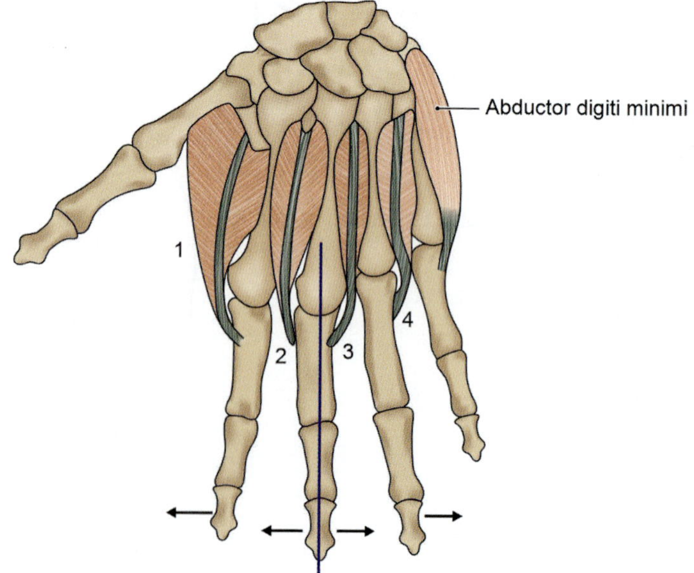

Fig. 1.31: Abduction of 2nd–5th digits

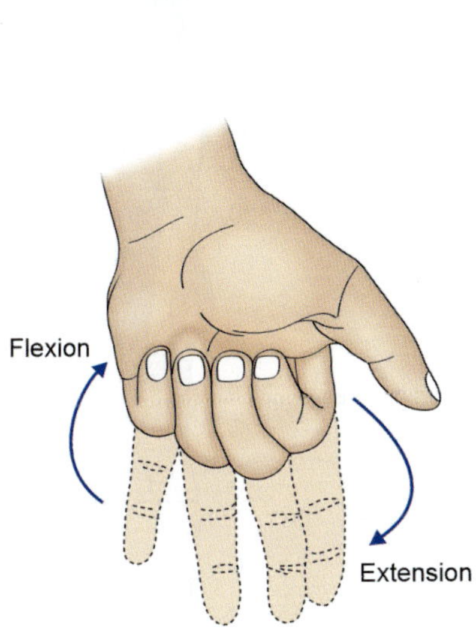

Fig. 1.32: Flexion and extension of metacarpophalangeal and interphalangeal joints

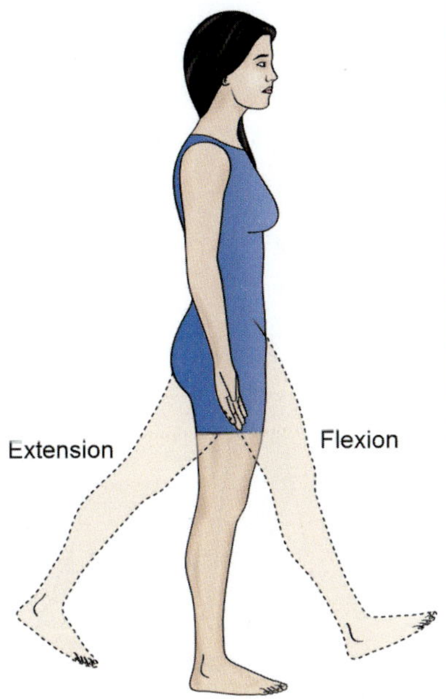

Fig. 1.33: Flexion and extension of thigh

- ***Flexion of knee:*** When back of thigh and back of leg come close to or are in opposition (Fig. 1.34a and b).
- ***Extension of knee:*** When thigh and leg are in straight line as in standing (Fig. 1.36).
- ***Dorsiflexion of foot:*** When dorsum of foot is brought close to front of leg and sole faces forwards (Fig. 1.37).
- ***Plantar flexion of foot:*** When sole of foot or plantar aspect of foot faces backwards.
- ***Inversion of foot:*** When medial border of foot is raised from the ground (Fig. 1.38).

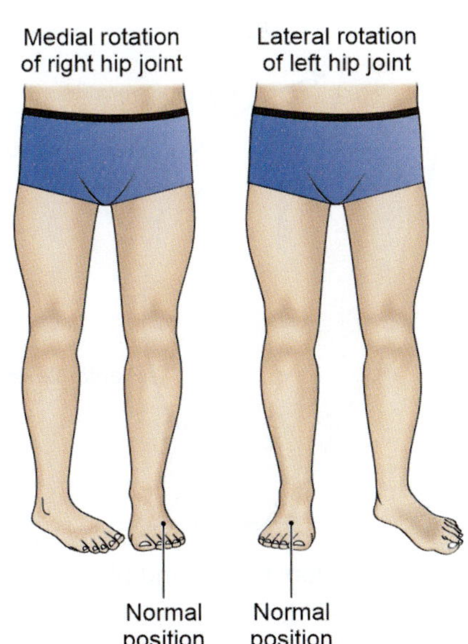

Fig. 1.34: Medial rotation and lateral rotation of thigh

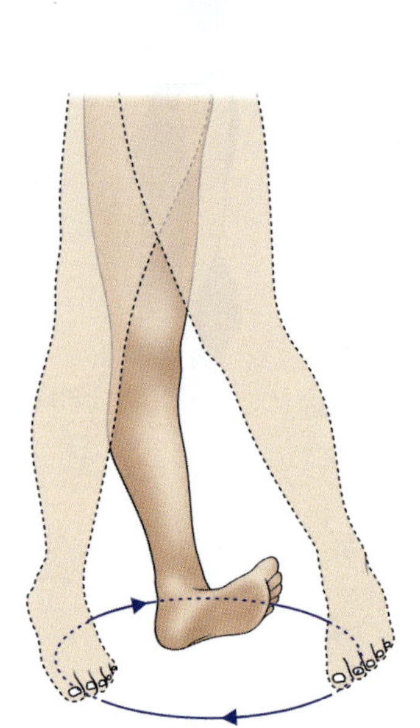

Fig. 1.35: Circumduction of lower limb

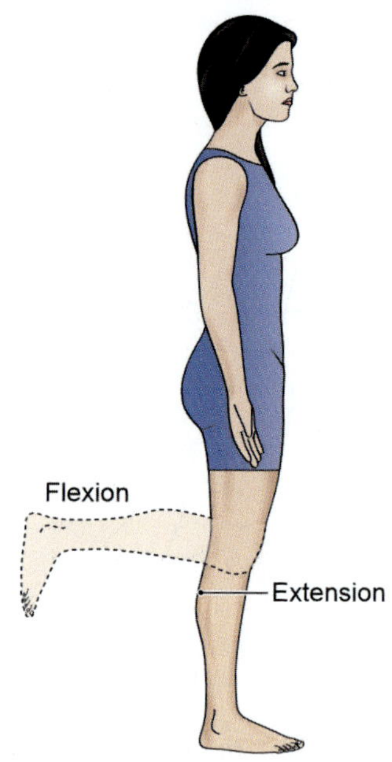

Fig. 1.36: Flexion and extension of knee joint

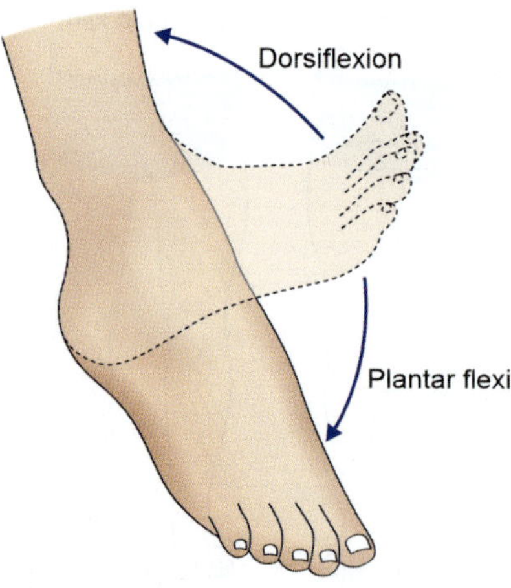

Fig. 1.37: Dorsiflexion and plantar flexion of foot

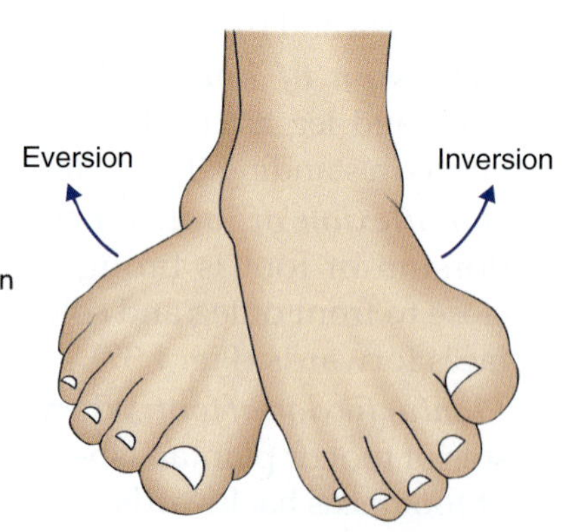

Fig. 1.38: Inversion and eversion of foot

- ***Eversion of foot:*** When lateral border of foot is raised from the ground.

In the Neck

- *Flexion:* When face comes closer to chest.
- *Extension:* When face is taken away from the chest (Fig. 1.39).
- *Lateral flexion:* When ear is brought close to shoulder (Fig. 1.40).
- *Rotation:* When neck rotates so that chin goes to opposite side.
- *Opening the mouth:* When lower jaw is lowered to open the mouth (Fig. 1.41).
- *Closure of the mouth:* When lower jaw is opposed to the upper jaw, closing the mouth (Fig. 1.42).
- *Protraction:* When lower jaw slides forwards in its socket in the temporal bone of skull (Fig. 1.43).
- *Retraction:* When lower jaw slides backwards in its socket in the temporal bone of skull (Fig. 1.44).

In the Trunk

- Backward bending is called *extension* (Fig. 1.39).
- Forward bending is *flexion*.
- Sideward movement *is lateral flexion* (Fig. 1.40)
- Sideward rotation is *lateral rotation*.

Terms used for Describing Muscles

a. *Origin:* The end of a muscle which is relatively fixed during its contraction (Fig. 1.45).

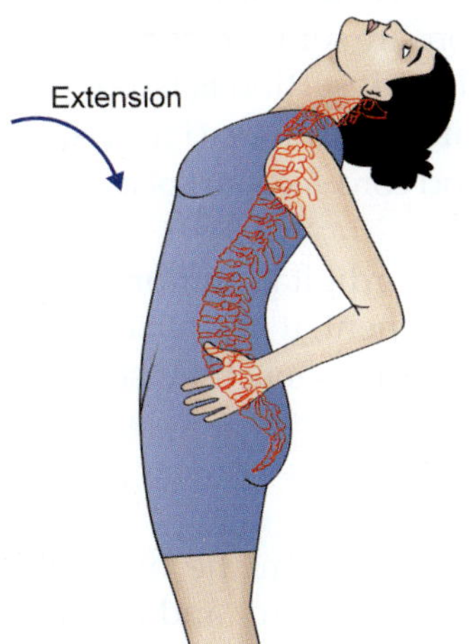

Fig. 1.39: Extension of neck and trunk

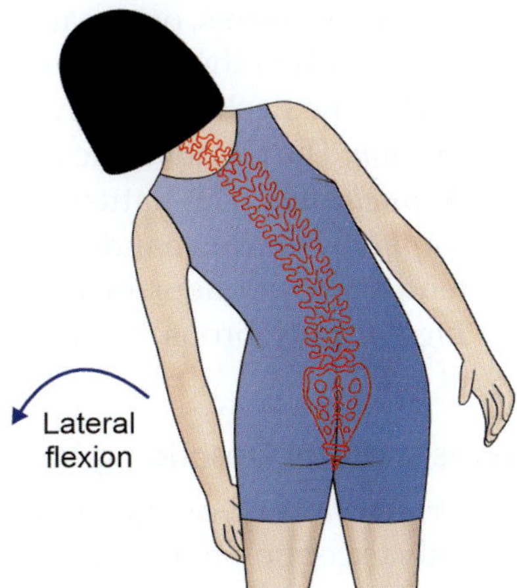

Fig. 1.40: Lateral flexion of neck and trunk

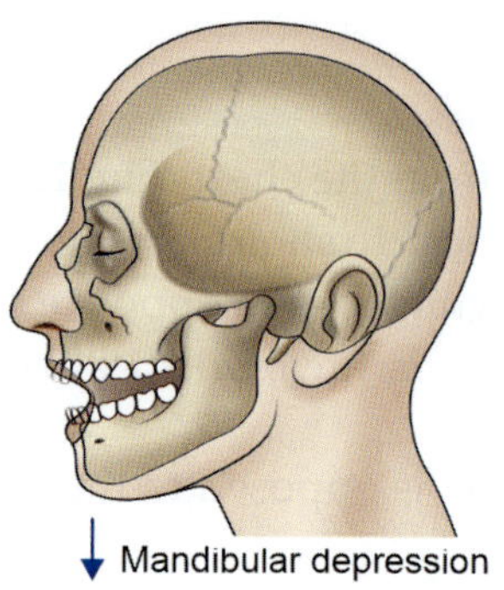

Fig. 1.41: Opening the mouth

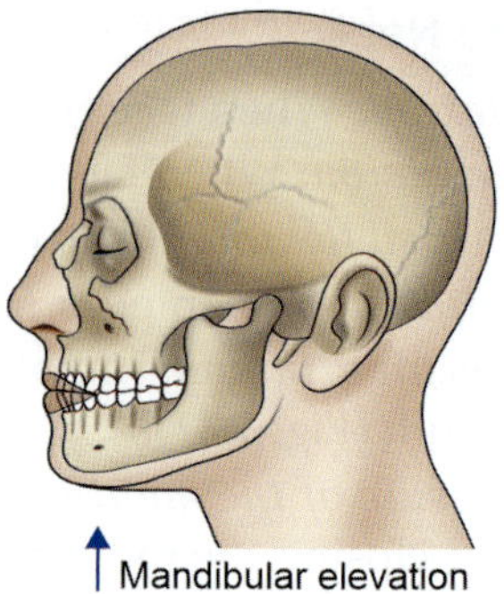

Fig. 1.42: Closing the mouth

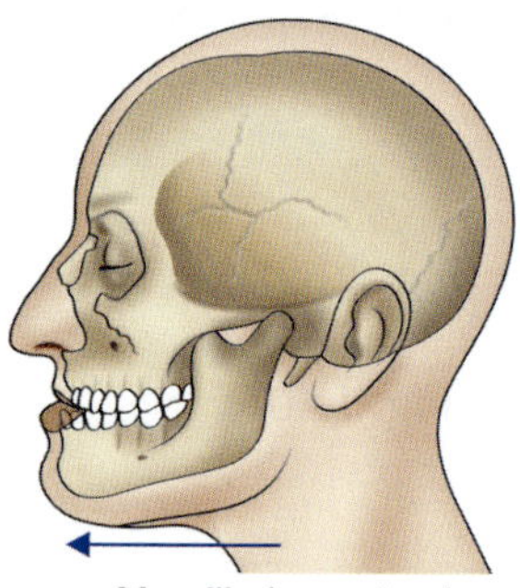

Fig. 1.43: Protraction of lower jaw

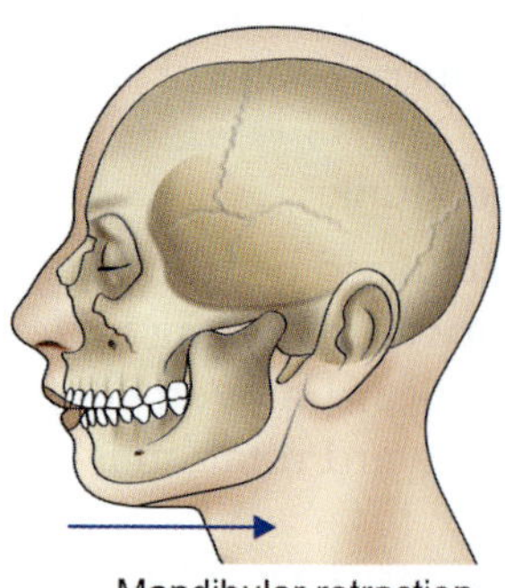

Fig. 1.44: Retraction of lower jaw

b. ***Insertion:*** The end of a muscle which moves during its contraction.

The two terms, origin and insertion, are sometimes interchangeable, when the origin moves and the insertion is fixed.

c. ***Belly:*** The fleshy and contractile part of a muscle (Fig. 1.45).
d. ***Tendon:*** The fibrous noncontractile and cord-like part of a muscle.
e. ***Aponeurosis:*** The flattened tendon.
f. ***Raphe:*** A fibrous band made up of interdigitating fibres of the tendons or aponeuroses. Unlike a ligament, it is stretchable.
g. ***Ligaments:*** Fibrous, inelastic bands which connect two segments of a joint.

Terms used for Describing Vessels

a. ***Arteries*** carry oxygenated blood away from the heart. The only exception to this remark are the pulmonary and umbilical arteries which carry deoxygenated blood. Arteries resemble trees because they have branches (arterioles) (Fig. 1.46).

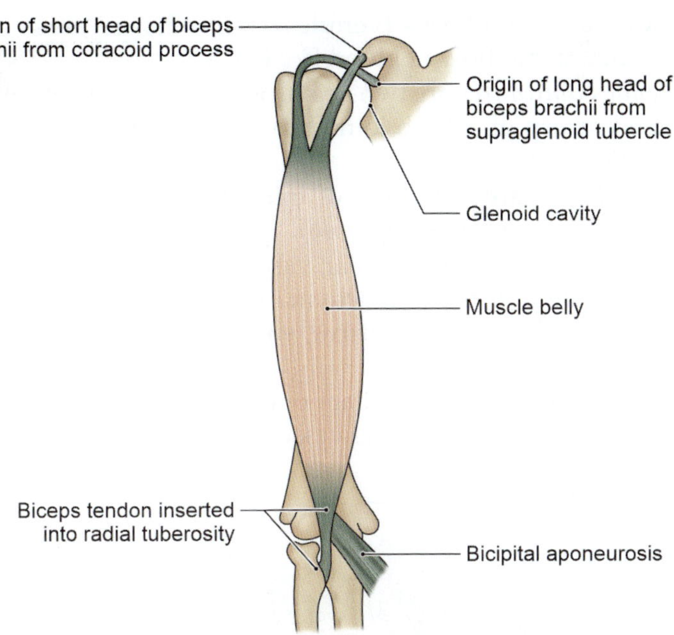

Fig. 1.45: Terms for describing muscles

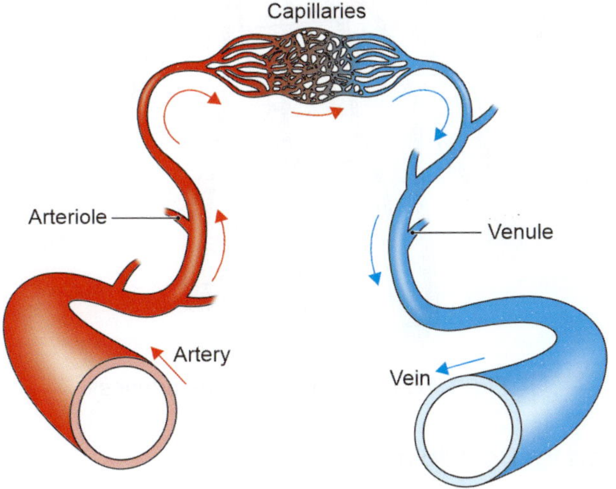

Fig. 1.46: Terms used for describing vessels

b. ***Veins*** carry deoxygenated blood towards the heart. The exception to this remark are the pulmonary and umbilical veins which carry oxygenated blood. Veins resemble rivers because they have tributaries (venules). Veins have valves to allow unidirectional flow of blood (*see* Fig. 5.8).

c. ***Venae comitantes*** are two veins, one on each side of a medium-sized artery of a limb joined to each other across the artery (*see* Fig. 5.11).

d. ***Capillaries*** are networks of microscopic vessels connecting arterioles to venules (Fig. 1.46).

e. ***Sinusoids*** are large, irregular, vascular spaces which are closely surrounded by the parenchyma of the organ. These are seen in liver, spleen, bone marrow, suprarenal glands, parathyroid glands.

f. ***Anastomoses*** are precapillary or postcapillary communications between the neighbouring vessels (Fig. 1.47).

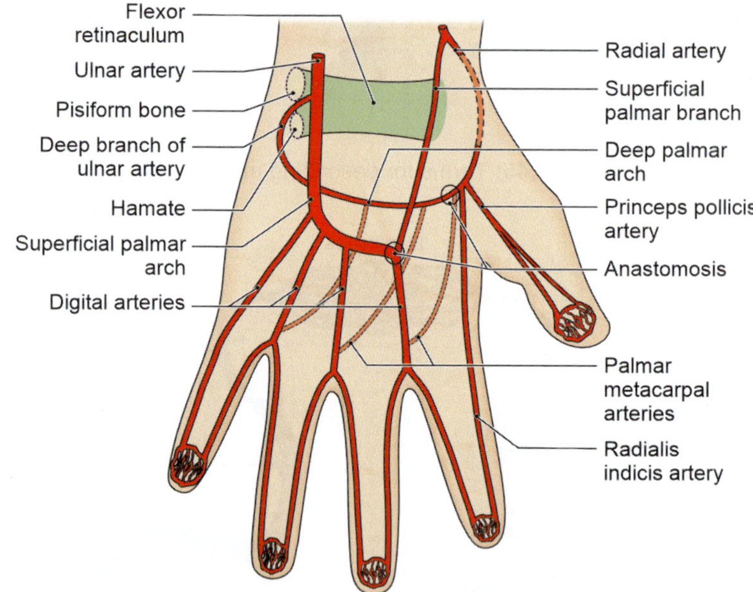

Fig. 1.47: Anastomoses of the arteries

Terms used for Describing Bone Features

Bone marking	*Example*
Linear elevation	
Line	Superior nuchal line and inferior nuchal line of the occipital bone (Fig. 1.48)

(Contd.)

Bone marking	*Example (Contd.)*
Crest	The illac crest of the hip bone, of spine of scapula (Fig. 1.49)
Ridge	The medial and lateral supracondylar ridges of the humerus (Fig. 1.50)
Rounded elevation	
Tubercle	Pubic tubercle, lesser and greater tubercles of humerus
Protuberance	External occipital protuberance (Fig. 1.48)
Tuberosity	Ischial tuberosity of the hip bone, deltoid tuberosity (Fig. 1.50)
Malleolus	Medial malleolus of the tibia, lateral malleolus of the fibula
Trochanter	Greater and lesser trochanters of the femur (Fig. 1.51)
Sharp elevation	
Spine or spinous process	Ischial spine, spine of vertebra, anterior superior iliac spine
Styloid process	Styloid process of temporal bone (Fig. 1.48)
Expanded ends for articulation	
Head	Head of humerus, head of femur, head of radius
Condyle	Medial and lateral condyles of femur (knuckle-like process Fig. 1.51)
Epicondyle (a prominence situated just above condyle)	Medial and lateral epicondyles of femur (Fig. 1.52), medial and lateral epicondyles of humerus (Fig. 1.50)
Small flat area for articulation	
Facet	Facet on head of rib for articulation with vertebral body
Depressions	
Notch	Greater sciatic notch and lesser sciatic notch of hip bone
Groove or sulcus	Bicipital groove of humerus (Fig. 1.50)
Fossa	Radial and coronoid fossae (Fig. 1.50) of humerus, acetabular fossa of hip bone
Openings	
Fissure	Superior orbital and inferior orbital fissures (Fig. 1.53)
Foramen	Infraorbital foramen of the maxilla
Canal	Carotid canal of temporal bone
Meatus	External acoustic meatus and internal acoustic meatus of temporal bone

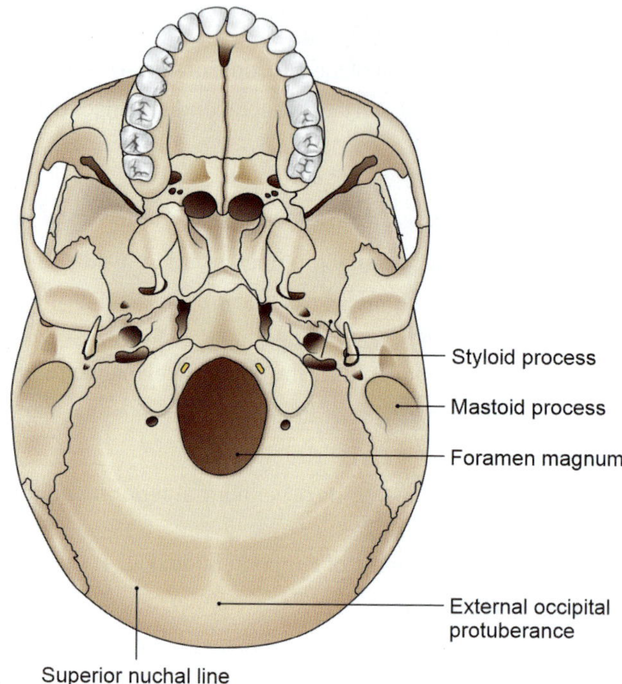

Fig. 1.48: Terms used for describing bone features

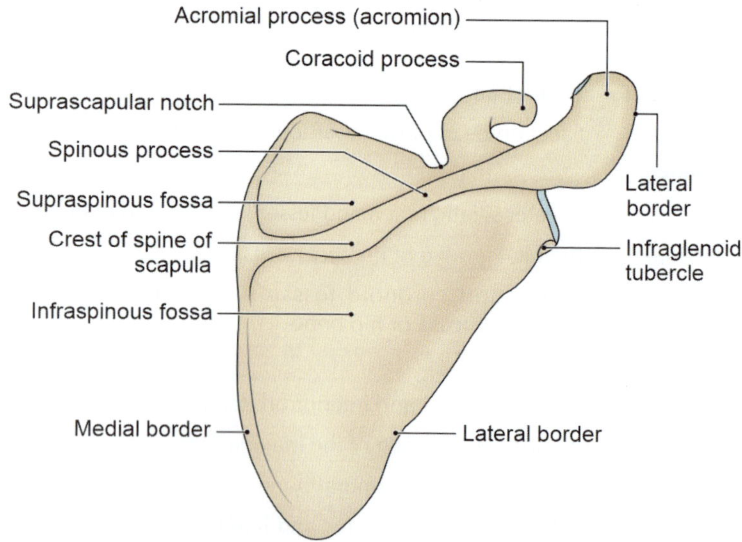

Fig. 1.49: Terms used for describing bone features

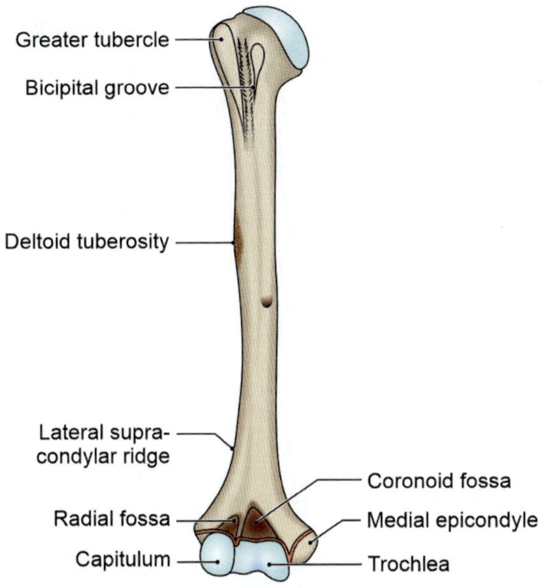

Fig. 1.50: Terms used for describing bone features

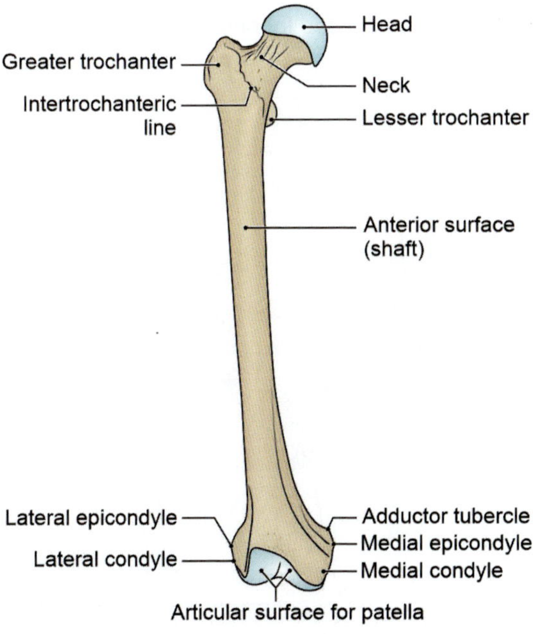

Fig. 1.51: Terms used for describing bone features

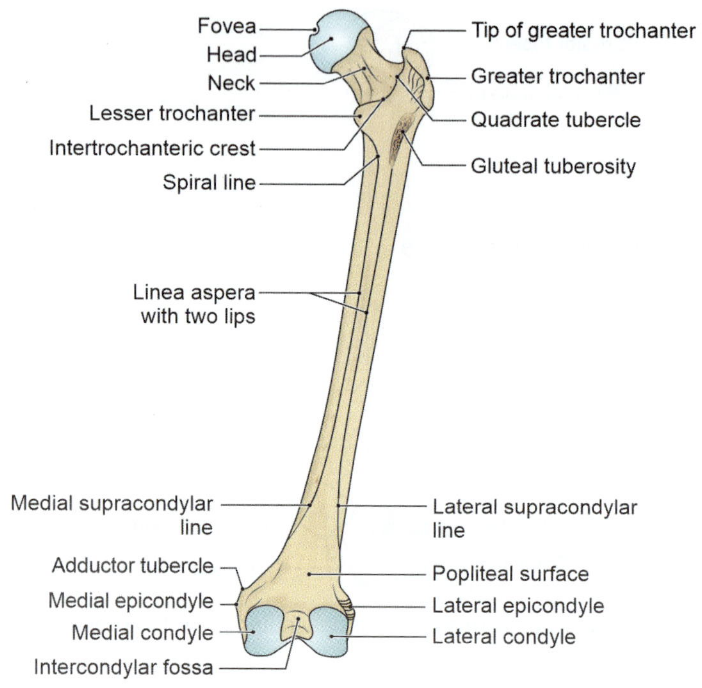

Fig. 1.52: Terms used for describing bone features

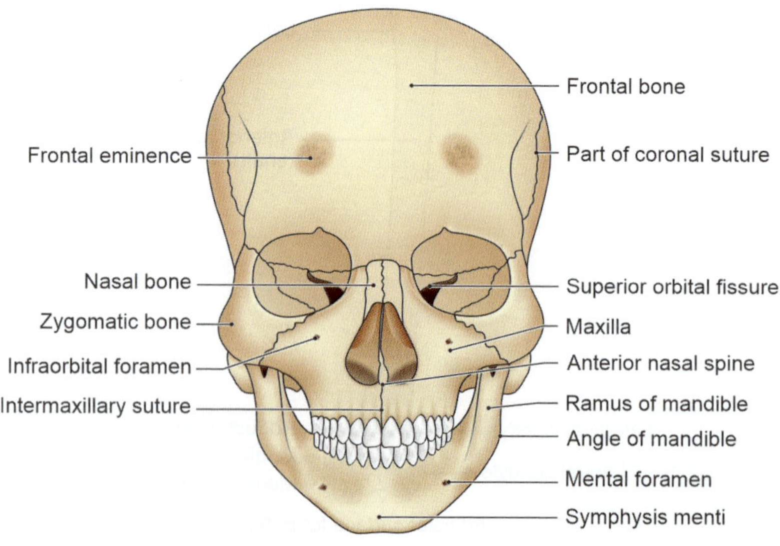

Fig. 1.53: Terms used for describing bone features

Systems of the Body

The study of anatomy can be divided into the following twelve major body systems. These body systems influence one another and work interdependently and independently to maintain health. These are as follows:

1. ***Respiratory system (pulmonology)*** consists of nose, nasopharynx, larynx, trachea, bronchi, bronchioles, alveoli and the main muscle is the diaphragm. These structures receive oxygen to oxygenate the venous blood and help in elimination of carbon dioxide (Fig. 1.54).
2. ***Articular system (arthrology)*** comprises various joints with their ligaments. Various types of movements take place at the synovial joints. Cartilaginous and fibrous joints are for growth of the bones. The joints provide integrity and stability to the adjoining bones (Fig. 1.55) and some form cavities for protection of organs.

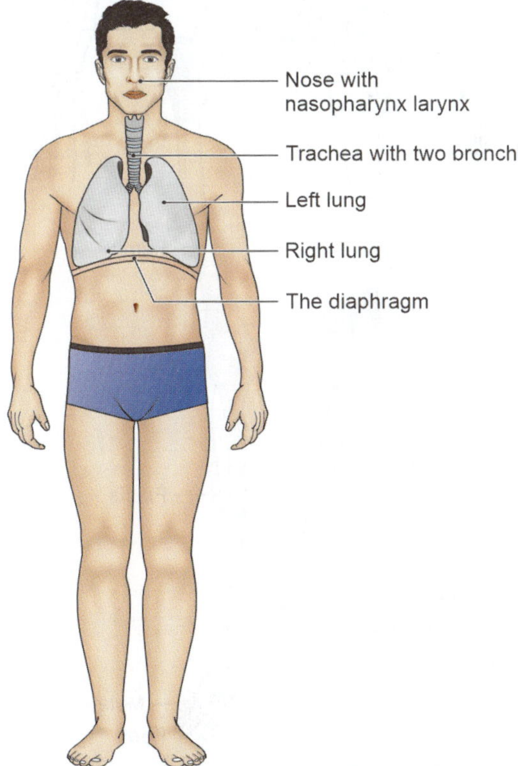

Fig. 1.54: Respiratory system

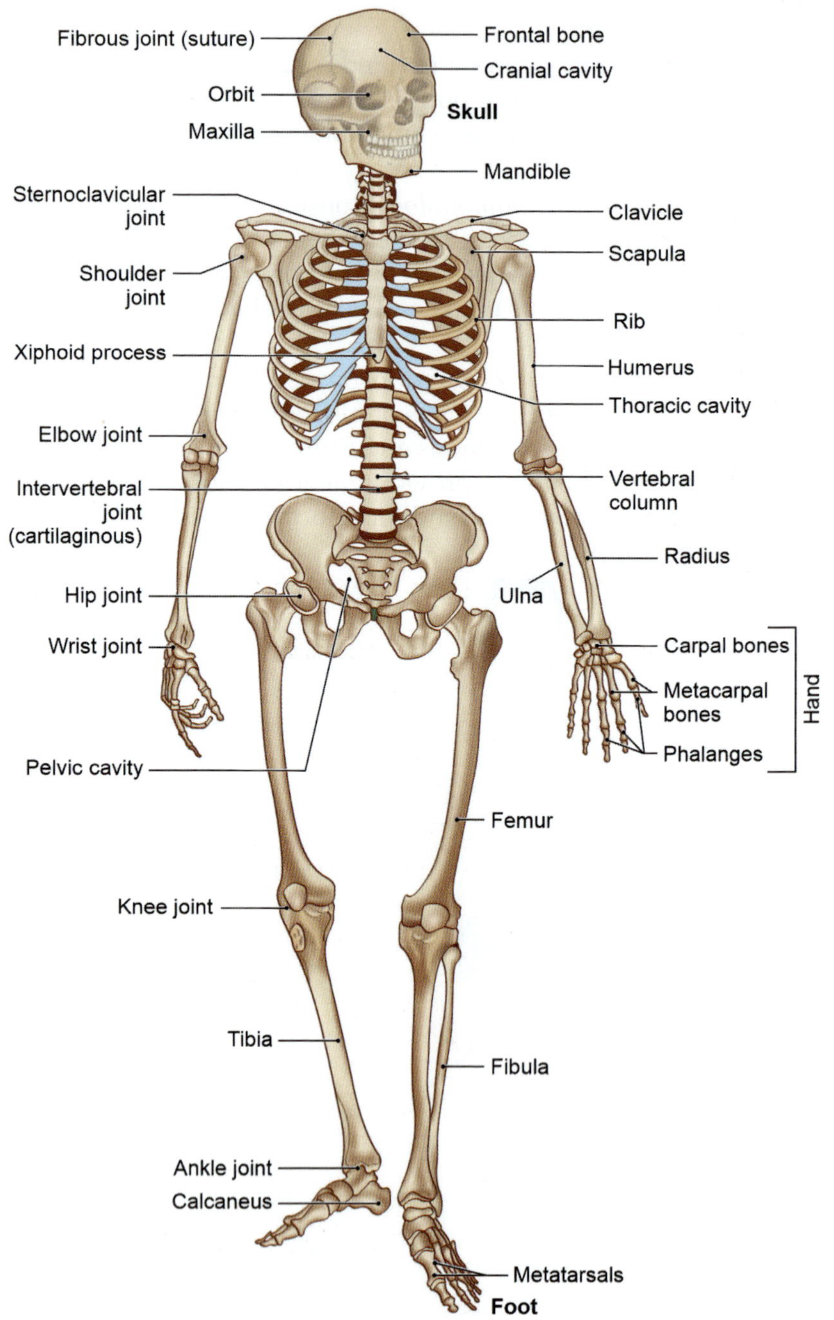

Fig. 1.55: Articular system

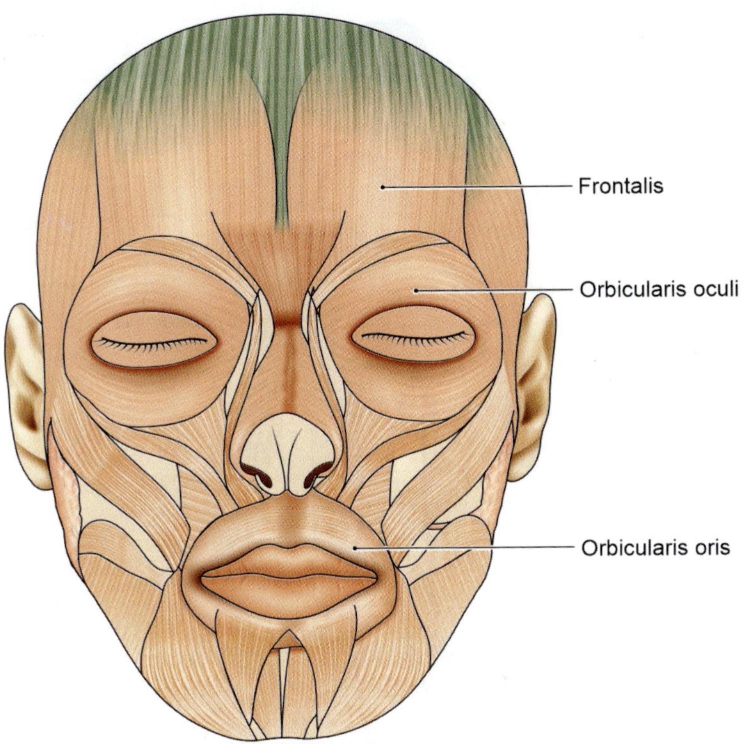

Fig. 1.56: Part of muscular system

3. ***Muscular system*** is the system which moves the various joints of the body and is responsible for activity, locomotion and facial expressions (Fig. 1.56).
4. ***Circulatory system (angiology)*** comprises cardiovascular system which consists of heart and blood vessels, i.e. arteries, veins and capillaries. Blood supplies nutrients and oxygen to cells and takes away carbon dioxide and wastes from cells and helps to regulate acid–base balance, temperature and water content of body fluids. Blood components help to defend against diseases and disease causing organisms (Fig. 1.57).
5. ***Lymphatic system*** comprises of various lymph vessels which withdraw excess tissue fluid with macromolecules, filters it through lymph nodes and returns it to the venous system (*see* Fig. 6.3).
6. ***Skeletal system (osteology)*** consists of numerous cartilages and bones, providing support and symmetry to the body. Cartilage

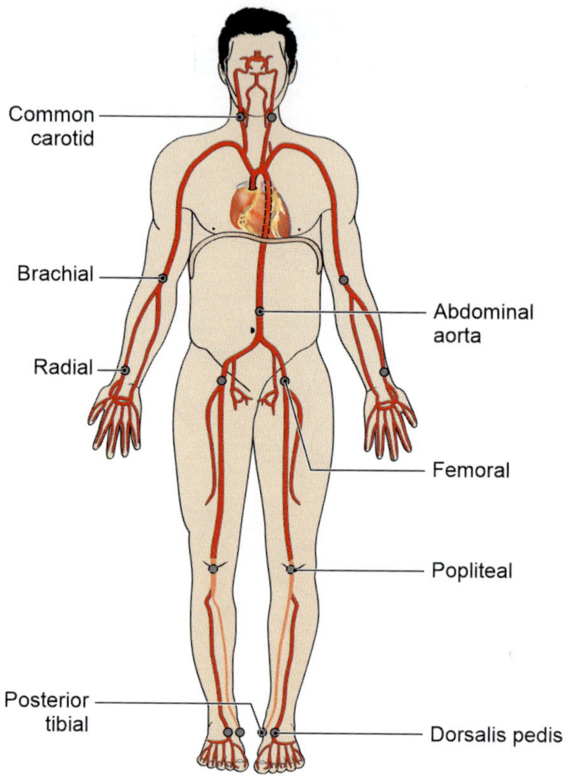

Fig. 1.57: Arterial system

keeps the respiratory pathway patent. Bones being the largest storehouse of calcium provide attachment to numerous skeletal muscles for locomotion. Bones also make cavities or cages for protection of organs like brain, spinal cord, heart, lungs, and reproductive organs (Fig. 1.55).

7. ***Integumentary system (dermatology)*** consists of the skin with its various appendages, i.e. hair, sweat gland, sebaceous gland and nail. Skin is the outermost protective and sensitive covering of the body (*see* Fig. 8.1).
8. ***Digestive system (gastroenterology)*** comprises various organs associated with ingestion, mastication, deglutition, digestion and absorption of food components. This system also eliminates the solid waste from the body through the anal canal. It is made up of a long tube from mouth to the anus and various associated

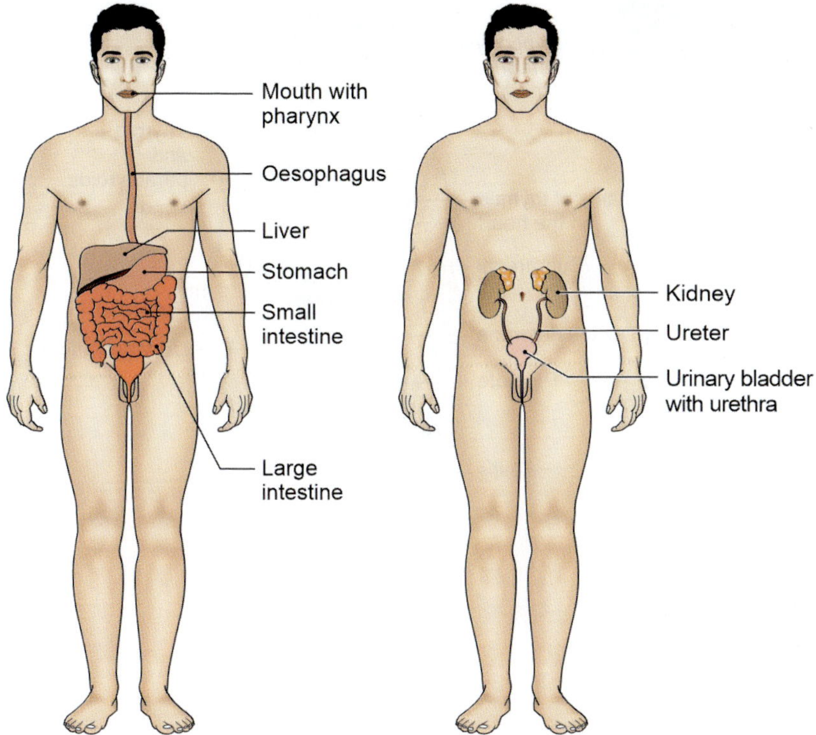

Fig. 1.58: Digestive system

Fig. 1.59: Urinary system

glands like salivary glands, liver, gallbladder, pancreas, gastric and intestinal glands (Fig. 1.58).

9. ***Urinary system (urology)*** helps in excretion of liquid waste from the body. This system comprises kidneys, ureters, urinary bladder and urethra. The kidneys filter the blood and produce, transport, store and expel the urine at frequent intervals (Fig. 1.59). Details can be learnt from 10th edition of *BD Chaurasia's Human Anatomy*, Volume 2, Chapter 24.
10. ***Reproductive system*** (***andrology*** in males and ***gynaecology*** in females) consists of different organs in males and females. In males these are testes, epididymes, vas deferens, ejaculatory ducts, urethra, prostate, seminal vesicles and penis (Fig. 1.60). In females the organs are ovaries, fallopian tubes, uterus and vagina (Fig. 1.61). These two sets of organs are responsible for the production of ova and spermatozoa which on fertilization, implantation and proper nourishment in the uterus develops

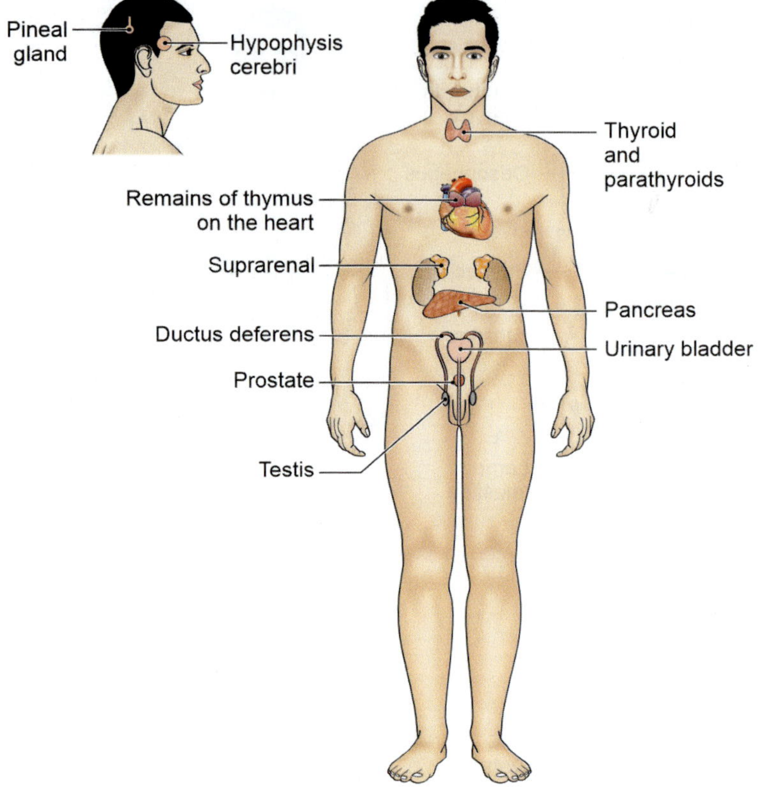

Fig. 1.60: Reproductive and endocrine systems in male

into a foetus. The foetus delivers out after nine months of pregnancy. Details can be seen from 10th edition of *BD Chaurasia's Human Anatomy*, Volume 2, Chapters 31 and 32.

11. ***Endocrine system (endocrinology)*** consists of ductless glands like hypothalamus, hypophysis cerebri, thyroid, parathyroid, suprarenal glands and islets of Langerhans in pancreas which produce hormones, that are carried to various target organs via blood. In male additional endocrine gland is testis, whereas in female it is replaced by ovary (Figs 1.60 and 1.61). These hormones influence metabolism and other processes like production of spermatozoa and the menstrual cycle.
12. ***Special senses*** include senses of taste, sight, smell, hearing, balance and touch. Taste is appreciated by the papillae present in the tongue, epiglottis and soft palate. Sense of sight is

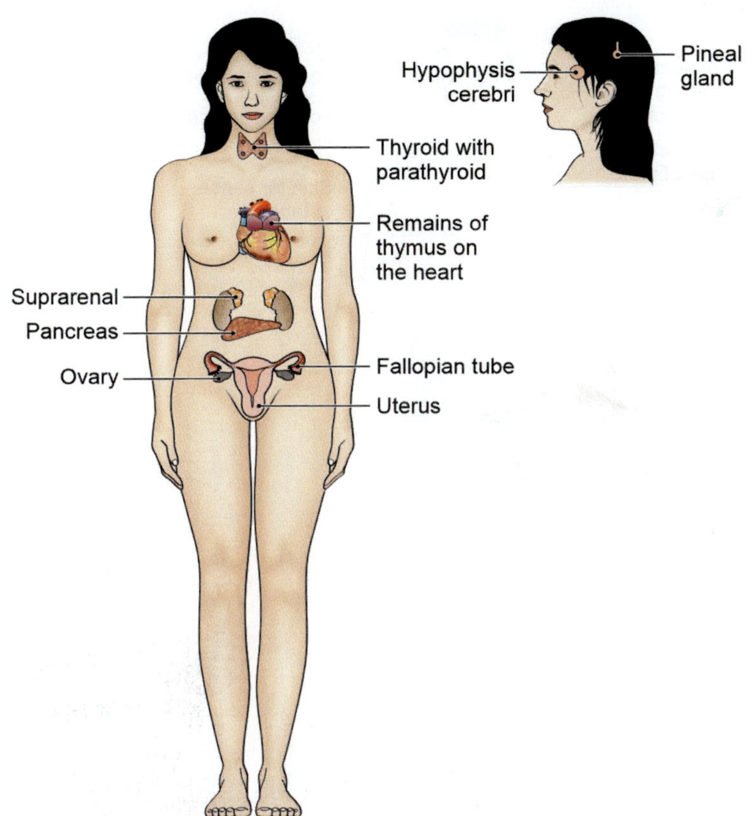

Fig. 1.61: Reproductive and endocrine systems in female

appreciated in the nervous layer, the retina, of the eyeball. Receptors of smell are only present in the mucous membrane of the upper part of the nasal cavity. Hearing and balance are compactly organised in the internal ear. Touch is perceived through the skin (Fig. 1.62).

13. ***Nervous system (neurology)*** consists of billions of neurons included in the central nervous system (brain and spinal cord) and peripheral nervous system (cranial and spinal nerves). This is the system which controls the whole body including its muscles, glands and organs. The nervous system controls both our voluntary and involuntary activities. The personality of the person is dependent on the integrity of the nervous system (Fig. 1.63). The details of the system can be available in 10th edition of *BD Chaurasia's Human Anatomy*, Volume 4.

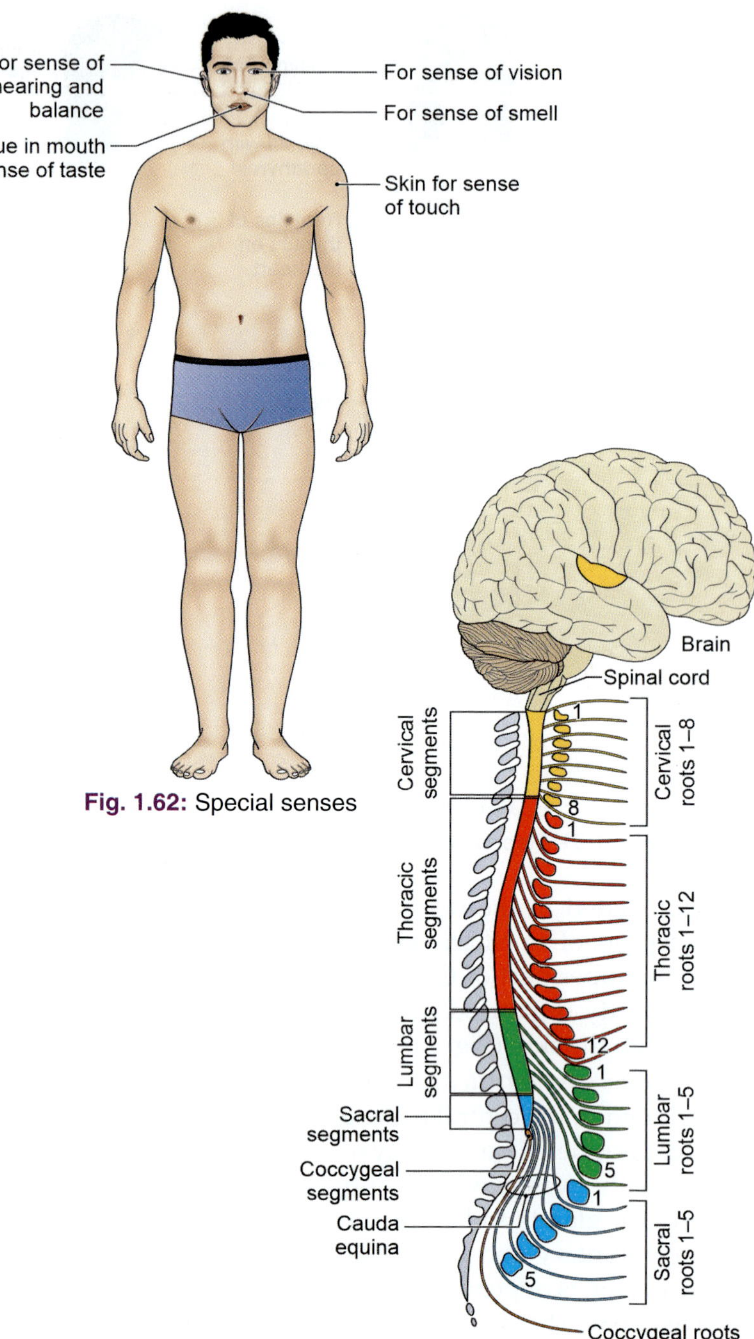

Fig. 1.62: Special senses

Fig. 1.63: Central nervous system

Clinical Anatomy

1. The *suffix*, '-itis', means inflammation, e.g. appendicitis, tonsillitis, arthritis, neuritis, dermatitis, etc.
2. The suffix, *'-ectomy'*, means removal from the body, e.g. appendicectomy, tonsillectomy, gastrectomy, nephrectomy, etc.
3. The suffix, *'-otomy'*, means to open and then close a hollow organ, e.g. laparotomy, hysterotomy, cystotomy, cystolithotomy, etc.
4. The suffix, *'-ostomy'*, means to open hollow organ and leave it open, e.g. cystostomy, colostomy, tracheostomy, etc.
5. The suffix, *'-oma'*, means a tumour, e.g. lipoma, osteoma, neurofibroma, haemangioma, carcinoma, etc.
6. *Puberty:* The age at which the secondary sexual characters develop, being 12–15 years in girls and 13–16 years in boys.
7. *Symptoms* are subjective complaints of the patient about his disease.
8. *Signs (physical signs)* are objective findings of the doctor on the patient.
9. *Diagnosis:* Identification of a disease, or determination of the nature of a disease.
10. *Prognosis:* Forecasting the probable course and ultimate outcome of a disease.
11. *Pyrexia:* Fever.
12. *Lesion:* Injury, or a circumscribed pathologic change in the tissues.
13. *Inflammation* is the local reaction of the tissues to an injury or an abnormal stimulation caused by a physical, chemical, or biologic agent. It is characterized by:
    a. Swelling
    b. Pain
    c. Redness
    d. Warmth or heat
    e. Loss of function.
14. *Oedema:* Swelling due to accumulation of fluid in the extracellular space.
15. *Thrombosis:* Intravascular coagulation (solidification) of blood.
16. *Embolism:* Occlusion of a vessel by a detached and circulating thrombus (embolus).
17. *Haemorrhage:* Bleeding which may be external or internal.
18. *Ulcer:* A localized breach (gap, erosion) in the surface continuity of the skin or mucous membrane.
19. *Sinus:* A blind track (open at one end) lined by epithelium.

20. ***Fistula:*** An abnormal passage usually between two internal organs or organ to surface of the body and lined by epithelium.
21. ***Necrosis:*** Local death of a tissue or organ due to irreversible damage to the nucleus.
22. ***Degeneration:*** A retrogressive change causing deterioration in the structural and functional qualities. It is a reversible process, but may end in necrosis.
23. ***Gangrene:*** A form of necrosis (death) combined with putrefaction.
24. ***Infarction:*** Death (necrosis) of a tissue due to sudden obstruction of its artery of supply (often an end-artery).
25. ***Atrophy:*** Diminution in the size of cells, tissue, organ, or a part due to loss of its nutrition.
26. ***Dystrophy:*** Diminution in the size due to defective nutrition.
27. Hypertrophy: Increase in the size without any increase in the number of cells.
28. ***Hyperplasia:*** Increase in the size due to increase in the number of cells.
29. ***Hypoplasia:*** Incomplete development.
30. ***Aplasia:*** Failure of development.
31. ***Syndrome:*** A group of diverse symptoms and signs constituting together the picture of a disease.
32. ***Paralysis:*** Loss of motor power (movement) of a part of body due to denervation or primary disease of the muscles.
33. ***Hemiplegia:*** Paralysis of one-half of the body.
34. ***Paraplegia:*** Paralysis of both the lower limbs.
35. ***Monoplegia:*** Paralysis of any one limb.
36. ***Quadriplegia:*** Paralysis of all the four limbs.
37. ***Anaesthesia:*** Loss of sensation.
38. ***Analgesia:*** Loss of the pain sensibility.
39. ***Thermanaesthesia:*** Loss of the temperature sensibility.
40. ***Hyperaesthesia:*** Abnormally increased sensibility.
41. ***Paraesthesia:*** Perverted feeling of sensations.
42. ***Coma:*** Deep unconsciousness.
43. ***Tumour (neoplasm):*** A circumscribed, noninflammatory, abnormal growth arising from the body tissues.
44. ***Benign:*** Mild illness or growth which does not endanger life.
45. ***Malignant:*** Severe form of illness or growth, which is resistant to treatment.

46. ***Carcinoma:*** Malignant growth arising from the epithelium (ectoderm or endoderm).
47. ***Sarcoma:*** Malignant growth arising from connective tissue (mesoderm).
48. ***Cancer:*** A general term used to indicate any malignant neoplasm which shows invasiveness and results in death of the patient, if not properly treated.
49. ***Metastasis:*** Spread of a local disease (like the cancer cells) to distant parts of the body.
50. ***Convalescence:*** The recovery period between the end of a disease and restoration to complete health.
51. ***Therapy:*** The treatment of disease.

ARRANGEMENT OF STRUCTURES IN THE BODY FROM WITHIN OUTWARDS

1. Bones form the supporting framework of the body.
2. Muscles are attached to bones.
3. Blood vessels, nerves and lymphatics form neurovascular bundles which course in between the muscles, along the fascial planes.
4. The thoracic and abdominal cavities contain several internal organs called viscera.
5. The whole body has three general coverings, namely (a) skin; (b) superficial fascia; and (c) deep fascia.

Points to Remember

- Hippocrates is the father of medicine.
- Leonardo da Vinci is the founder of modern anatomy.
- Dr Inderjit Dewan researched on osteology and anthropology.
- Anatomical position is the most important position for understanding anatomy.
- Median plane is only one plane in the trunk.
- Pronation and supination of forearm are special movements which permit "picking up of food (pronation)" and "putting it in the mouth (supination)".
- Big toe being in the same plane as rest of the toes is unique to human.

- Inversion and eversion of the foot help in its adjustment to the rough ground.
- There are 12 systems in the body. Medical students learn anatomy as regional anatomy, whereas nursing students learn it as systemic anatomy.
- Median/midsagittal plane divides the body into right and left halves.
- Coronal plane divides the body/any part into anterior and posterior parts.
- Transverse/horizontal plane divides the body/part into upper and lower portions.

Multiple Choice Questions

1. Name the founder of modern anatomy:

a. Vesalius b. Herophilus
c. Galen d. Leonardo da Vinci

2. Name the father of medicine:

a. Herophilus b. Galen
c. Hippocrates d. Vesalius

3. Name the father of anatomy:

a. Henry Gray b. Hippocrates
c. Galen d. Herophilus

4. Phylogeny is the developmental history of a human:

a. Through evolution b. Through life
c. Before birth d. From birth to death

5. Ontogeny is the developmental/history of a human:

a. Through evolution b. Before birth
c. From fertilization till death d. After birth

6. Anatomical position has following features *except*:

a. Person standing erect b. Forearms are pronated
c. Feet together d. Eyes looking forwards

7. Which statement about the coronal plane is incorrect:

a. Divides the body into anterior half and posterior half
b. Lies at right angle to sagittal plane
c. Lies at right angle to transverse plane
d. Divides the body into right half and left half

8. Define abduction:
- a. Movement away from central axis
- b. Movement towards central axis
- c. Approximation of the ventral surfaces
- d. Approximation of the dorsal surfaces

9. What is the position of forearms in the anatomical position?
- a. Pronated
- b. Supinated
- c. Midprone
- d. None of the above

10. Plane at right angle to the long axis of body/body part is called:
- a. Sagittal
- b. Coronal
- c. Transverse/horizontal
- d. Oblique

11. The term cranial means:
- a. Towards the head
- b. Towards the back
- c. Towards the tail
- d. Towards the front

12. Preaxial border of upper limb is:
- a. Its inner border
- b. Its outer border
- c. Its anterior median line
- d. Its posterior median line

Answers

1. d **2.** c **3.** d **4.** a **5.** c **6.** b **7.** d **8.** a
9. b **10.** c **11.** a **12.** b

Chapter 2

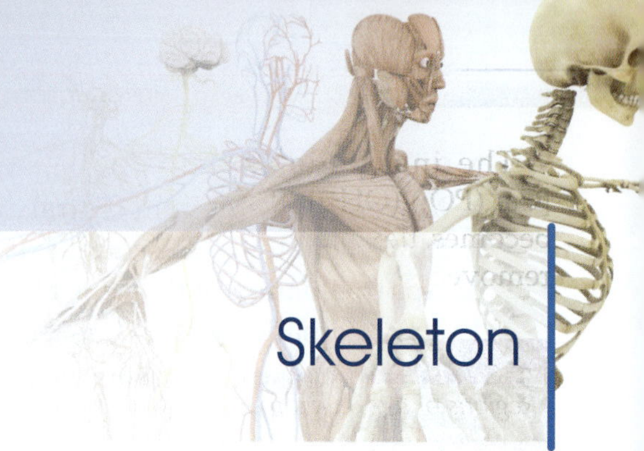

Skeleton

One quarter of what you eat keeps you alive; the three quarters keep doctors alive.

Skeleton includes bones and cartilages. It forms the main supporting framework of the body, and is primarily designed for a more effective production of movements by the attached muscles.

BONES

Synonyms

1. Os (L)
2. Osteon (G).

Compare with the terms, osteology, ossification, osteomyelitis, osteomalacia, osteoma, osteotomy, etc.

> *Competency achievement:* The student should be able to:
> AN 1.2 Describe composition of bone and bone marrow

Definition and Composition

Bone is one-third connective tissue. It is impregnated with calcium salts which constitute the remaining two-thirds part.

The inorganic calcium salts (mainly calcium phosphate, partly calcium carbonate, and traces of other salts) make it hard and rigid, which can afford resistance to compressive forces of weight-bearing and impact forces of jumping. The organic connective tissue (collagen fibres) makes it tough and resilient (flexible), which can afford resistance to tensile forces. In strength, bone is comparable to iron and steel.

The inorganic calcium salt is calcium hydroxy-apatite [$Ca_{10}(PO_4)_6(OH)_2$]. If it is removed by putting the bone in acid, it becomes flexible and can be tied as a 'knot'. If organic tissue is removed by burning, the bone crumples into small pieces.

Divisions of the Skeletal System (Fig. 2.1)

Regions of the skeleton	*Number of bones*	*Cranial and facial bones (mnemonic is A–Z)*	
AXIAL SKELETON			
Skull			
Cranium	8	**A–D**	–
Face	14	Ethmoid	1
Hyoid	1	Frontal	1
Auditory ossicles (3 in each ear):	6	**G–H**	–
(Malleus, incus, stapes)		Inferior nasal	
Vertebral column	26	choncha	2
Thorax		**J–K**	–
Sternum	1	Lacrimal	2
Ribs	24	Maxilla	2
APPENDICULAR SKELETON		Mandible	1
Pectoral (shoulder) girdles		Nasal	2
Clavicle	2	Occipital	1
Scapula	2	Parietal	2
Upper extremities		Palatine	2
Humerus	2	**Q–R**	–
Ulna	2	Sphenoid	1
Radius	2	Temporal	2
Carpals	16	**U**	–
Metacarpals	10	Vomer	1
Phalanges	28	**W–Y**	–
Pelvic (hip) girdle		Zygomatic	2
Pelvic, or hip bone	2		
Lower extremities			
Femur	2		
Fibula	2		
Tibia	2		
Patella	2		
Tarsals	14		
Metatarsals	10		
Phalanges	28		
	–		
Total	**206**		

Despite its hardness and high calcium content the bone is very much a living tissue. It is highly vascular, with a constant turnover of its calcium content. It shows a characteristic pattern of growth. It is subjected to disease and heals after a fracture. It has greater regenerative power than any other tissue of the body, except blood. It can mould itself according to changes in stress and strain it bears. It shows disuse atrophy and overuse hypertrophy.

Functions

1. Bones give shape and support to the body, and resist any forms of stress (Fig. 2.1a).
2. These provide surface for the attachment of muscles, tendons, ligaments, etc.
3. These serve as levers for muscular actions.
4. The skull, vertebral column and thoracic cage protect brain, spinal cord, thoracic and some abdominal viscera, respectively (Fig. 2.1b).
5. Bone marrow manufactures blood cells (Fig. 2.17).
6. Bones store 97% of the body calcium and phosphorus.
7. Bone marrow contains reticuloendothelial cells which are phagocytic in nature and take part in immune responses of the body.
8. The larger paranasal air sinuses, e.g. ethmoidal sinuses affect the timbre of the voice (Fig. 2.9).

CLASSIFICATION OF BONES

A. According to Shape

1. ***Long bones:*** Each long bone has an elongated shaft (diaphysis) and two expanded ends (epiphyses) which are smooth and articular (Fig. 2.2). The shaft typically has 3 surfaces separated by 3 borders, a central medullary cavity, and a nutrient foramen directed away from the growing end. Examples:
   a. *Typical long bones:* These are humerus, radius, ulna, femur, tibia and fibula; with two secondary epiphyses.
   b. *Miniature or short long bones:* Have only one epiphysis like metacarpals, metatarsals (Fig. 2.3) and phalanges.
   c. *Modified long bones:* Have medullary cavity in medial 2/3rd part like clavicle (Fig. 2.4). It transmits weight from appendicular skeleton to axial skeleton.

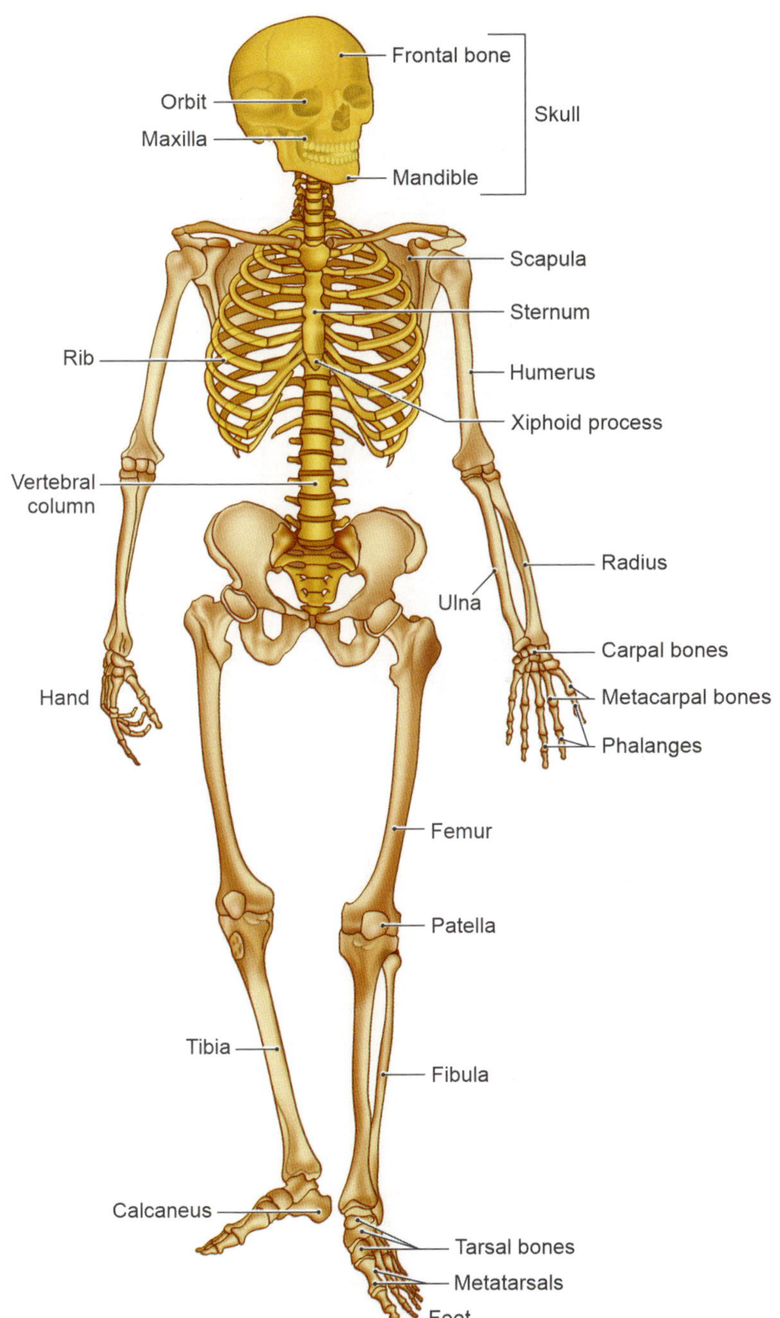

Fig. 2.1a: Anterior view of skeleton. Axial skeleton is colored

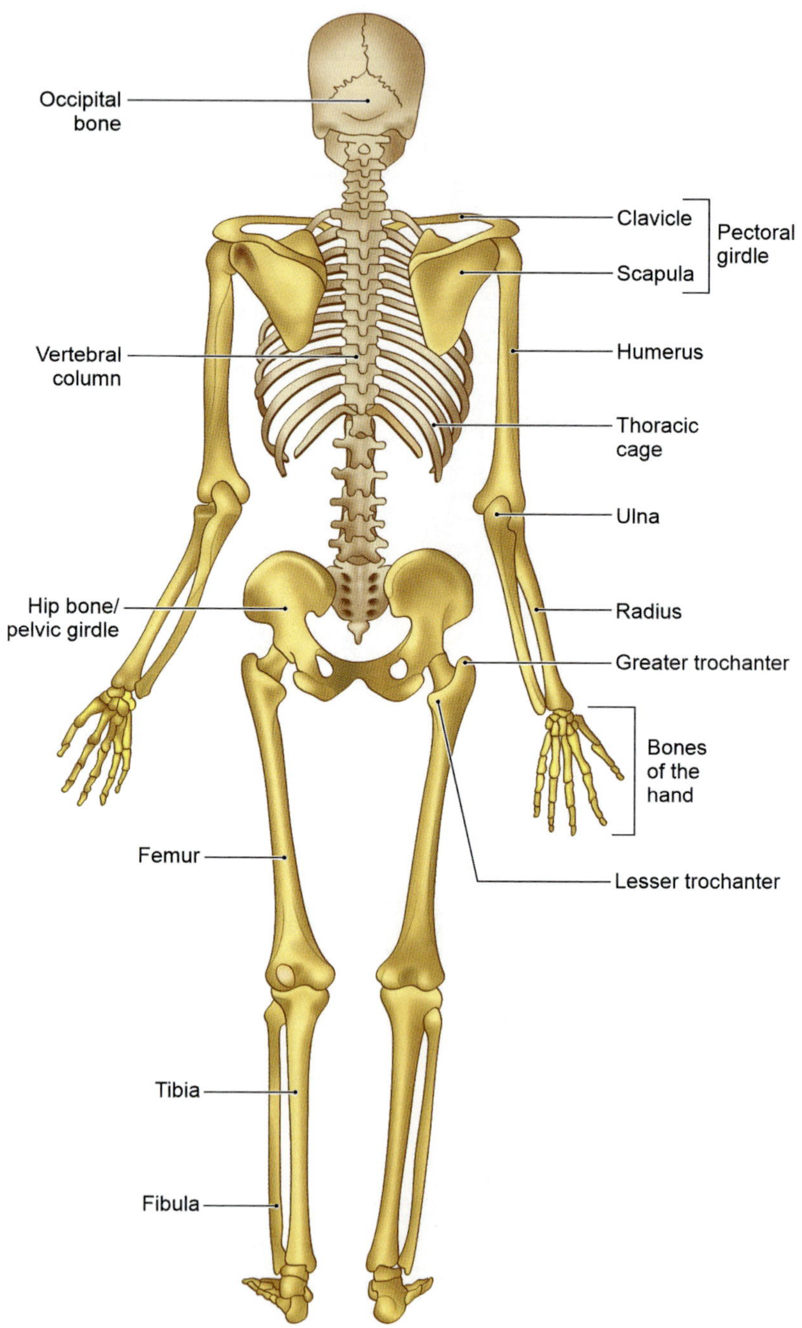

Fig. 2.1b: Posterior view of skeleton. The appendicular skeleton is colored

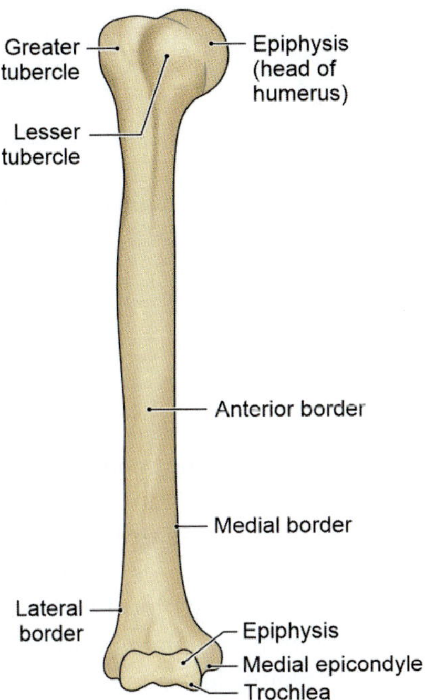

Fig. 2.2: Typical long bone—humerus

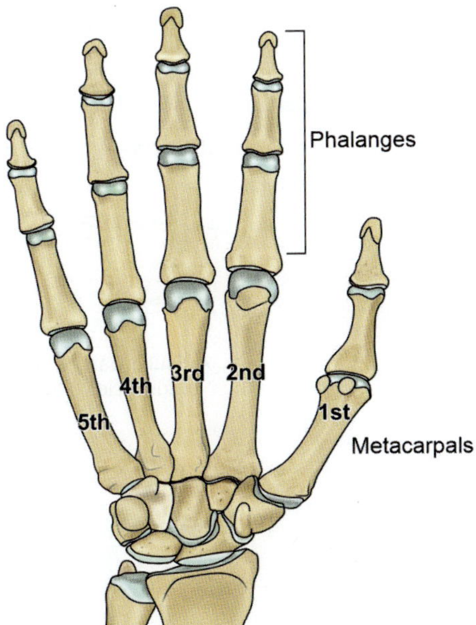

Fig. 2.3: Short long bones of hand

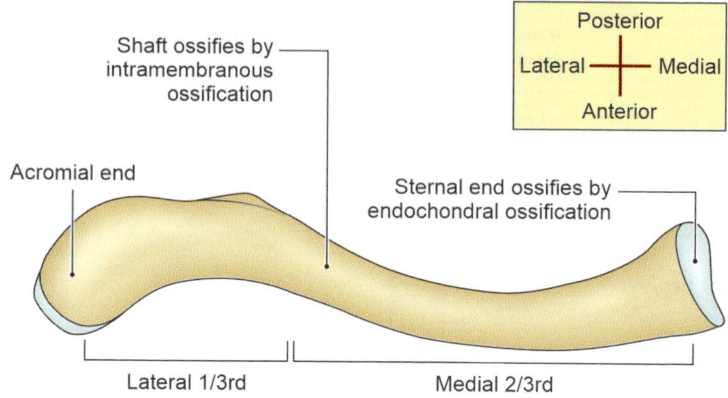

Fig. 2.4: Modified long bone-clavicle

2. ***Short bones:*** Their shape is usually cuboid, (like a cube) or scaphoid (boat shaped). Examples: Tarsal and carpal bones (Fig. 2.1a). These are pierced by blood vessels.
3. ***Flat bones:*** Resemble shallow plates and form boundaries of certain body cavities. Examples: Bones in the vault of the skull, sternum, ribs, and scapula (Figs 2.5 and 2.6).
4. ***Irregular bones:*** Examples: Hip bone (Fig. 2.1b) and bones in the base of the skull, e.g. sphenoid and first and second cervical vertebrae (Figs 2.7 and 2.8).

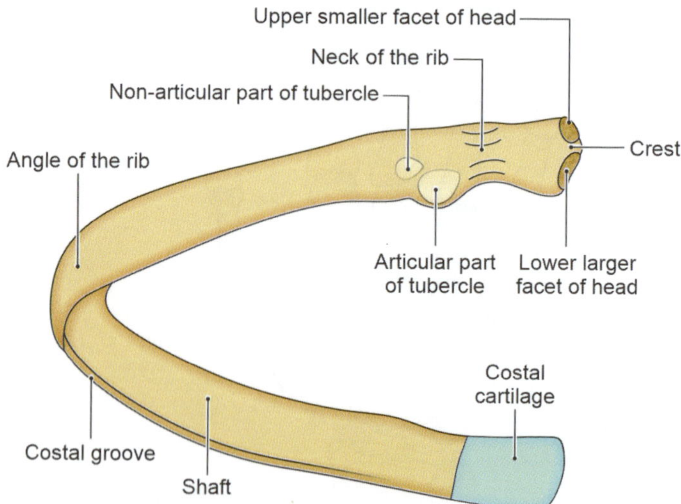

Fig. 2.5: Flat bone-rib

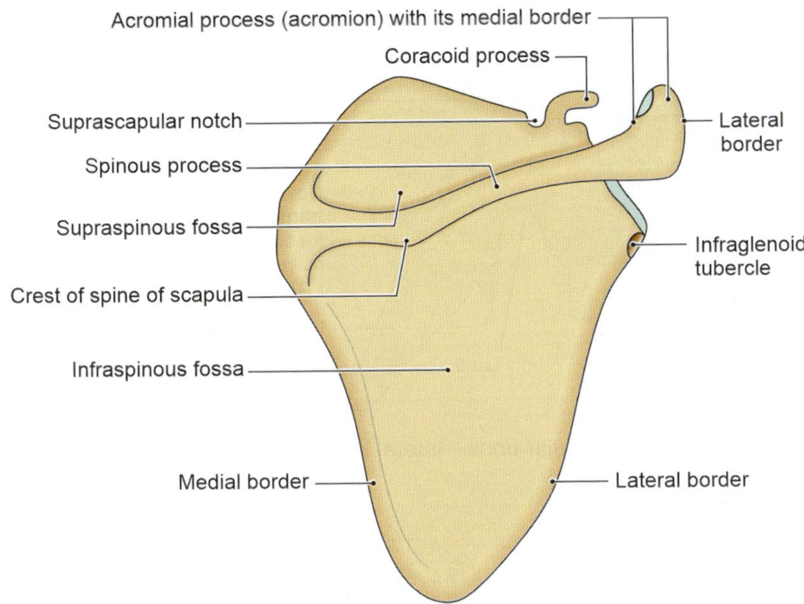

Fig. 2.6: Flat bone-scapula

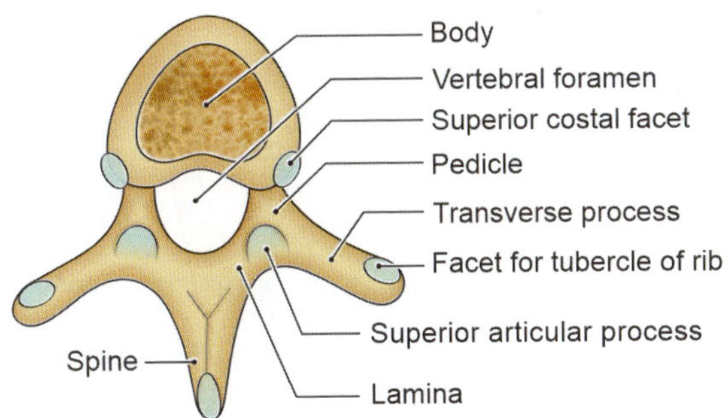

Fig. 2.7: Irregular bone—superior view of thoracic vertebra

5. ***Pneumatic bones:*** Certain irregular bones contain large air spaces lined by epithelium. Examples: Maxilla, sphenoid, ethmoid (Fig. 2.9), etc. They make the skull (a) light in weight, (b) help in resonance of voice, and (c) act as air conditioning chambers for the inspired air. (d) It improves timbre (quality) of the voice.

Competency achievement: The student should be able to:
AN 2.3 Enumerate special features of a sesamoid bone

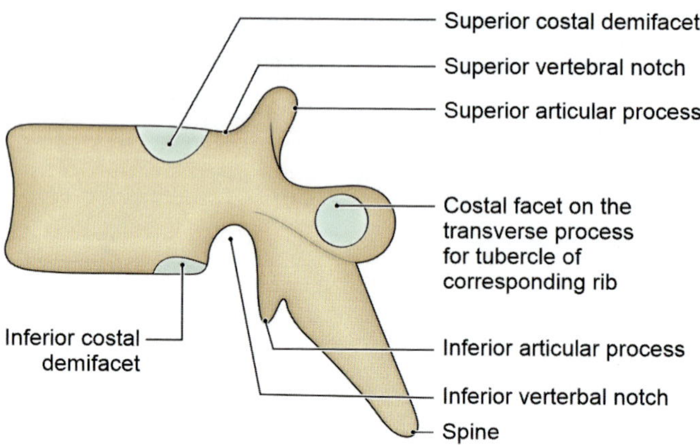

Fig. 2.8: Irregular bone—lateral view of thoracic vertebra

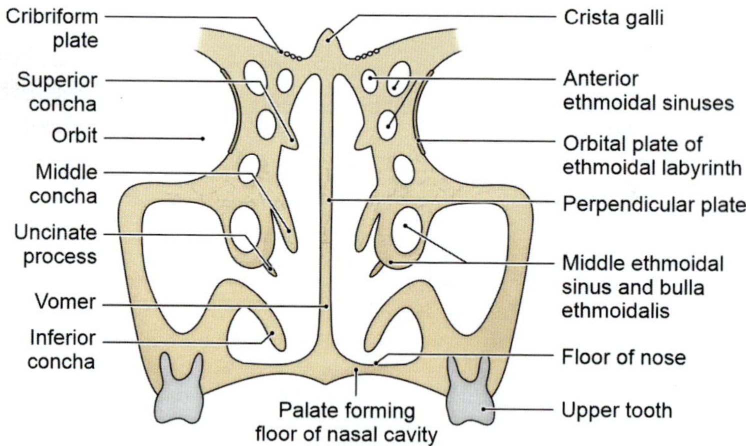

Fig. 2.9: Pneumatic bone—ethmoid

6. ***Sesamoid bones:*** These are bony nodules found embedded in the tendons or joint capsules. They have no periosteum and ossify after birth. They are related to an articular or nonarticular bony surface, and the surfaces of contact are covered with hyaline cartilage and lubricated by a bursa or synovial membrane. Examples: Patella in the tendon of quadriceps femoris (Fig. 2.10), pisiform, in the tendon of flexor carpi ulnaris, flabella in the tendon of lateral head of gastrocnemius, riders bone developed in tendon of adductor longus in professional

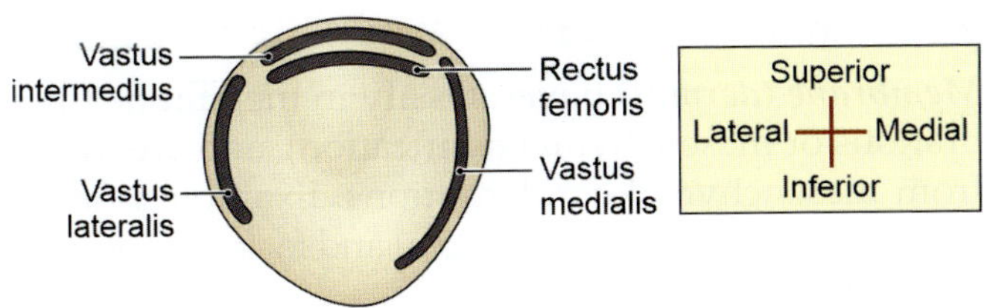

Fig. 2.10: Sesamoid bone—patella

riders. These do not have medullary cavity, haversian system, or periosteum.

Functions of the sesamoid bones are:

a. to resist pressure;
b. to minimise friction;
c. to alter the direction of pull of the muscle; and
d. to maintain the local circulation, protect the vessels and nerves.

7. ***Accessory (supernumerary) bones*** are not always present. These may occur as ununited epiphyses developed from extra centres of ossification. Examples: Sutural bones of the skull, cervical ribs, lumbar ribs. The sutural/wormian bone is mostly seen in the region of lambda (Fig. 2.11). These can be present at asterion and pterion as well. Such bones are common in hydrocephalic skulls.

In medicolegal practice, accessory bones may be mistaken for fractures. However, these are often bilateral, and have smooth surfaces without any callus.

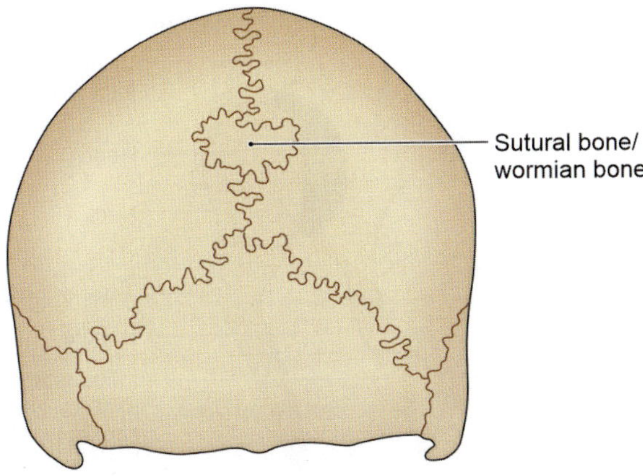

Fig. 2.11: Sutural bone/wormian bone in the skull

B. Developmental Classification

1. • ***Membrane (dermal) bones:*** Ossify in membrane (intramembranous or mesenchymal ossification), and are thus derived from mesenchymal condensations. Examples: Bones of the vault of skull like frontal, parietal and facial bones like maxilla (Fig. 2.1a).
   • ***Cartilaginous bones:*** Ossify in cartilage (intracartilaginous or endochondral ossification), and are thus derived from replacement of preformed cartilaginous models. Examples: Bones of limbs like humerus, femur, vertebral column and thoracic cage (Fig. 2.1b).
   • ***Membrano-cartilaginous bones:*** Ossify partly in membrane and partly in cartilage. Examples: Clavicle (sternal end ossifies by endochondral ossification while the rest of the bone ossifies by intramembranous ossification) (Fig. 2.4), mandible, occipital, temporal, sphenoid.
2. • ***Somatic bones:*** Most of the bones are somatic.
   • ***Visceral bones:*** These are a few and develop from pharyngeal arches. Examples are hyoid bone, part of mandible (Fig. 2.1a) and ear ossicles (Fig. 2.12).

C. Regional Classification

1. ***Axial skeleton:*** Includes skull, vertebral column, and thoracic cage (Fig. 2.1a).
2. ***Appendicular skeleton:*** Includes bones of the limbs, e.g. pectoral girdle, free upper limb and pelvic girdle, free lower limb (Fig. 2.1b).

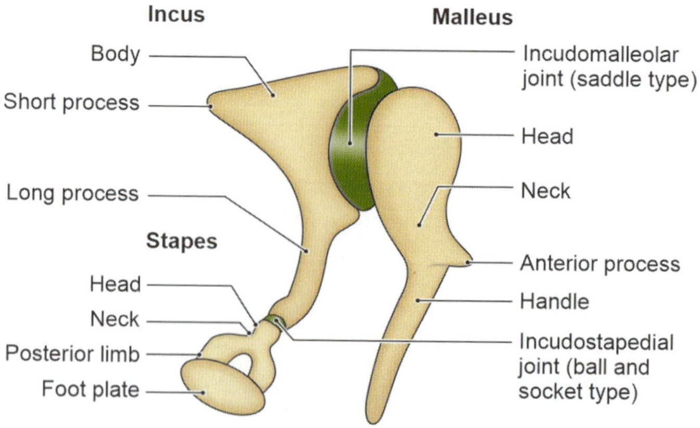

Fig. 2.12: Visceral bones—ear ossicles with their joints

D. Structural Classification

I. *Macroscopically*, the architecture of bone may be compact or cancellous (Fig. 2.13).

1. Compact bone is dense in texture like ivory, but is extremely porous. It is best developed in the cortex of the long bones. This is an adaptation to bending and twisting forces (a combination of compression, tension and shear).

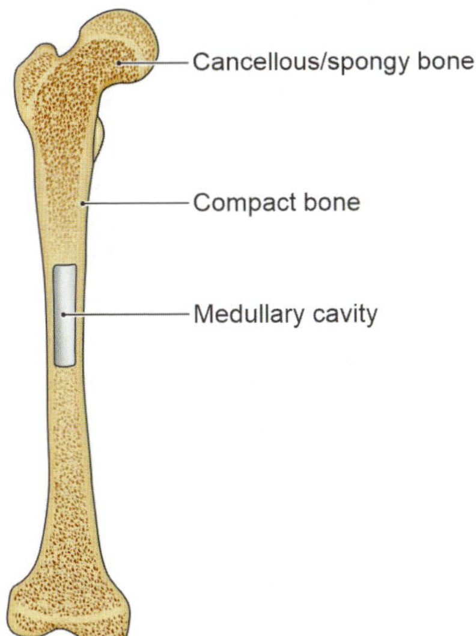

Fig. 2.13: Structure of bone

2. Cancellous or spongy or trabecular bone is open in texture, and is made up of a meshwork of trabeculae (rods and plates) between which are marrow containing spaces. The trabecular meshworks are of three primary types, namely:
   a. meshwork of rods,
   b. meshwork of rods and plates, and
   c. meshwork of plates.

   Cancellous bone is an adaptation to compressive forces.

Bones are marvellously constructed to combine strength, elasticity and lightness in weight. Though the architecture of bone may be modified by mechanical forces, the form of the bone is primarily determined by heredity (Table 2.1).

Table 2.1: Comparison of compact and cancellous bones

	Compact bone	*Cancellous (spongy) bone*
Location	In shaft (diaphysis) of long bone	In the epiphyses of long bone
Lamellae	Arranged to form Haversian system	Arranged in a meshwork, so Haversian systems are not present
Bone marrow	Yellow which stores fat after puberty. It is red before puberty	Red, produce RBCs, granular series of WBC and platelets
Nature	Hard and ivory like	Spongy

According to *Wolff's law* (Trajectory Theory of Wolff, 1892), the bone formation is directly proportional to stress and strain. There are two forces, tensile force and compressive force. Both the tensile and compressive forces can stimulate bone formation under proper conditions.

The architecture of cancellous bone is often interpreted in terms of the trajectorial theory. Thus the arrangement of bony trabeculae (lamellae) is governed by the lines of maximal internal stress in the bone.

Compression lamellae are arranged parallel to the line of weight transmission, whereas *tension lamellae* are arranged at right angles to pressure lamellae. The compact arrangement of pressure lamellae forms bony buttress, for additional support, like calcar femorale (Fig. 2.14).

II. *Microscopically*, the bone is of five types, namely lamellar (including both compact and cancellous), woven, fibrous, dentine and cement.

1. ***Lamellar bone:*** Most of the mature human bones, whether compact or cancellous, are composed of thin plates of bony tissue called lamellae. These are arranged as branching curved plates in the cancellous bone, but in concentric cylinders (Haversian system or secondary osteon) in a compact bone (Fig. 2.15).

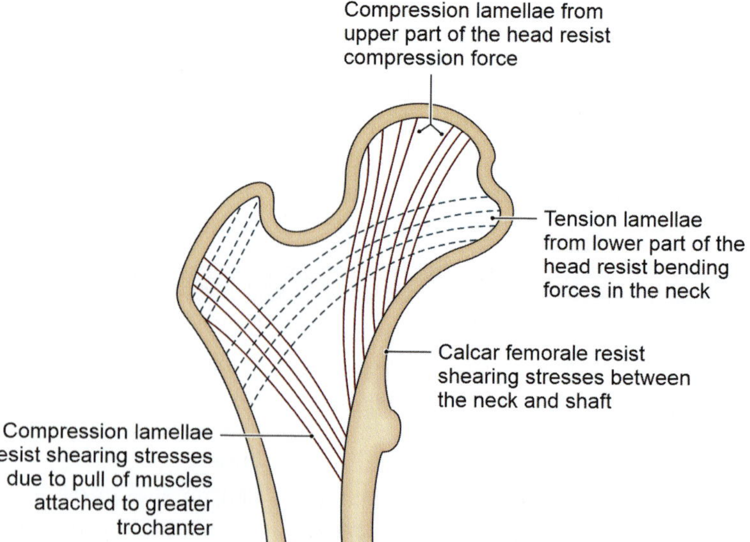

Fig. 2.14: Types of lamellae and calcar femorale

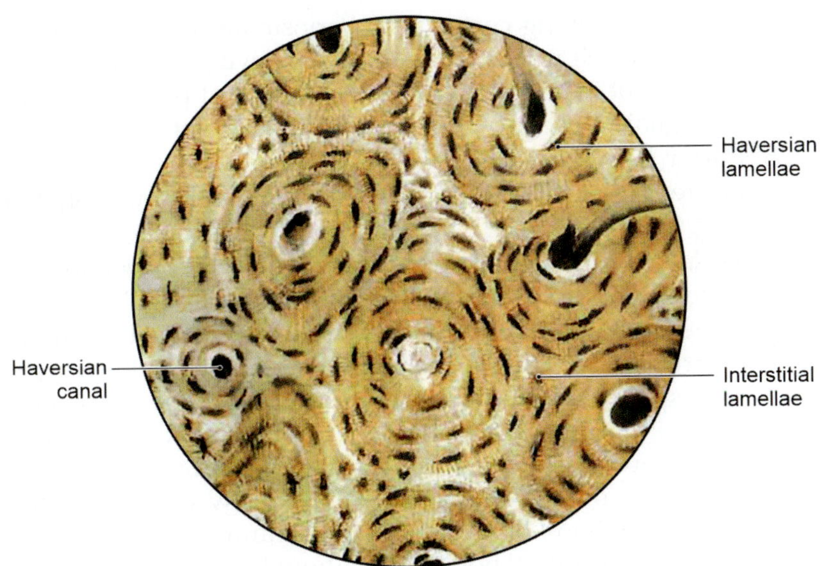

Fig. 2.15: Microscopic structure of compact bone

2. ***Woven bone:*** Seen in fetal bone, fracture repair and in cancer of bone. The collagen fibres and bone crystals are arranged randomly.
3. ***Fibrous bone*** is found in young foetal bones, but are common in reptiles and amphibia.
4. ***Dentine*** and
5. ***Cement*** occur in teeth.

GROSS STRUCTURE OF AN ADULT LONG BONE

Naked eye examination of the longitudinal and transverse sections of a long bone shows the following features.

1. ***Shaft:*** From without inwards, it is composed of periosteum, cortex and medullary cavity (Fig. 2.16a).
   a. *Periosteum* is a thick fibrous membrane covering the external surface of the bone. It is made up of an outer fibrous layer, and an inner cellular layer which is osteogenic in nature. Periosteum is united to the underlying bone by Sharpey's fibres, and the union is particularly strong over the attachments of tendons, and ligaments. At the articular margin the periosteum is continuous with the capsule of the joint. The abundant periosteal arteries nourish the outer part

of the underlying cortex also. Periosteum has a rich nerve supply which makes it the most sensitive part of the bone. It is absent in sesamoid bones. Functions of periosteum are osteogenic, bone growth, bone repair and protective.

b. *Cortex* is made up of a compact bone which gives it the desired strength to withstand all possible mechanical strains (Fig. 2.16b).

c. *Medullary cavity* is lined by endosteum. The osteoblasts in endosteum help in bone repair and remodelling of bone.

The medullary cavity is filled with red or yellow bone marrow. At birth the marrow is red everywhere with widespread active haemopoiesis. As the age advances, the red marrow at many places atrophies and is replaced by yellow, fatty marrow which stores calories and with no power of haemopoiesis. Red marrow persists in the cancellous ends of long bones, sternum, ribs, iliac crest, vertebrae and skull bones throughout life. The sites of bone marrow in adult are shown in Fig. 2.17.

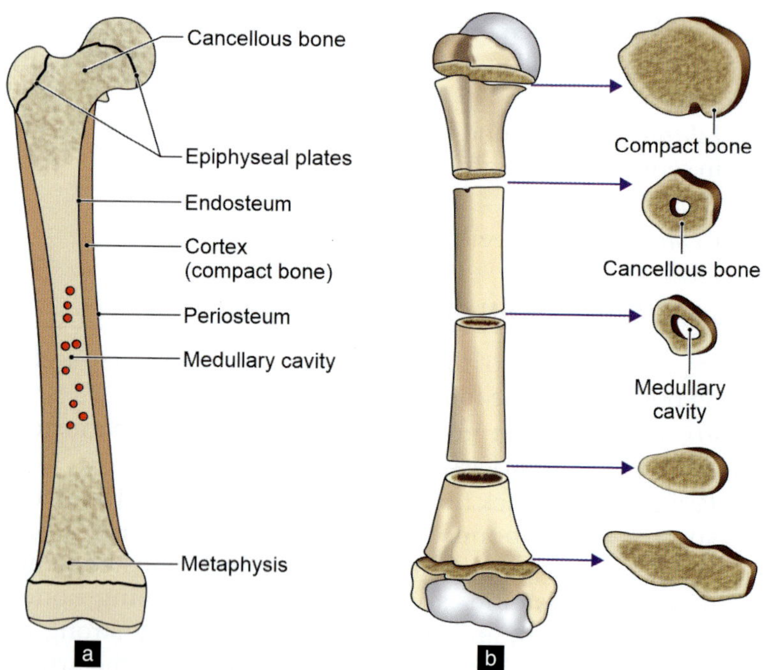

Fig. 2.16: (a) Components of long bone and (b) Transverse sections of a bone at different levels

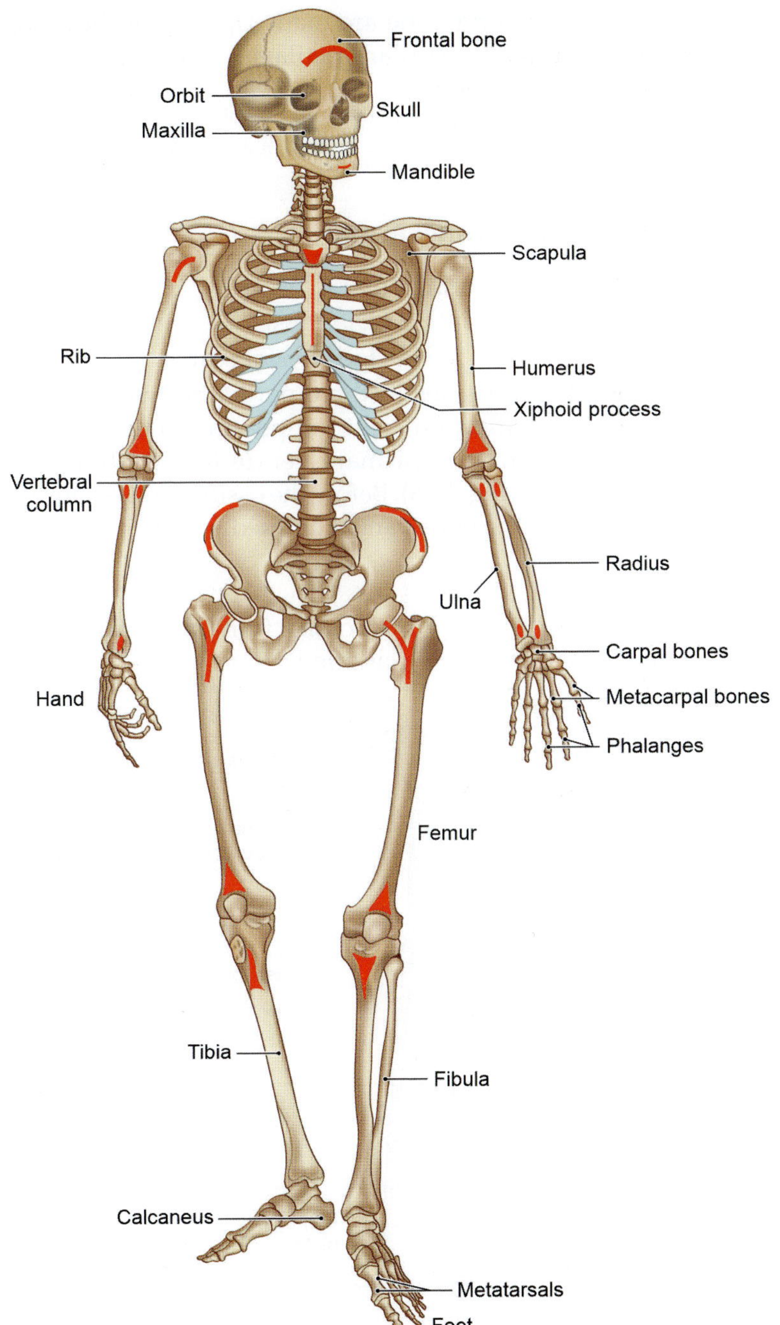

Fig. 2.17: Sites of red bone marrow in an adult

2. The **two ends** of a long bone are made up of cancellous bone covered with hyaline (articular) cartilage.

Competency achievement: The student should be able to:
AN 2.1 Describe parts, blood and nerve supply of a long bone

PARTS OF A YOUNG GROWING BONE

There are four parts of a young bone:

1. Epiphysis
2. Diaphysis
3. Metaphysis
4. Epiphysial plates

A typical long bone ossifies in three parts, the two ends form secondary centres (ossification centre appearing after birth), and the intervening shaft from a primary centre (ossification centre appearing before birth) (Fig. 2.18). Before the ossification is complete, the following parts of the bone can be defined.

1. Epiphysis

The ends and tips of a bone which ossify from secondary centres are called epiphyses. These are classified as:

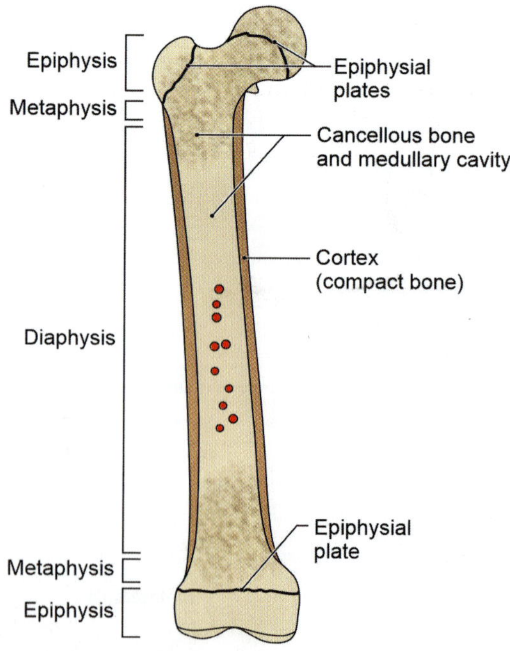

Fig. 2.18: Parts of a young growing bone

1. **According to number of epiphysis:**
   a. ***Simple:*** Ends of long bones develop from many epiphyses. These fuse independently with shaft, e.g. femur.
   b. ***Compound:*** The ends of bones develop from many centres, which unite to form a single epiphysis. The single epiphysis fuses with the shaft, e.g. humerus.
2. **Based on function:**
   a. ***Pressure epiphysis:*** It is articular and takes part in transmission of the weight. Examples: Head of humerus; lower end of radius, etc. (Fig. 2.19)
   b. ***Traction epiphysis:*** It is nonarticular and does not take part in the transmission of the weight. It always provides attachment to one or more tendons which exert a traction on the epiphysis. The traction epiphyses ossify later than the pressure epiphyses. Examples: Trochanters of femur and tubercles of humerus (Figs 2.1b and 2.2).
   c. ***Atavistic epiphysis:*** It is phylogenetically an independent bone which in human becomes fused to another bone.
   Examples: Coracoid process of scapula (Fig. 2.19a) and os trigonum or lateral tubercle of posterior process of talus (Fig. 2.19b).
   d. ***Aberrant epiphysis:*** It is not always present. Examples: Epiphysis at the head of the first metacarpal and at the bases of other metacarpal bones.
   e. ***Compound epiphysis:*** In some bones 2–3 smaller epiphyses join to form a compound epiphysis before these join the shaft, e.g. at upper end of humerus, epiphysis of head, greater and lesser tubercles join to form a compound epiphysis. Then this compound epiphysis joins the shaft. Similar events occur at the lower end of humerus also.

2. Diaphysis

It is the elongated shaft of a long bone which ossifies from a primary centre of ossification (Fig. 2.18). It receives blood supply from nutrient artery.

3. Metaphysis

The epiphysial ends of a diaphysis are called metaphyses. Each metaphysis is the zone of active growth. Before epiphysial fusion, the metaphysis is richly supplied with blood through end arteries forming 'hair-pin' bends (Fig. 2.20).

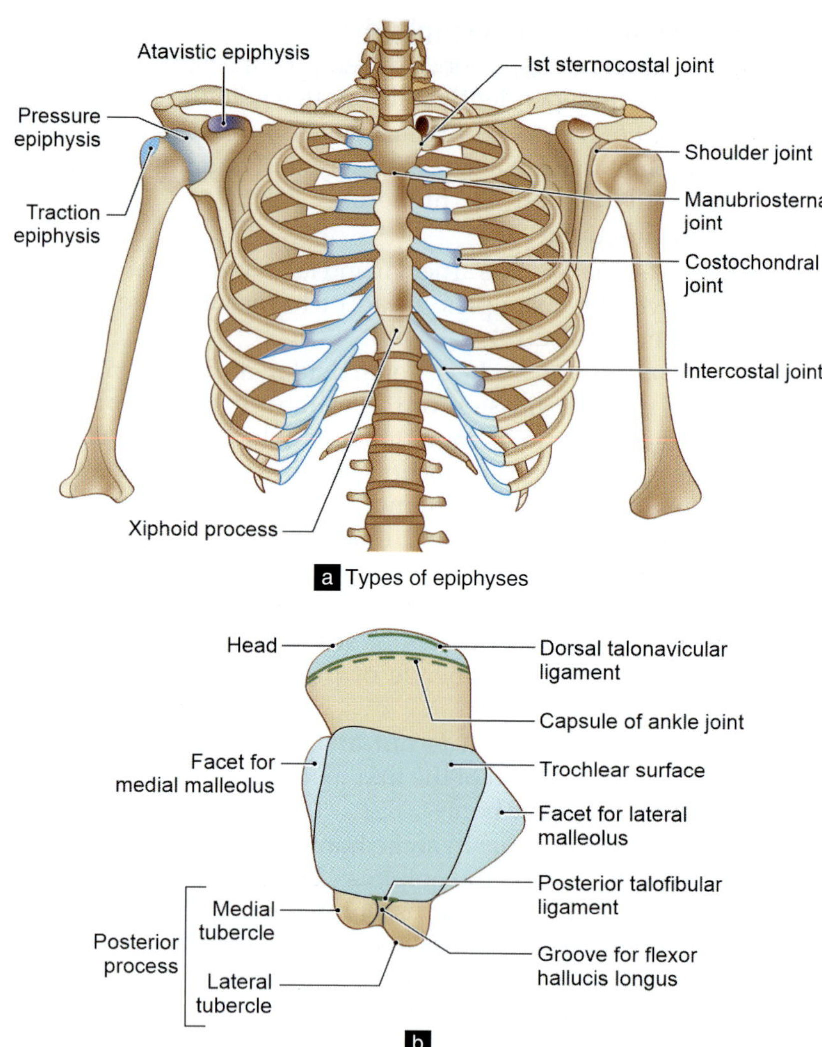

Fig. 2.19: Atavistic epiphysis—lateral tubercle

Thus metaphysis is the common site of osteomyelitis in children because the bacteria or emboli are easily trapped in the hair-pin bends, causing infarction. After the epiphysial fusion, vascular communications are established between the metaphysial and epiphysial arteries. Now the metaphysis contains no more end-arteries and is no longer subjected to osteomyelitis. Metaphysis may be (i) intracapsular, e.g. both ends of humerus, (ii) extracapsular, e.g. upper and lower ends of radius and tibia.

4. Epiphysial Plate of Cartilage

Epiphysial plate separates epiphysis from metaphysis.

Proliferation of cells in this cartilaginous plate is responsible for lengthwise growth of a long bone.

After the epiphysial fusion, the bone can no longer grow in length.

The growth cartilage is nourished by both the epiphysial and metaphysial arteries.

BLOOD SUPPLY OF BONES

Arterial Supply

1. Young Long Bones

The arterial supply of a long bone is derived from the following sources (Fig. 2.20).

a. ***Nutrient artery***

- It enters the shaft through the nutrient foramen, runs through the cortex, and divides into ascending and descending branches which turn down to form hair pin bends.
- Each branch divides into a number of small parallel channels which terminate in the adult metaphysis by anastomosing with the epiphysial, metaphysial and periosteal arteries.

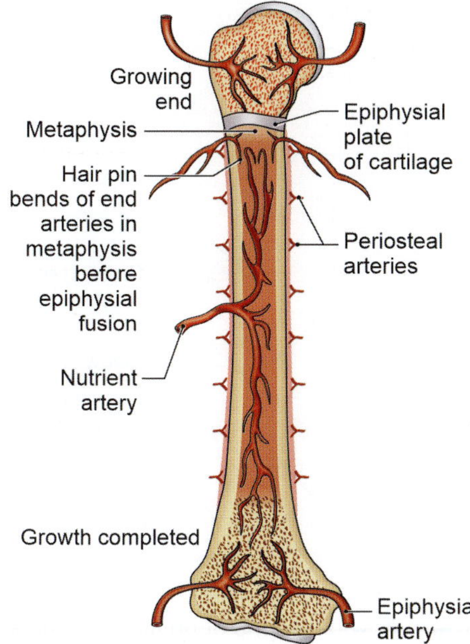

Fig. 2.20: Arterial supply of a long growing bone

- The nutrient artery supplies medullary cavity, inner 2/3rd of cortex and metaphysis.
- The growing ends of bones in upper limb are upper end of humerus and lower ends of radius and ulna. In lower limb, the lower end of femur and upper end of tibia are the growing ends.
- The *nutrient foramen* is directed away from the growing end of the bone. Their directions are indicated by a jingle, *'To the elbow I go, from the knee I flee'* (Fig. 2.21).
- Infection in blood produces small emboli. These may block the nutrient artery at the site of hair pin bend; resulting in osteomyelitis.

b. ***Periosteal arteries***
- These are especially numerous beneath the muscular and ligamentous attachments.
- They ramify beneath the periosteum and enter the Volkmann's canals to supply the outer 1/3rd of the cortex.

c. ***Epiphysial arteries***
- These are derived from periarticular vascular arcades (circulus vasculosus) found on the nonarticular bony surface.
- Out of the numerous vascular foramina in this region, only a few admit the arteries (epiphysial and metaphysial), and the rest are venous exits.

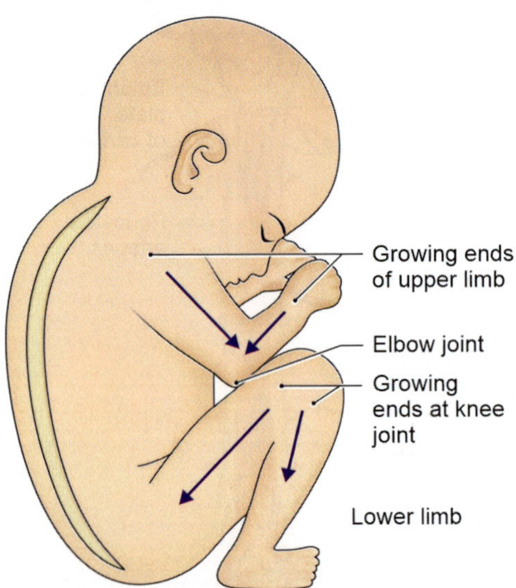

Fig. 2.21: Blue arrows show directions of nutrient foramina, seen away from the growing ends of bones

- The number and size of these foramina may give an idea of the relative vascularity of the two ends of a long bone (Tandon, 1964).

d. ***Metaphysial arteries***
- These are derived from the neighbouring systemic vessels.
- They pass directly into the metaphysis and reinforce the metaphysial branches from the primary nutrient artery.

In miniature long bones (metacarpals), the infection begins in the middle of the shaft rather than at the metaphysis because, the nutrient artery breaks up into a plexus immediately upon reaching the medullary cavity. In the adults, however, the chances of infection are minimized because the nutrient artery is mostly replaced by the periosteal vessels.

2. Long Short Bones

Nutrient artery enters the middle of shaft and divides to form a plexus. Periosteal artery supplies major part of bone and may replace the nutrient artery.

3. Short Bones

Short bones are supplied by numerous periosteal vessels which enter their nonarticular surfaces.

4. Vertebra

In a vertebra, the body is supplied by anterior and posterior vessels; and the vertebral arch by large vessels entering the bases of transverse processes. Its red marrow is drained by two large basivertebral veins. These foramina lie on the posterior aspect of the body of the vertebra.

5. Rib

A rib is supplied by: (a) The nutrient artery which enters it just beyond the tubercle and (b) the periosteal arteries.

Venous Drainge

Veins are numerous and large in the cancellous red marrow containing bones (e.g. basivertebral veins). In the compact bone, they accompany arteries in the Volkmann's canals.

Lymphatic Drainage

Lymphatics have not been demonstrated within the bone, although some of them do accompany the periosteal blood vessels, which drain to the regional lymph nodes.

NERVE SUPPLY OF BONES

Nerves accompany the blood vessels. Most of them are sympathetic and vasomotor in function.

A few of them are sensory which are distributed to the articular ends and periosteum of the long bones, to the vertebra, and to large flat bones.

> *Competency achievement:* The student should be able to:
> AN 2.2 Enumerate laws of ossification

DEVELOPMENT AND OSSIFICATION OF BONES

Bones are first laid down as mesodermal (connective tissue) condensations. Replacement of mesodermal models into bone is called *intramembranous* or *mesenchymal ossification*, and the bones are called membrane (dermal) bones.

However, mesodermal stage may pass through cartilaginous stage by chondrification during 2nd month of intrauterine life. Replacement of cartilaginous model into bone is called *intracartilaginous* or *endochondral ossification*, and such bones are called cartilaginous bones.

Ossification takes place by centres of ossification, each one of which is a point where laying down of lamellae (bone formation) starts by the osteoblasts situated on the newly formed capillary loops. The centres of ossification may be primary or secondary. The *primary centres* appear before birth, usually during 8th week of intrauterine life. The *secondary centres* appear after birth during childhood with a few exceptions of lower end of femur and upper end of tibia which appear during 9th month of intrauterine life. Many secondary centres appear during puberty (Fig. 2.22a).

A primary centre forms diaphysis, and the secondary centres form epiphyses. Fusion of epiphysis with the diaphysis starts at puberty and is complete by the age of 25 years, after which no more bone growth can take place. The *law of ossification* states that secondary centres of ossification which appear first are last to unite. Exception is lower end of fibula. The end of a long bone where epiphysial fusion occur later is called the *growing end of the bone*.

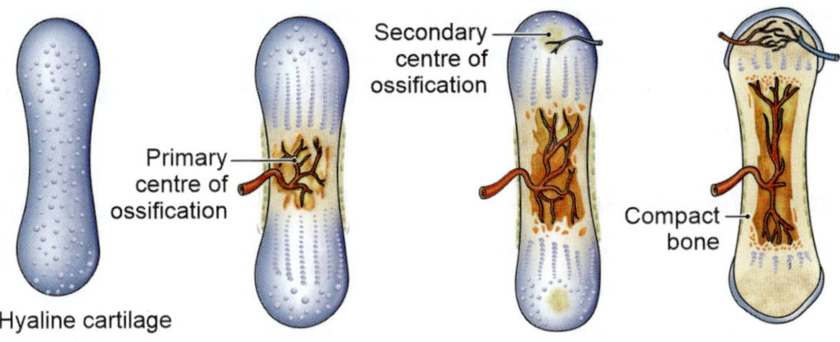

Fig. 2.22a: Intracartilaginous ossification

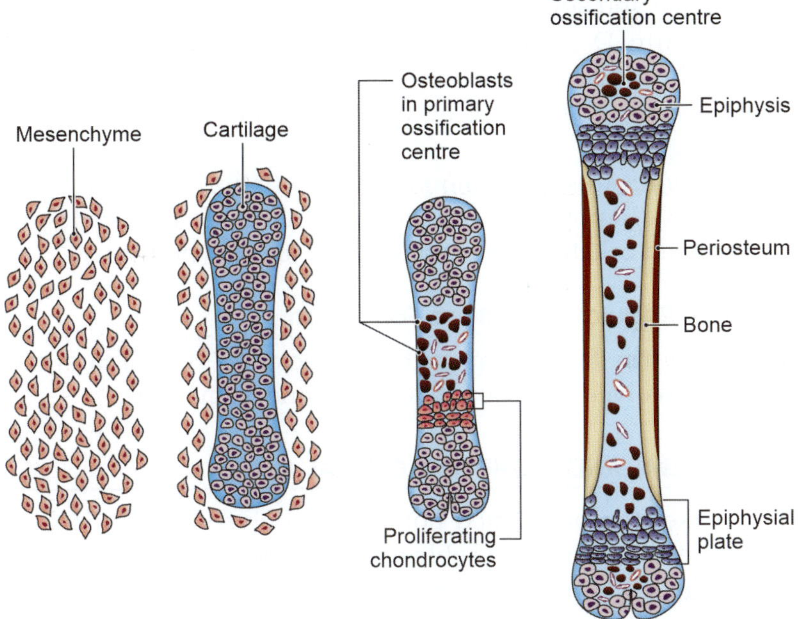

Fig. 2.22b: Development, ossification and growth of a long bone

GROWTH OF A LONG BONE

1. Bone grows in length by multiplication of cells in the epiphysial plate of cartilage (Fig. 2.22b).
2. Bone grows in thickness by multiplication of cells in the deeper layer of periosteum.
3. Bones grow by deposition of new bone on the surface and at the ends. This process of bone deposition by osteoblasts is called

appositional growth or surface accretion. However, in order to maintain the shape, the unwanted bone must be removed. This process of bone removal by osteoclasts is called *remodelling*. This is how marrow cavity increases in size.

Factors Affecting Growth

Adequate amounts of proteins, carbohydrates, minerals, vitamins and hormones are necessary for proper growth of bones.

1. ***Vitamins:*** Vitamin A controls the activity, co-ordination and distribution of osteoblasts and osteoclasts. Lack of vitamin A decreases the activity of osteoclasts leading to reduction in size of cranial and spinal foramina.

   Vitamin D is necessary for the absorption of calcium and phosphorus from intestines, which helps in proper ossification. Vitamin C is necessary for maintenance of organic matrix.
2. ***Hormonal:*** Adequate amounts of growth hormone of anterior pituitary (hypophysis cerebri), parathormone of parathyroid gland and calcitonin of thyroid gland are also necessary.

Molecular Regulation of Bone Formation

Members of the transforming growth factor-β (TGF-β) family of genes are involved in various stages of bone formation.

MEDICOLEGAL AND ANTHROPOLOGICAL ASPECTS

When a skeleton or isolated bones are received for medicolegal examination, one should be able to determine:

a. whether the bones are human or not;
b. whether they belong to one or more persons;
c. the age of the individual;
d. the sex;
e. the stature; and
f. the time and cause of death.

1. Estimation of Skeletal Age

Up to the age of 25 years, the skeletal age can be estimated to within 1–2 years of correct age by the state of dentition and ossification, provided the whole skeleton is available.

From 25 years onwards, the skeletal age can be estimated to within ± 5 years of the correct age by the state of cranial sutures and of the bony surfaces of symphysis pubis.

In general, the appearance of secondary centres and fusion of epiphyses occur about one year earlier in females than in males.

These events are also believed to occur 1–2 years (Bajaj et al. 1967) or 2–3 years (Pillai, 1936) earlier in India than in Western countries. However, Jit and Singh (1971) did not find any difference between the eastern and western races.

2. Estimation of Sex

Gender can be determined after the age of puberty.

Gender differences are best marked in the pelvis and skull, and accurate determination of gender can be done in over 90% cases with either pelvis or skull alone.

However, gender sexual dimorphism has been worked out in a number of other bones, like sternum (Jit et al, 1980), atlas (Halim and Siddiqui, 1976), and most of the limb bones.

3. Estimation of Stature (Height)

It is a common experience that trunk and limbs show characteristic ratios among themselves and in comparison with total height.

Thus a number of regression formulae have been worked out to determine height from the length of the individual limb bones (Siddiqui and Shah, 1944; Singh and Sohal, 1952; Jit and Singh, 1956; Athawale, 1963; Kolte and Bansal, 1974; Kate and Majumdar, 1976).

Height can also be determined from parts of certain long bones (Mysorekar et al), from hand length (Saxena et al, 1981), and from foot measurements (Charnalia, 1961; Qamra et al, 1980).

Crown-rump (CR) length has been correlated with diaphysial length of foetal bones (Vare and Bansal, 1977) and with the neonatal and placental parameters (Jeya Singh et al, 1980; Saxena et al, 1981).

4. Estimation of Race

It is of interest to anthropologists. A number of metrical (like cranial and facial indices) and nonmetrical features of the skull, pelvis, and certain other bones are of racial significance (Krogman, 1962; Berry, 1975).

Competency achievement: The student should be able to:
AN 2.4 Describe various types of cartilage with its structure and distribution in body

CARTILAGE

Synonyms

1. Chondros (G) and 2. Gristle. Compare with the terms chondrification, chondrodystrophy, synchondrosis, etc.

Definition

Cartilage is a connective tissue composed of cells (chondrocytes) and fibres (collagen or yellow elastic) embedded in a firm, gel-like matrix which is rich in a mucopolysaccharide. It is much more elastic than bone.

General Features

1. Cartilage has no blood vessels or lymphatics. The nutrition of cells diffuses through the matrix.
2. Cartilage has no nerves. It is, therefore, insensitive.
3. Cartilage is surrounded by a fibrous membrane, called perichondrium, which is similar to periosteum in structure and function. The articular cartilage has no perichondrium, so that its regeneration after injury is inadequate.
4. When cartilage calcifies, the chondrocytes die and the cartilage is replaced by bone like tissue.

   Table 2.2 shows the comparison between bone and cartilage.

Table 2.2: Comparison between bone and cartilage

Bone	*Cartilage*
1. Bone is hard	Cartilage is firm
2. Matrix has inflexible material called ossein	It has chondroitin providing flexibility
3. Matrix possesses calcium salt	Calcium salts not present
4. Bone has rich nerve supply. It is vascular in nature	It does not have nerve supply. It is avascular in nature
5. Bone marrow is present	Bone marrow is absent
6. Growth is only by apposition (by surface deposition)	Growth is both appositional and interstitial (from within)

Types of Cartilage

There are three types of cartilages:

1. Hyaline cartilage (Fig. 2.23)
2. Fibrocartilage (Fig. 2.24)
3. Elastic cartilage (Fig. 2.23)

Table 2.3 reveals the comparison among three types of cartilages.

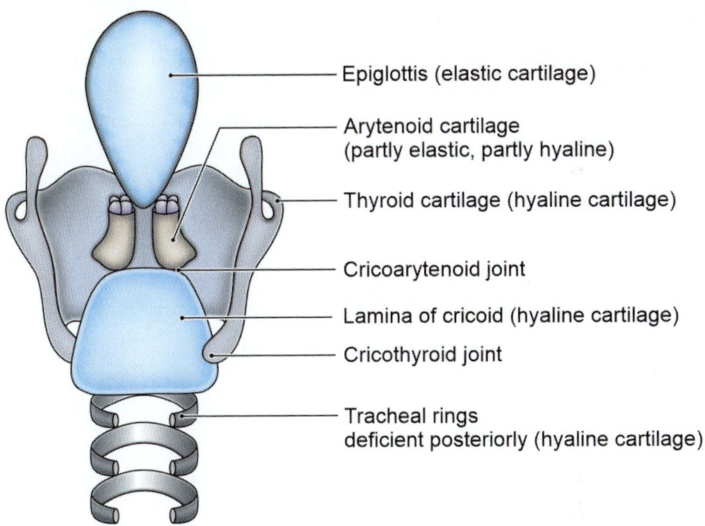

Fig. 2.23: Hyaline and elastic cartilages

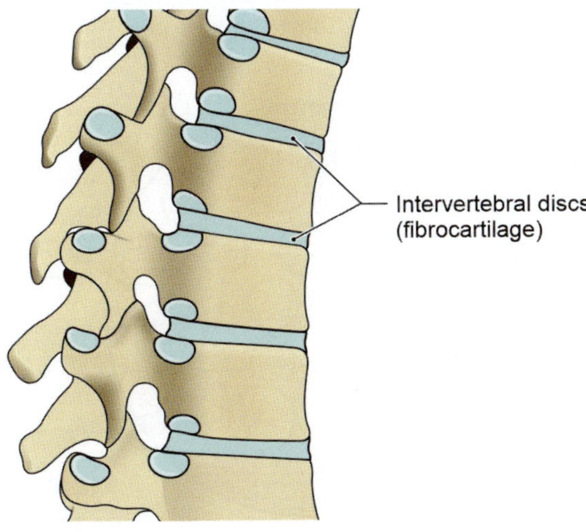

Fig. 2.24: Fibrocartilage in intervertebral disc

Table 2.3: Comparison of three types of cartilages

	Hyaline cartilage	*Fibrocartilage*	*Elastic cartilage*
Location	In the articular cartilages of long bones, epiphysial plates, nasal cartilages, thyroid, cricoid, most of arytenoid, trachea, bronchi and costal cartilages (Fig. 2.25a)	In the intervertebral disc, interpubic disc of symphysis pubis, articular discs of temporomandibular joints (TMJ), sterno-clavicular joint and inferior radioulnar joint. Articular cartilages of TMJ and sternoclavicular joint (Fig. 2.25b)	In the pinna, external auditory meatus, Eustachian tubes, epiglottis, vocal process of arytenoid cartilage, corniculate and cuneiform cartilages (Fig. 2.25c)
Colour	Bluish white	Glistening white	Yellowish
Appearance	Shiny or translucent	Opaque	Opaque
Fibres	Very thin, having same refractive index as matrix, so these are not seen	Numerous white fibres	Numerous yellow fibres
Elasticity	Flexible	More firm strongest	Most flexible
Perichon-drium	Present	Absent	Present
Cells	Maximum	Minimum, squeezed between fibres	Moderate

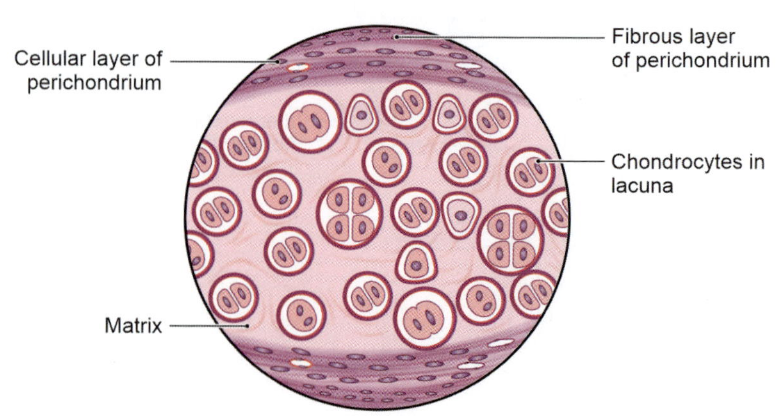

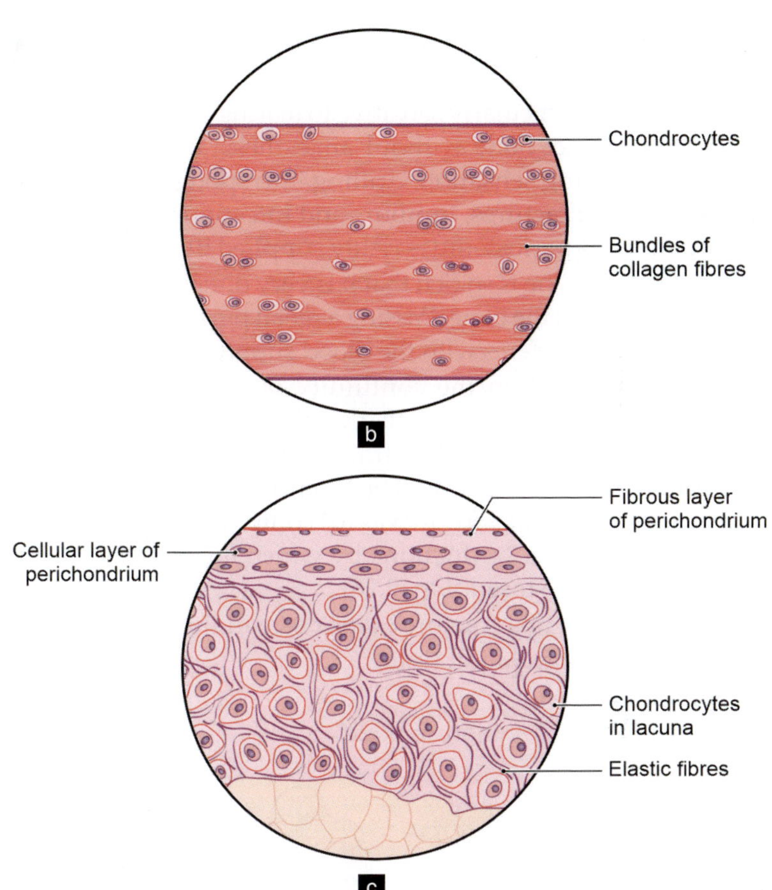

Fig. 2.25a to c: Types of cartilages: (a) Hyaline cartilage, (b) fibrocartilage and (c) elastic cartilage

Clinical Anatomy of Skeleton

- A defect in membranous ossification causes a rare syndrome called *cleidocranial dysostosis*. It is characterized by three cardinal features:
  a. Varying degrees of aplasia of the clavicles
  b. Increase in the transverse diameter of cranium
  c. Retardation in fontanelle ossification (Srivastava et al. 1971). It may be hereditary or environmental in origin.
- A defect in endochondral ossification causes a common type of dwarfism called *achondroplasia*, in which the limbs are short, but

the trunk is normal. It is transmitted as a Mendelian dominant character.

- Periosteum is particularly sensitive to tearing or tension. Drilling into the compact bone without anaesthesia causes only mild pain or an aching sensation; drilling into spongy bone is much more painful. Fractures, tumours and infections of the bone are very painful as periosteum is richly supplied by somatic nerves.
- *Blood supply* of bone is so rich that it is very difficult to interrupt it, sufficiently to kill the bone. Passing a metal pin into the medullary cavity hardly interferes with the blood supply of the bone.
- *Fracture* is a break in the continuity of a bone. The fracture which is not connected with the skin wound is known as simple (closed) fracture. The fracture line may be (a) spiral or (b) horizontal or (c) oblique. The fracture which communicates with the skin wound is known as (d) compound (open) fracture. A fracture requires "reduction" by which the alignment of the broken ends is restored (Fig. 2.26).

  Healing (repair) of a fracture takes place in three stages:

  a. Repair by granulation tissue
  b. Union by callus
  c. Consolidation by mature bone.

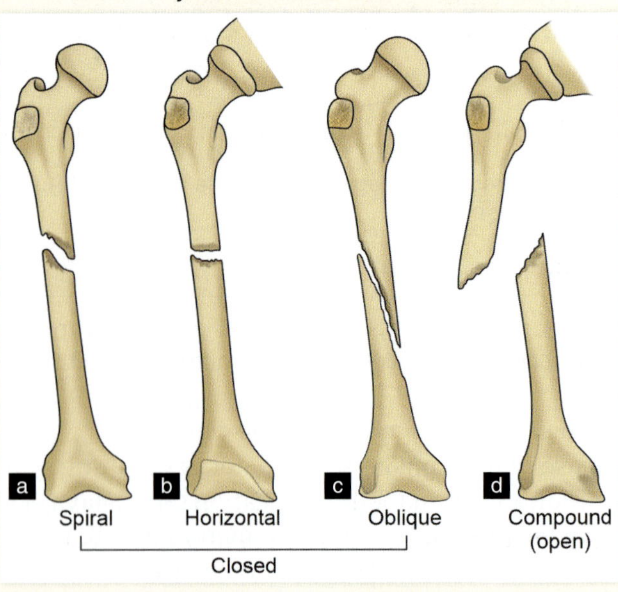

Fig. 2.26: Types of fractures

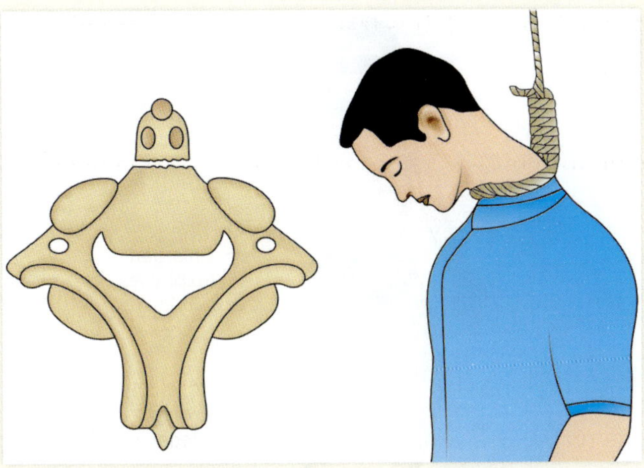

Fig. 2.27: Hanging leading to fracture of dens of axis vertebra

- Axis or 2nd cervical vertebra may get fractured. If dens of axis gets separated from the body (as in hanging), it hits the vital centres in the medulla oblongata causing instantaneous death (Fig. 2.27). Even fracture of laminae may cause death.
- In **rickets** (deficiency of vitamin D), calcification of cartilage fails and ossification of the growth zone is disturbed. Rickets affects the growing bones and, therefore, the disease develops during the period of most rapid growth of skeleton, i.e. 3 months to 3 years. Osteoid tissue is formed normally and the cartilage cells proliferate freely, but mineralization does not take place. This results in craniotabes, rachitic rosary at the costochondral junctions, Harrison's sulcus at the diaphragmatic attachments, enlarged epiphyses in limb bones and the spinal and pelvic deformities.
- For proper development of bones, a child requires adequate amounts of proteins, calcium, vitamin D, etc. Deficiency of calcium and vitamin D in growing children leads to widening of ends of bones with inadequate ossification. This condition is called rickets (Fig. 2.28).
- In scurvy (deficiency of vitamin C), formation of collagenous fibres and matrix is impaired. Defective formation of the intercellular cementing substances and lack of collagen cause rupture of capillaries and defective formation of new capillaries. Haematoma in the muscles and bones (subperiosteal) cause

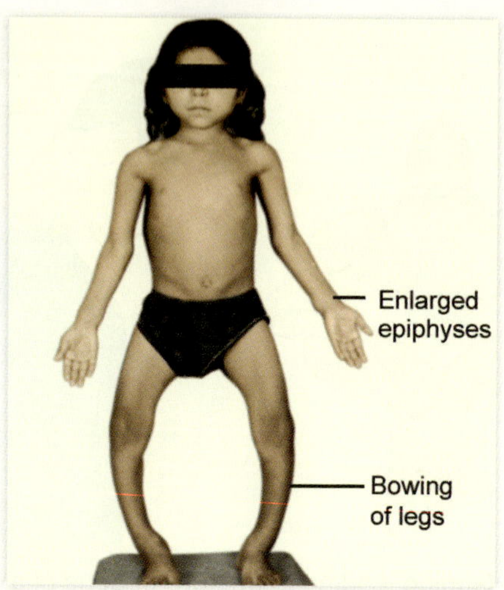

Fig. 2.28: Some deformities in rickets

severe pain and tenderness. The normal architecture at the growing ends of the bones is lost.

- Many skeletal defects are caused by genetic factors, or by a combination of genetic, hormonal, nutritional factors.
- (a) The vertebral arch or laminae of the vertebral column are mostly normal. (b) The spinal cord may be covered just by skin, i.e. spina bifida occulta. (c) There may be protrusion of the meninges surrounding the spinal cord placed in the vertebral canal, i.e. meningocele (d) There may be protrusion of the spinal cord as well as meninges, i.e. meningo-myelocele (Fig. 2.29).
- If deficiency of calcium and vitamin D occurs in adult life, it leads to *osteomalacia*. The bones on X-rays examination reveal thick uncalcified osteoid. Osteoporosis shows thin and small trabeculae. Table 2.4 shows the comparison between osteoporosis and osteomalacia.

  Deficiency of calcium in bones in old age leads to osteoporosis, seen both in females and males. Due to osteoporosis, there is forward bending of the vertebral column, leading to kyphosis (Fig. 2.30).
- Nerves are closely related to bones in some areas. Fracture of the bones of those areas may lead to injury to the nerve, leading to paralysis of muscles supplied, including the sensory loss (Fig. 2.31).

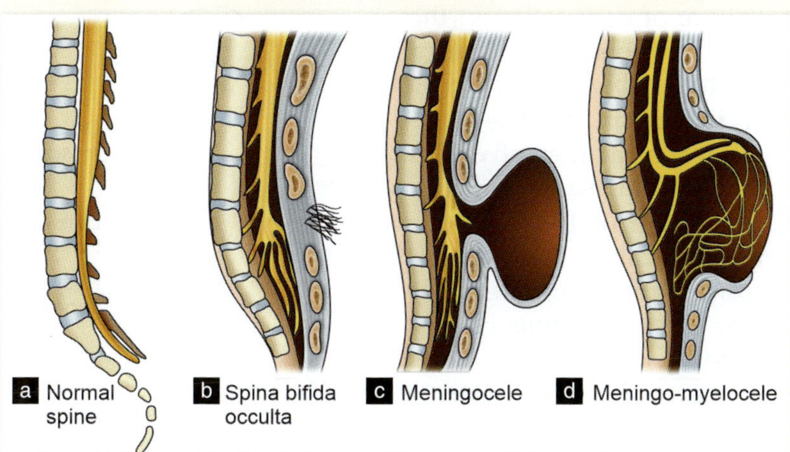

Fig. 2.29: Normal spine and defective spines

Table 2.4: Comparison of osteoporosis and osteomalacia

	Calcium and phosphate	*Alkaline phosphatase*	*Osteoblast*	*Trabeculae*
Osteoporosis	Normal	Normal	Normal	Thin and small
Osteomalacia	May be low	Raised	Increased	Thick uncalcified osteoid

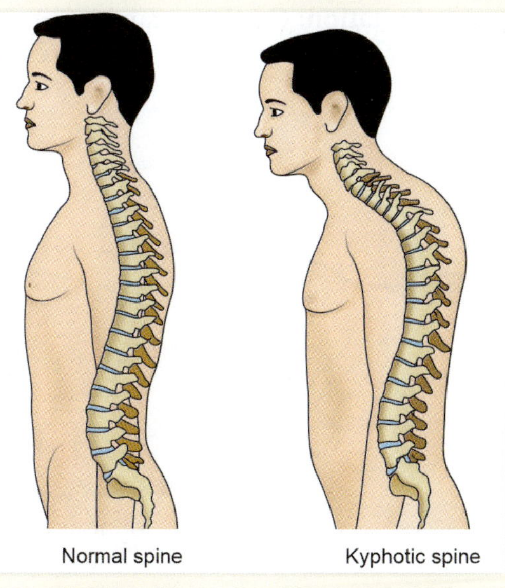

Fig. 2.30: Normal and kyphotic spines

- Failure of ossification in the sesamoid bone is mistaken for fracture of bone, e.g. patella.
- If infection reaches the intracapsular metaphysis, it may result in septic arthritis.
- **Bone marrow biopsy:** Bone marrow can be taken either from manubrium sterni or iliac crest in various clinical conditions (Fig. 2.32).
- **Bone tumour:** Benign or malignant tumours can occur in the bone (Fig. 2.33).
- **Rupture of the cartilage:** The medial meniscus of knee joint is mostly affected. It is treated by replacement.
- **Tumors of cartilage:** The tumor may be benign or malignant. These are called chondromas and chondrosarcomas respectively.
- **Cartilage transplantation:** Cartilage can be transplanted from one person to other. The matrix of cartilage prevents the entry of antigens.

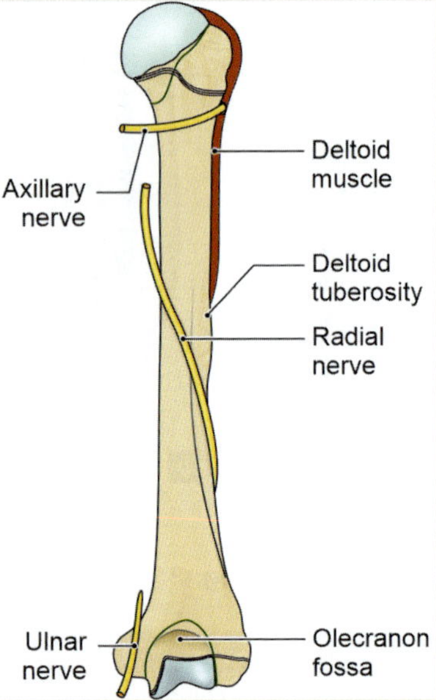

Fig. 2.31: Sites of close relations of nerves on posterior surface of humerus

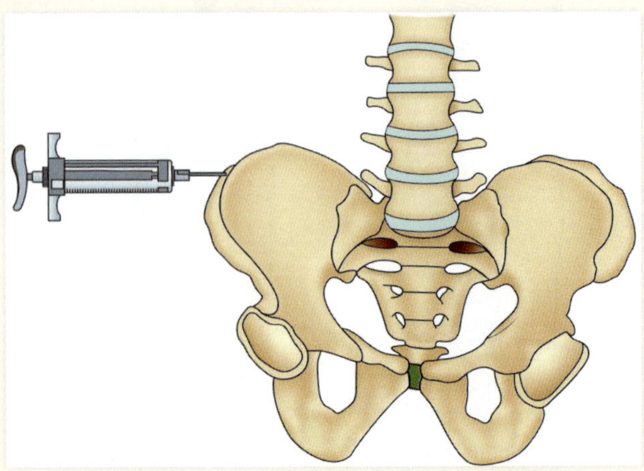

Fig. 2.32: Bone marrow biopsy from iliac crest

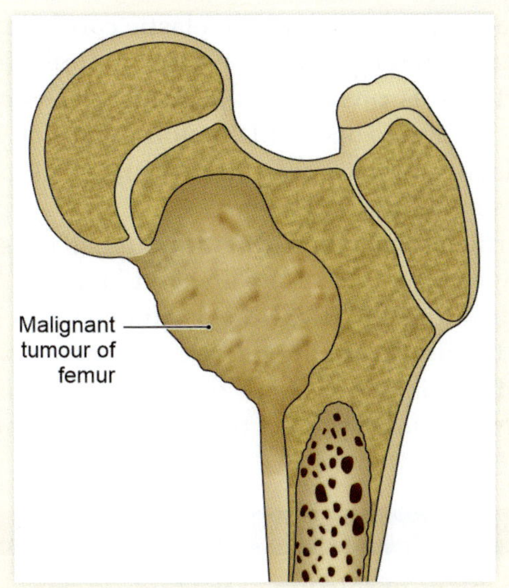

Fig. 2.33: Malignant tumour of femur

Points to Remember

- Inorganic calcium salt as calcium hydroxy-apatite $[Ca_{10}(PO_4)_6(OH)_2]$ is present in the bone.
- Femur is the longest and strongest bone.
- Stapes of the middle ear is the shortest bone.
- Three bony ossicles of middle ear are fully developed at birth.
- Hyoid bone, mandible and 3 bony ossicles of middle ear develop from branchial cartilages. Hyoid bone does not articulate with any other bone.
- Fibula does not follow the "law of ossificiation".
- Clavicle is a long, horizontally placed bone.
- Periosteum does not cover the sesamoid bones and the 3 bony ossicles of middle ear.
- Most common site of osteomyelitis is the metaphysis region of long bone.
- Bone marrow puncture is done in iliac crest in children and in manubrium sterni in adult.
- Bone fractures are seen more often in persons without adequate protein, calcium and vitamin D.

- External ear or pinna is made of elastic cartilage. Its size does not increase even if it is pulled as part of punishment.
- Elastic cartilage is present in epiglottis and vocal process of arytenoid cartilage. This cartilage does not calcify/ossify.
- Fibrocartilage gives strength to the site of its presence. It is chiefly present in midline joints.
- Hyaline cartilage is maximum in the body. All the somatic bones initially were composed of hyaline cartilage.
- Intramembranous ossification is quicker one step process compared to intracartilaginous, two step process.
- Bones of the cranial vault are ossified by intramembranous ossification to quickly protect the developing brain.

Multiple Choice Questions

1. What percentage of calcium of the body is stored in the bones?

a. 90% b. 80%
c. 97% d. 75%

2. Proportion of inorganic matter to organic matter in the bones is:

a. 3 : 1 b. 2 : 1
c. 1 : 1 d. 4 : 1

3. The cartilaginous model of bone arises from:

a. Ectoderm b. Mesoderm
c. Endoderm d. Neuroectoderm

4. Length of the bone increases by multiplication of cells at:

a. Periosteum b. Epiphysis
c. Epiphyseal plate d. Diaphysis

5. Ossification of long bones begins in intrauterine life at:

a. First week b. Fifth week
c. Eighth week d. Twelfth week

6. Which cartilage has no perichondrium?

a. Hyaline b. Elastic
c. White fibro d. All of the above

7. The first bone to start ossifying is:

a. Mandible b. Femur
c. Clavicle d. Humerus

8. Which one is not a traction epiphysis?
- a. Lesser tubercle of humerus
- b. Greater trochanter of femur
- c. Head of humerus
- d. Lesser trochanter of femur

Answers

1. c **2.** a **3.** b **4.** c **5.** c **6.** c **7.** c **8.** c

Chapter

3

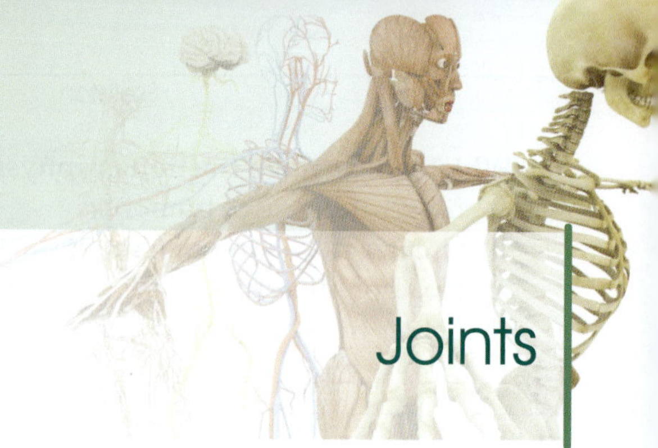

Joints

What I hear, I forget, What I see, I remember, What I do, I understand

Related Terms

1. Arthron (G a joint). Compare with the terms arthrology, synarthrosis, diarthrosis, arthritis, arthrodesis, etc.
2. Articulatio (L a joint); articulation (NA).
3. Junctura (L a joint).
4. Syndesmology (G syndesmosis = ligament) is the study of ligaments and related joints.

Definition and Functions

Joint is a junction between two or more bones or cartilages. It is a device to permit *movements*.

However, immovable joints are primarily meant for growth. Primary cartilaginous joints of long bones increase length of bone. A newborn baby is about 15 inches long and length increases to 60–70 inches in an adult due to growth at these joints. Fontanelles of skull may permit moulding during childbirth.

There are more joints in a child than in an adult because as growth proceeds some of the bones fuse together, e.g. the ilium, ischium and pubis to fuse form the pelvic bone. The two halves of the infant frontal bone, and of the infant mandible also fuse to form single frontal and mandible bone respectively. The five sacral vertebrae fuse to form sacrum and the four coccygeal vertebrae join to form coccyx.

Joints help to form *cavities* like cranial, thoracic, abdominal and pelvic cavities including vertebral canal where the respective organs are safely kept. Joints of thoracic cage help in increasing transverse and anteroposterior diameters of the cage, helping in *respiration*. Joints of larynx help in speech. Joints transmit weight of the body to the ground.

Competency achievement: The student should be able to:
AN 2.5 Describe various joints with subtypes and examples

CLASSIFICATION OF JOINTS

A. Structural Classification

1. Fibrous Joints

a. Sutures b. Syndesmosis c. Gomphosis

2. Cartilaginous Joints

a. Primary cartilaginous joints or synchondrosis
b. Secondary cartilaginous joints or symphysis or amphiarthrosis

3. Synovial Joints

a. Ball-and-socket or spheroidal joints
b. Sellar or saddle joints
c. Condylar or bicondylar joints
d. Ellipsoid joints
e. Hinge joints
f. Pivot or trochoid joints
g. Plane joints

B. Functional Classification (According to the Degree of Mobility)

1. Synarthroses (immovable), like sutures of the fibrous joints (Fig. 3.1).
2. Amphiarthroses (slightly movable), like secondary cartilaginous joints (Fig. 3.2).
3. Diarthroses (freely movable), like synovial joints (Fig. 3.3).

Synarthroses are fixed joints at which there is no movement. The articular surfaces are joined by tough fibrous tissue. Often the edges of the bones are dovetailed into one another as in the sutures of the skull.

Amphiarthroses are joints at which slight movement is possible. The articulating bones are covered by hyaline cartilage. A pad of fibrocartilage lies between the bone surfaces, and there are fibrous

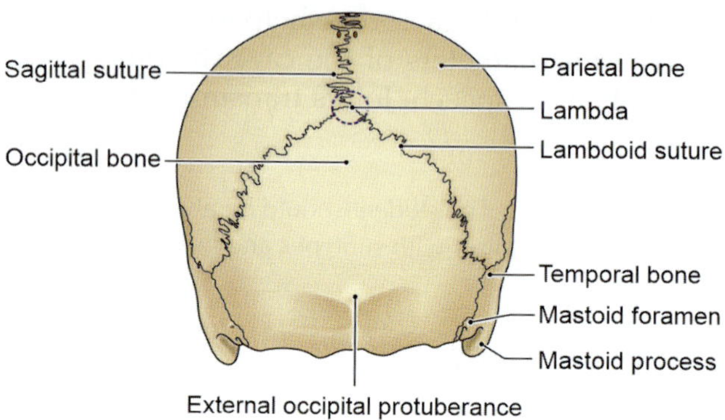

Fig. 3.1: Fibrous joint—sutures

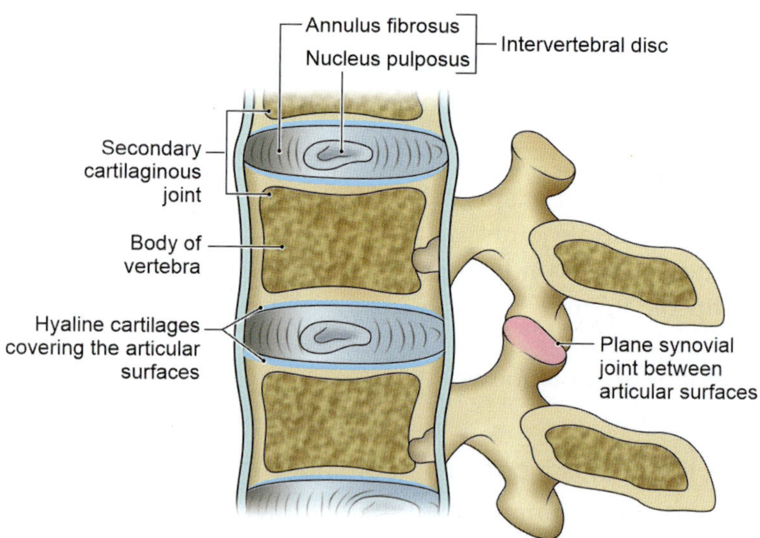

Fig. 3.2: Secondary cartilaginous joints (symphysis) and plane synovial joint

ligaments to hold the bones and cartilages in place. The cartilages of such joints also act as shock absorbers, e.g. the intervertebral discs between the bodies of the vertebrae (Fig. 3.2).

Diarthroses or synovial joints are known as freely movable joints, though at some of them the movement is restricted by the shape of the articulating surfaces and by the ligaments which hold the bones together. These ligaments are of elastic connective tissue.

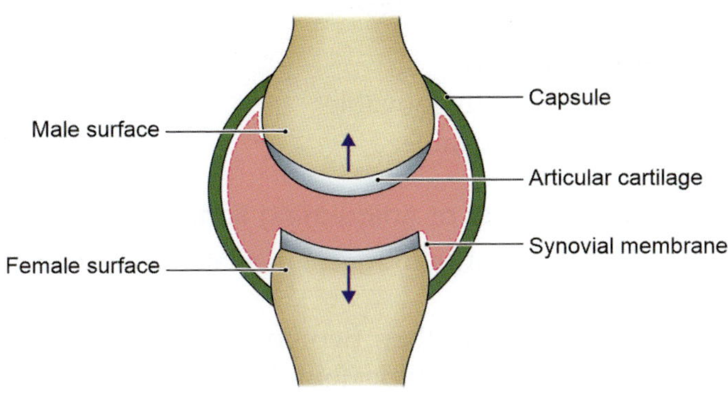

Fig. 3.3: Structure of a simple synovial joint

A synovial joint has a fluid-filled cavity between articular surfaces which are covered by articular cartilages. The fluid, known as synovial fluid, is produced by the synovial membrane. The synovial membrane lines the cavity except for the actual articular surfaces. It covers any ligaments or tendons which pass through the joint. Synovial fluid acts as a lubricant.

The form of the articulating surfaces controls the type of movement which takes place at any joint.

The movements possible at synovial joints are:

Angular	flexion	:	Decreasing the angle between two bones or two parts
	extension	:	Increasing the angle between two bones or two parts
	abduction	:	Moving the part away from the mid-line
	adduction	:	Bringing the part towards the mid-line
Rotatory	rotation	:	Rotating along the vertical axis
	circumduction	:	Moving the extremity or the part round in a circle so that the whole part inscribes a cone. When flexion, abduction, extension and adduction occur in sequence, the movement is called the circumduction
Gliding	one part slides on another.		

C. Regional Classification

1. ***Skull type:*** Immovable
2. ***Vertebral type:*** Slightly movable
3. ***Limb type:*** Freely movable

D. According to Number of Articulating Bones

1. ***Simple joint:*** When only two bones articulate, e.g. interphalangeal joints (Fig. 3.4).
2. ***Compound joint:*** More than two bones articulate within one capsule, e.g. elbow joint, wrist joint (Fig. 3.4).
3. ***Complex joint:*** When joint cavity is divided by an intra-articular disc, e.g. temporomandibular joint (Fig. 3.17), sternoclavicular joint. Figure 3.5 is diagrammatic representation of complex joint.

The *structural* classification is most commonly followed, and will be considered in detail in the following paragraphs.

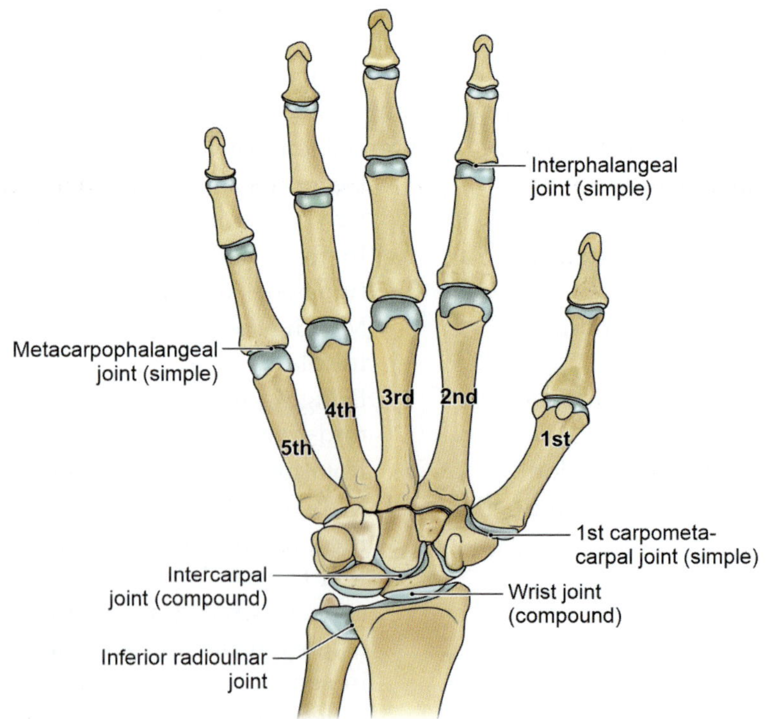

Fig. 3.4: Some simple and compound joints

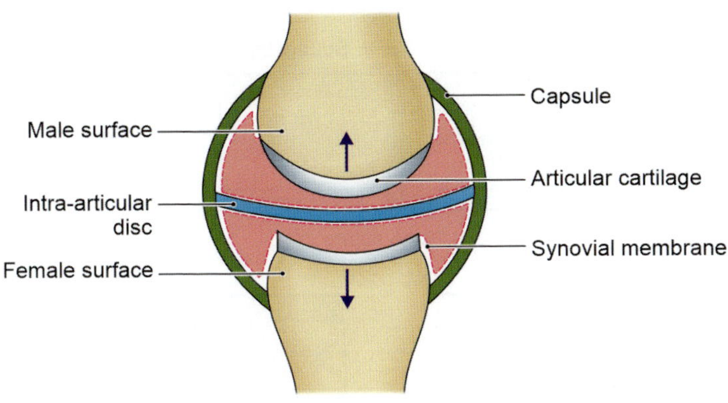

Fig. 3.5: Complex joint

FIBROUS JOINTS

In fibrous joints the bones are joined by fibrous tissue. These joints are either immovable or permit a slight degree of movement. These can be grouped in the following three subtypes.

1. ***Sutures:*** Sutures are present only in skull. Two bones are separated by connective tissue. The sutural side of each bone is covered by a layer of osteogenic cells/cambial layer, covered by capsular layer which is continuous with the periosteum. The area between the bones decreases with age, so that osteogenic surfaces become opposed. Sutures may synostose and get obliterated as age advances.

   Sutures are peculiar to skull, and are immovable. According to the shape of bony margins, the sutures can be:

   i. Plane, e.g. internasal suture (Fig. 3.6)
   ii. Serrate, e.g. interparietal sagittal suture
   iii. Squamous, e.g. temporo-parietal suture
   iv. Denticulate, e.g. lambdoid suture between parietal and occipital
   v. Schindylesis type (Fig. 3.6), e.g. between rostrum of sphenoid and upper border of vomer.

   Neonatal skull reveals fontanelles (widened sutures) which are temporary in nature, permit moulding (overlapping of bones, temporarily) during normal (vaginal) childbirth. At six specific points on the sutures (in newborn skull) are membrane filled gaps called "fontanelles". These also allow the underlying

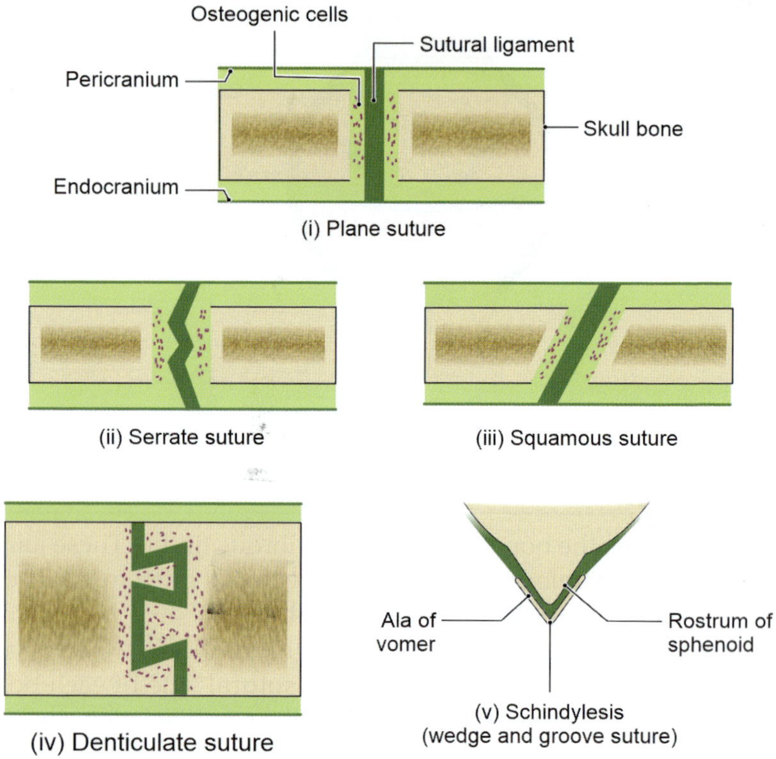

Osteogenic cells
Sutural ligament
Pericranium
Skull bone
Endocranium
(i) Plane suture
(ii) Serrate suture
(iii) Squamous suture
(iv) Denticulate suture
Ala of vomer
Rostrum of sphenoid
(v) Schindylesis (wedge and groove suture)

Fig. 3.6: Types of sutures

Anterior fontanelle
Anterolateral or sphenoidal fontanelle
Posterior fontanelle
Posterolateral or mastoid fontanelle

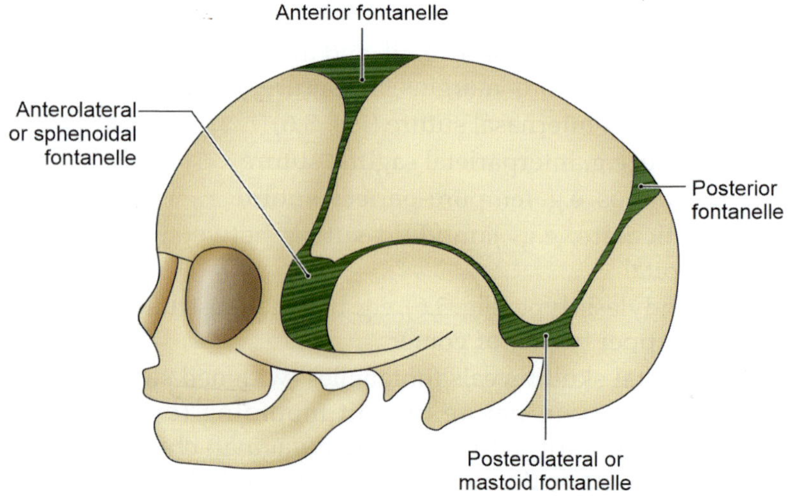

Fig. 3.7: Fontanelles of skull of a newborn baby

brain to increase in size. Anterior fontanelle is used to judge the hydration of the infant. All these fontanelles become bone by 18 months (Fig. 3.7). Fontanelles represent intra-membranous ossification in progress.

2. ***Syndesmosis:*** It is a fibrous union between bones. It may be represented as interosseous ligament as in inferior tibiofibular joint (Fig. 3.8) or a tense membrane as in posterior part of sacroiliac joint, or as interosseous talocalcanean ligament (Fig. 3.8).
3. ***Gomphosis:*** It is a peg and socket junction between the tooth and its socket. The periodontal ligament connects the dental element to the alveolar bone. Actually gomphosis is an articulation between two bones (Fig. 3.9).

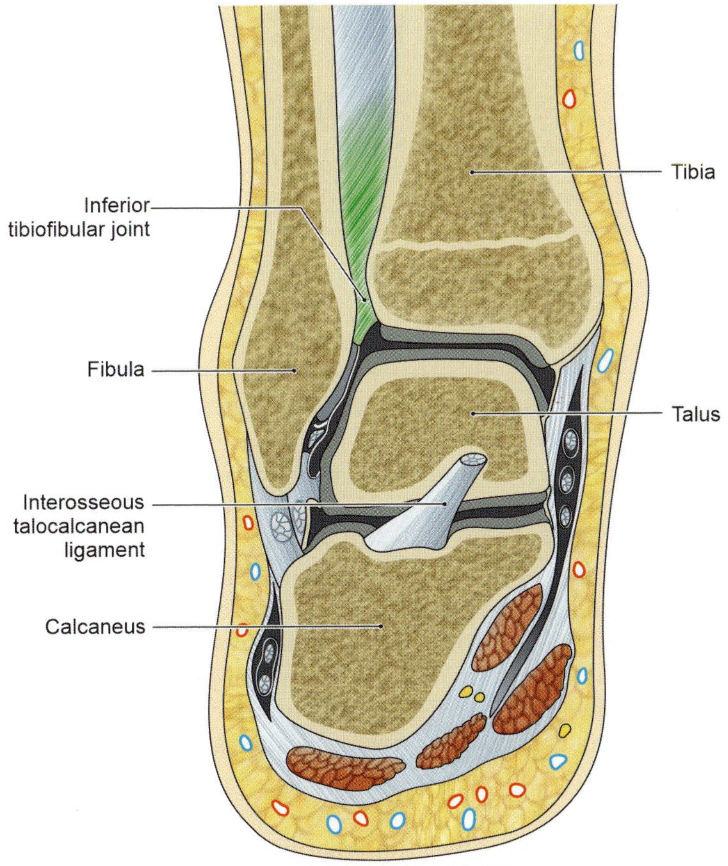

Fig. 3.8: Syndesmosis

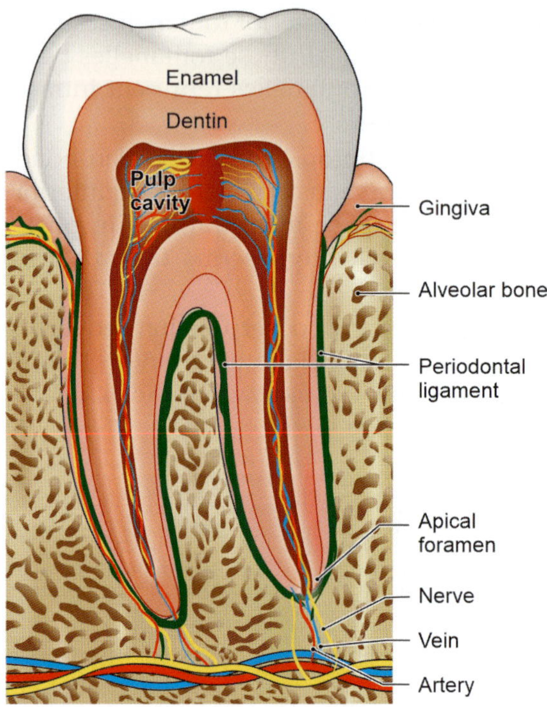

Fig. 3.9: Gomphosis

CARTILAGINOUS JOINTS

In this type of joints the bones are joined by cartilage. These are of the following two types:

1. ***Primary cartilaginous joints*** (synchondrosis, or hyaline cartilage joints): The bones are united by a plate of hyaline cartilage so that the joint is immovable and strong.

   These joints are temporary in nature because after a certain age the cartilaginous plate is replaced by bone (synostosis). These are seen in between epiphysis and diaphysis of long bone. These are associated with growth or epiphysial plates and increasing length of the bone (*see* Fig. 2.18). Primary cartilaginous joints or synchondrosis become synostosed after some age and are not identifiable.

   Examples:

   a. Joint between epiphysis and diaphysis of a growing long bone (Fig. 3.10a)

3

b. Spheno-occipital joint
c. First chondrosternal joint
d. Costochondral joints (Fig. 3.12)
e. Xiphisternal

2. ***Secondary cartilaginous joints*** (symphyses or fibrocartilaginous joints): The articular surfaces are covered by a thin layer of hyaline cartilage, and united by a disc of fibrocartilage.

These joints are permanent and persist throughout life. In this respect symphysis menti is a misnomer as it is a synostosis. Typically the secondary cartilaginous joints occur in the median plane of the body, and permit limited movements due to compressible pad of fibrocartilage such as in the pubic symphysis (Fig. 3.10b) and manubriosternal joints (Fig. 3.12a).

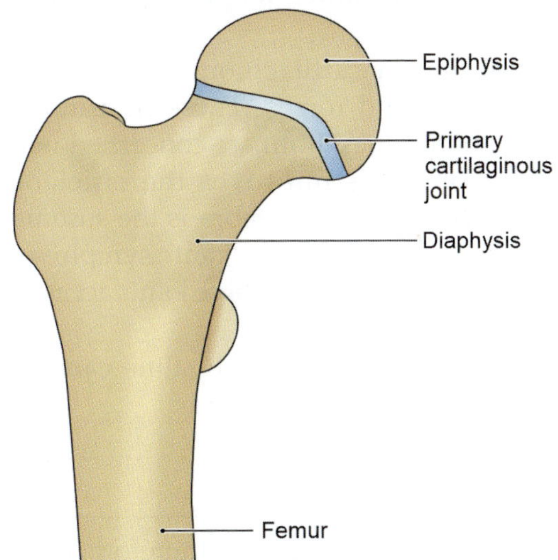

Fig. 3.10a: Primary cartilaginous joint

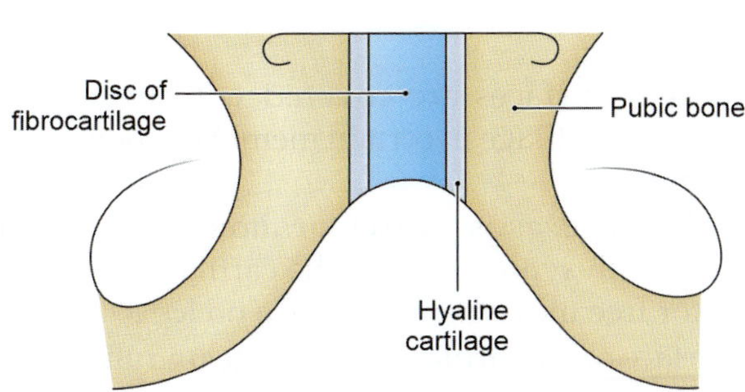

Fig. 3.10b: Symphysis pubis

The thickness of fibrocartilage is directly related to the range of movement. Secondary cartilaginous joints may represent an intermediate stage in the evolution of synovial joints.

Examples:

a. Symphysis pubis (Fig. 3.10b)
b. Manubriosternal joint (Fig. 3.12)
c. Intervertebral joints between the vertebral bodies (Fig. 3.2).

The disc varies from a few mm to 10 mm and there is dense connective tissue with a few chondrocytes. Collagen ligaments extend from the periostea of articulating bones across symphysis to blend with perichondria of hyaline cartilage. Complete capsule is not formed, but plexuses of afferent nerve terminals are seen. It can withstand stress of compression, tension, shear, etc. Range of motion is limited.

Primary and secondary cartilaginous joints are concerned with strength and to withstand forces. These transmit weight/force. Growth occurs in both types. Both are concerned with movement. Rigidity of synchondrosis improves the efficiency of nearby synovial joint. Movement of a vertebra is the summation effect of synchondrosis (primary cartilaginous joint), symphysis and synovial joints associated with the vertebra. These joints act as shock absorber and help in weight transmission.

Synchondrosis allows growth of hyaline cartilaginous plates where endochondral ossification extends.

SYNOVIAL JOINTS

Synovial joints are most evolved, and, therefore, most mobile type of joints (Table 3.1).

Characters

1. The articular surfaces are covered with hyaline (articular) cartilage (fibrocartilage in certain membrane bones) like clavicle and mandible.

   Articular cartilage is avascular, non-nervous and elastic. Lubricated with synovial fluid, the cartilage provides slippery surfaces for free movements, like 'ice on ice'.

   The surface of the cartilage shows fine undulations filled with synovial fluid.

Table 3.1: Classification of synovial joints and their movements

Type of Joint	*Movement*
A. Plane or gliding type	Gliding movements
B. Uniaxial joints	
1. Hinge joint	Flexion and extension
2. Pivot joint	Rotation only
C. Biaxial joints	
1. Condylar joint	Flexion, extension, and limited rotation
2. Ellipsoid joint	Flexion, extension, abduction, adduction, and circumduction
D. Multiaxial joints	
1. Saddle joint	Flexion and extension, abduction, adduction, and conjunct rotation
2. Ball-and-socket (spheroidal) joint	Flexion and extension, abduction and adduction, circumduction, medial and lateral rotation

2. Between the articular surfaces there is a *joint cavity* filled with synovial fluid. The cavity may be partially or completely subdivided by an articular disc or meniscus (Fig. 3.5).
3. The joint is surrounded by an *articular capsule* which is made up of a fibrous capsule lined by synovial membrane.

   Because of its rich nerve supply, the *fibrous capsule* is sensitive to stretches imposed by movements. This sets up appropriate reflexes to protect the joint from any sprain. This is called the 'watchdog' action of the capsule.

   The fibrous capsule is often reinforced by:
   a. *Capsular* or *true ligaments* representing thickenings of the fibrous capsule.
   b. The *accessory ligaments* (distinct from fibrous capsule) which may be intra- or extracapsular.

      The *synovial membrane* lines whole of the interior of the joint, except for the articular surfaces covered by articular cartilages.

      The membrane secretes a slimy viscous fluid called the synovia or *synovial fluid* which lubricates the joint and nourishes the articular cartilage. The viscosity of fluid is due to hyaluronic acid secreted by cells of the synovial membrane.
4. Varying degrees of movements are always permitted by the synovial joints.

Classification of Synovial Joints

1. Plane Synovial Joints

Articular surfaces are more or less flat (plane). They permit gliding movements (translations) in various directions.

Examples:

a. Intercarpal joints (Fig. 3.4)
b. Intertarsal joints (Fig. 3.18)
c. Joints between articular processes of vertebrae (Fig. 3.2)
d. Cricothyroid joint (Fig. 2.23)
e. Cricoarytenoid joint (Fig. 2.23)
f. Superior tibiofibular (Fig. 3.29)
g. Interchondral joint (5–9 ribs) (Fig. 3.12a)
h. Costovertebral
i. Costotransverse
j. Acromioclavicular with intra-articular disc (Fig. 3.17)
k. Carpometacarpal (except first) (Fig. 3.4)
l. Tarsometatarsal (Fig. 3.12a)
m. Intermetacarpal (Fig. 3.4)
n. Intermetatarsal
o. Chondrosternal (except first)
p. Sacroiliac (Fig. 3.12a)

2. Hinge Joints (Ginglymi)

Articular surfaces are pulley-shaped. There are strong collateral ligaments. Movements are permitted in one plane around a transverse axis.

Examples:

a. Elbow joint (Fig. 3.11a and b)
b. Ankle joint (Fig. 3.12a)
c. Interphalangeal joints (Fig. 3.16)

3. Pivot (Trochoid) Joints

Articular surfaces comprise a central bony pivot (peg) surrounded by an osteoligamentous ring. Movements are permitted in one plane around a vertical axis.

Examples:

a. Superior and inferior radioulnar joints (Fig. 3.12b)
b. Median atlantoaxial joint (Fig. 3.13 and Table 3.2)

4. Condylar (Bicondylar) Joints

Articular surfaces include two distinct condyles (convex male surfaces) fitting into reciprocally concave female surfaces (which are also, sometimes, known as condyles, such as in tibia). These joints permit movements mainly in one plane around a transverse axis, but partly in another plane (rotation) around a vertical axis.

Table 3.2: Comparison between median atlantoaxial and superior radioulnar joints

Joints	*Median atlantoaxial*	*Superior radioulnar*
Bones	Between anterior arch of atlas and odontoid process of axis	Head of radius and radial notch of ulna
Ring	Transverse ligament of atlas	Annular ligament
Ring (moving fixed)	Ring moves	Ring fixed
Axis	Fixed (dens)	Radius moves
Movements	"NO" movements	Supination, pronation
Clinical	Rupture of trans. ligament of the joint as in "hanging"	Subluxation of the joint

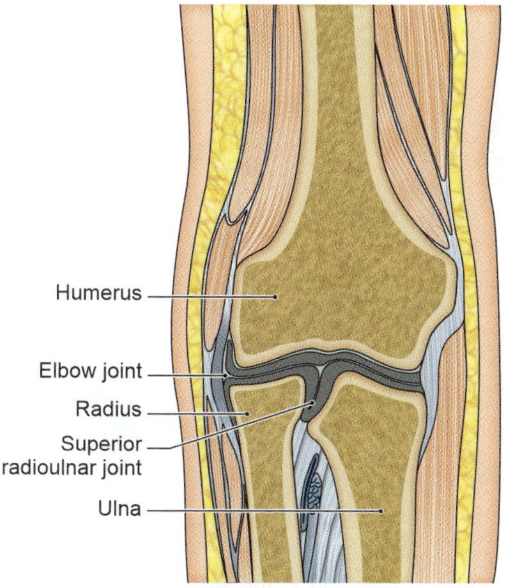

Fig. 3.11a: Elbow joint and superior radioulnar joint (anterior aspect)

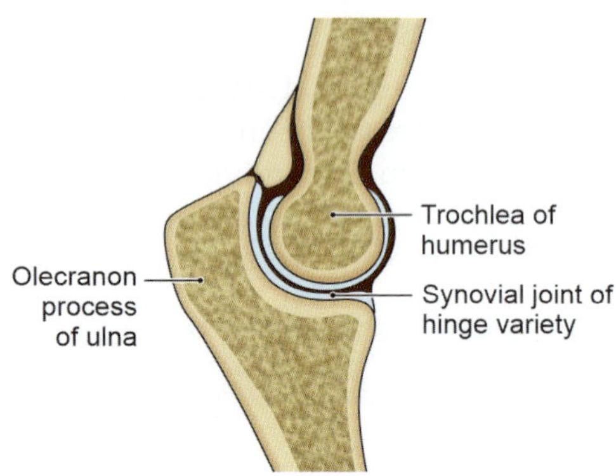

Fig. 3.11b: Elbow joint (medial aspect)

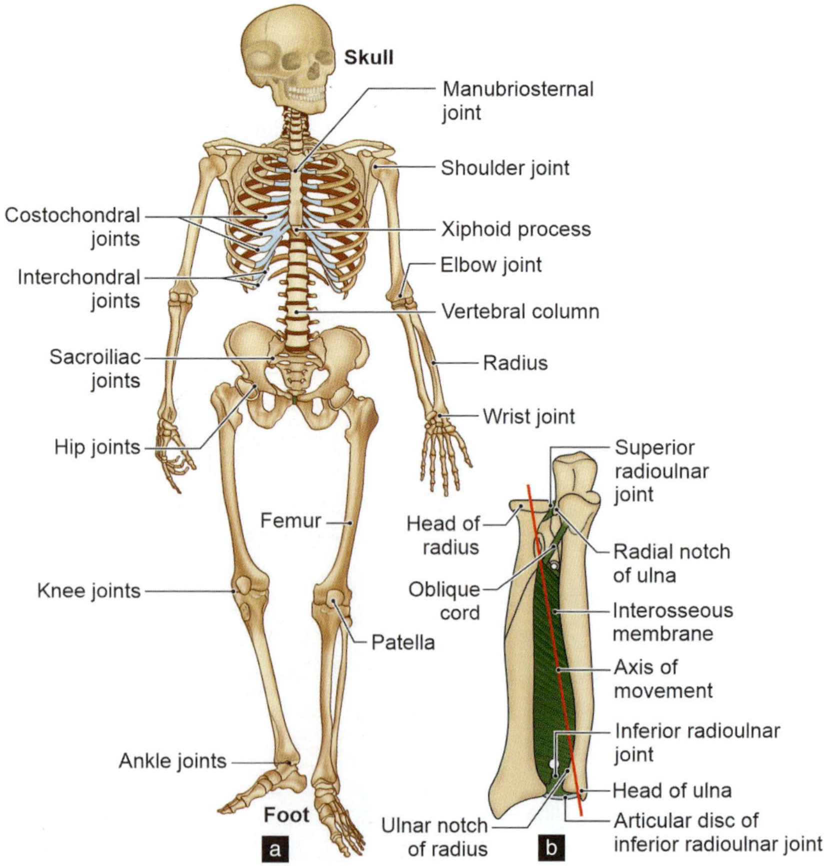

Fig. 3.12: (a) Skeleton showing some joints and (b) superior and inferior radioulnar joints

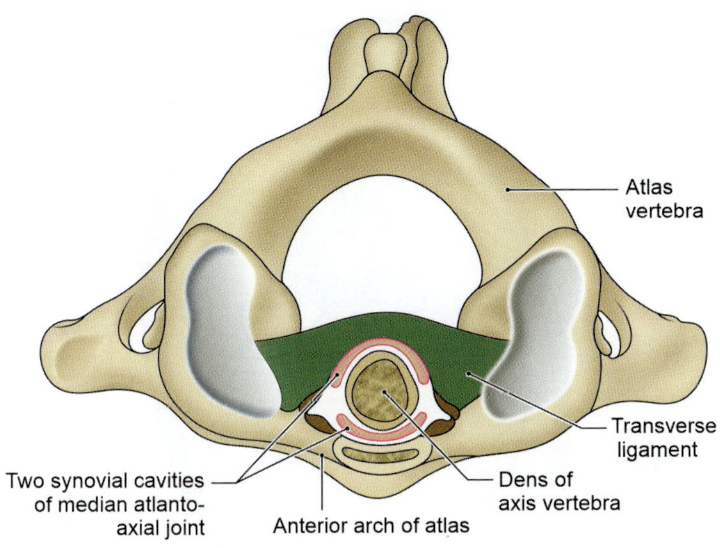

Fig. 3.13: Median atlantoaxial joint

Examples:

a. Knee joint (Fig. 3.14)
b. Right and left jaw joints or temporomandibular joint (Fig. 3.15).

5. Ellipsoid Joints

Articular surfaces include an oval, convex, male surface fitting into an elliptical, concave female surface. Free movements are permitted around both the axes; flexion and extension around the transverse axis, and abduction and adduction around the anteroposterior axis. Combination of movements produces circumduction. Typical rotation around a third (vertical) axis does not occur.

Examples:

a. Atlanto-occipital joints.
b. Wrist joint (Fig. 3.4)
c. Metacarpophalangeal joints (Fig. 3.16)

6. Saddle (Sellar) Joints

Articular surfaces are reciprocally concavoconvex. Movements are similar to those permitted by an ellipsoid joint, with addition of some rotation (conjunct rotation) around a third axis which, however, cannot occur independently.

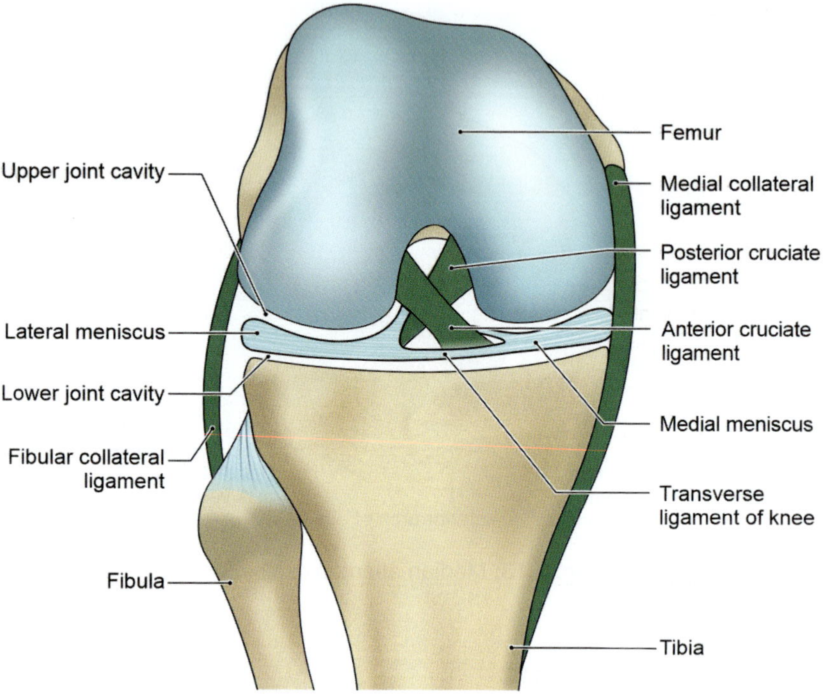

Fig. 3.14: Condylar joint: Knee joint

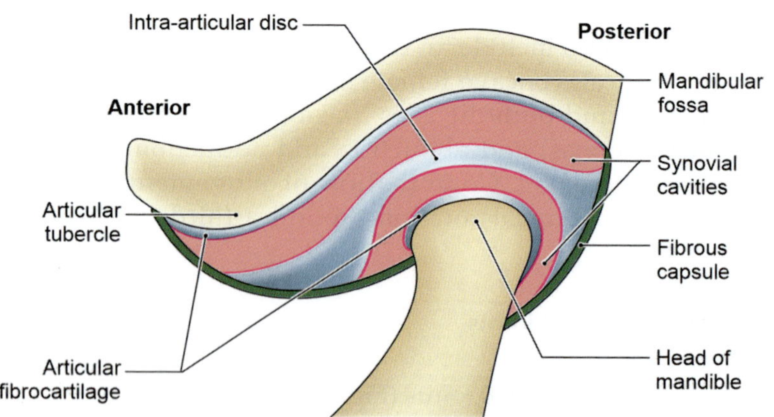

Fig. 3.15: Condylar joint: Temporomandibular joint

Examples:

a. First carpometacarpal joint (Fig. 3.16a and b)
b. Sternoclavicular joint (Fig. 3.17)

c. Calcaneocuboid joint (Fig. 3.18)
d. Incudomalleolar joint (*see* Fig. 2.12)
e. Between femur and patella (Fig. 3.12a).

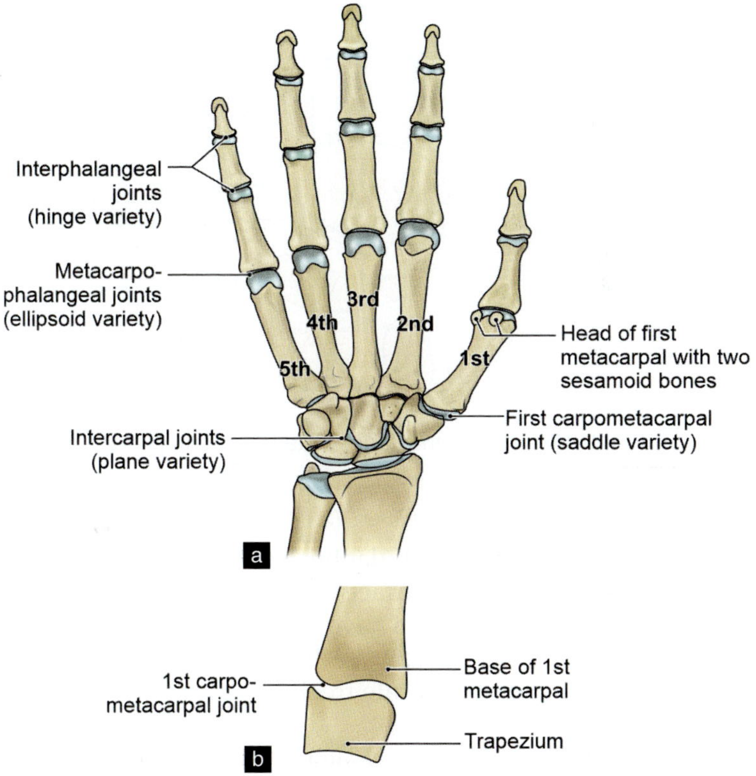

Fig. 3.16: (a) Joints of hand and (b) magnified 1st carpometacarpal joint of right side

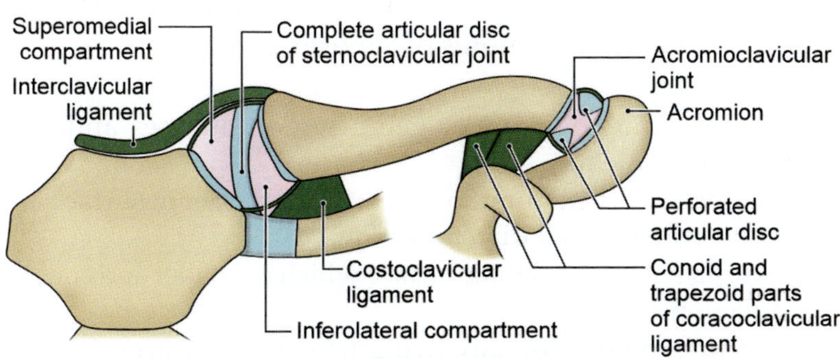

Fig. 3.17: Sternoclavicular and acromioclaviclar joints

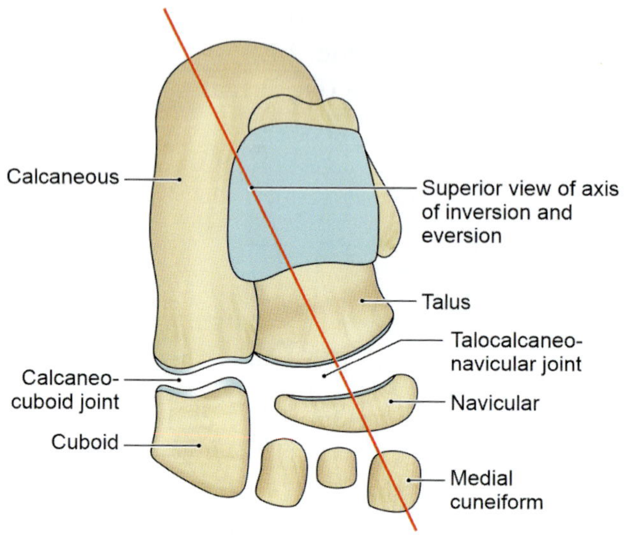

Fig. 3.18: Tarsal bones and some intertarsal joints

7. Ball-and-Socket (Spheroidal) Joints

Articular surfaces include a globular head (male surface) fitting into a cup-shaped socket (female surface). Movements occur around an indefinite number of axes which have one common centre. Flexion, extension, abduction, adduction, medial rotation, lateral rotation, and circumduction, all occur quite freely.

Examples:

a. Shoulder joint (Fig. 3.12)
b. Hip joint (Fig. 3.19)
c. Talocalcaneonavicular joint (Figs 3.18 and 3.20a)
d. Incudostapedial joint (*see* Fig. 2.12)

Classification and Movements of Synovial Joints

1. Terminology and Definition

Human Kinesiology: Study of geometry of surfaces and their associated movements.

Male surface: An articulating surface which is larger in surface area and always convex in all directions (Fig. 3.3).

Female surface: An articulating surface which is smaller and concave in all directions (Fig. 3.3).

Simple joints: Joints with only two articulating surfaces, i.e. male and female (Fig. 3.3).

3

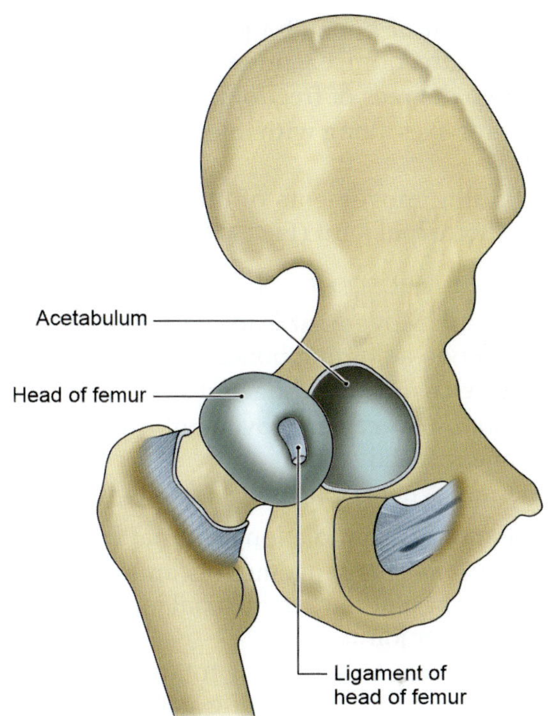

Fig. 3.19: Hip joint

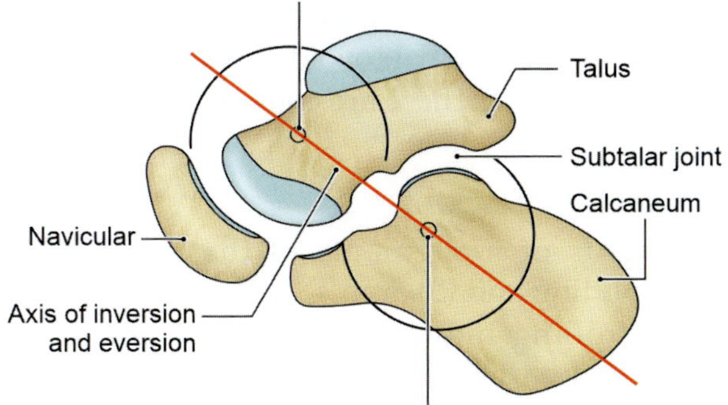

Fig. 3.20a: Side view of axis of movements of inversion and eversion

Compound joints: Joint possessing more than one pair of articulating surfaces, e.g. wrist joint (Fig. 3.16a).

Degrees of freedom: Number of axes at which the bone in a joint can move.

Uniaxial: Movement of bone at a joint is limited to one axis, i.e. with one degree of freedom, e.g. interphalangeal joints (Fig. 3.16a).
Biaxial: With two degrees of freedom, e.g. wrist joint.
Multi-axial: Three axes along with intermediate positions also, e.g. shoulder joint
Translation: Sliding movements of one articulating surface over the other, e.g. intercarpal joint (Fig. 3.16a).

2. Movements and Mechanism of Joints

Angular movement: Movement leading to diminution or increase in angle between two adjoining bones. They are of two types:

a. ***Flexion and extension:*** Bending and straightening respectively.
b. ***Abduction and adduction:*** Movement away and towards the median plane respectively.
   Circumduction: When a long bone circumscribes a conical space.

Rotation: Bone moves around a longitudinal axis.

a. ***Adjunct rotation:*** This movement is an independent rotation, e.g. movement at median atlantoaxial joint and rotation at hip joint and shoulder joint.
b. ***Conjunct rotation:*** This type of rotation accompanies other movements at the joint, e.g. locking and unlocking of knee joint and movements at first carpometacarpal joint (of thumb).

3. Shape of Articular Surface

The common articular surface shapes are:

a. ***Ovoid:*** When concave–female ovoids. When convex–male ovoids.
b. ***Sellar/saddle-shaped:*** These are convex in one plane, concave in the perpendicular plane.

4. Components of Movement

Basic components of movements of the synovial joints are: (1) Rolling, (2) Sliding and (3) Spin.

1. ***Rolling:*** In rolling movement, one end of the mechanical axis moves in a particular direction and the other end moves in opposite direction. The transverse axis of movement is almost fixed. The resultant movement is rolling along an arc. Rolling and sliding occur together in knee joint (Fig. 3.20b).

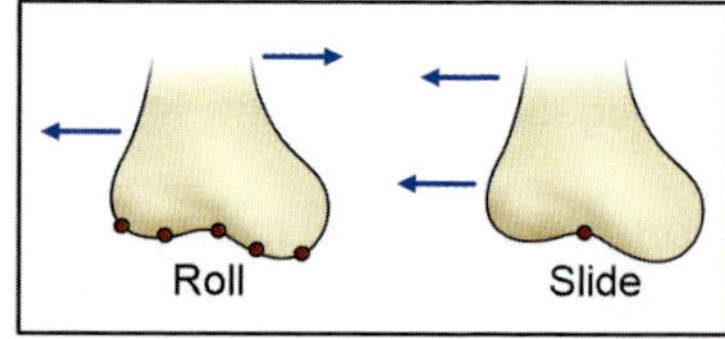

Fig. 3.20b: Showing roll and slide movements

2. *Slide:* During sliding movement, the mechanical axis of the joint and both ends of a moving bone move in the same direction. The transverse axis of movement is not fixed and it undergoes gliding or translation or linear movement.
3. *Spin:* It occurs around a fixed mechanical axis.

Muscles classified according to force of contraction.

These may spurt and shunt muscles

Spurt muscle, e.g. brachialis

- Its origin is at a distance from the joint where it acts.
- It is a prime mover.
- Its insertion is near the joint where it acts (*see* Fig. 4.8i).

Shunt muscle, e.g. brachioradialis

- Its origin is near the joint where it acts.
- It is a synergist.
- Its insertion is away from the joint where it acts (*see* Fig. 4.4).

Joint Positions

Close packed position: When the joint surfaces become completely congruent, their area of contact is maximal and they are tightly compressed.

In this position fibrous capsule and ligaments are maximally spiralized and tense; no further movement is possible; surfaces cannot be separated by disruptive forces; articular surfaces are liable to trauma. Table 3.3 shows the closed packed positions of various joints.

Loose packed: All other positions of incongruency.

Swing: Cardinal and arcuate.

Cardinal: The mechanical axis moves in the shortest pathway when bone moves.

Arcuate: The mechanical axis moves in the longest pathway while bone moves.

Limitation of Movement

Factors

- Reflex contraction of antagonistic muscles
- Due to stimulation of mechanoreceptors in articular tissue
- Ligaments get taut
- Approximation of soft parts

Table 3.3: Close packed positions of the joints	
Joint	*Close packed position*
Temporomandibular	Clenched teeth
Spine	Extension
Shoulder	Abduction and lateral rotation
Elbow	Extension
Wrist	Extension with radial deviation
Trapeziometacarpal	• Opposition (thumb)
Metacarpophalangeal	• Flexion (finger)
Interphalangeal of hand	• Extension
Hip	Extension and medial rotation
Knee	Extension with locking
Ankle	Dorsiflexion
Subtalar and mid-tarsal	Inversion
Metatarsophalangeal	Extension
Interphalangeal of foot	Extension

Mechanism of Lubrication

1. ***Synovial fluid:*** Secreted by synovial membrane, is sticky and viscous due to hyaluronic acid (a mucopolysaccharide). It serves the main function of lubrication of the joint. It also nourishes the articular cartilages.
2. ***Hyaline cartilage:*** Covering the articular surfaces possesses inherent slipperiness, like that of the ice.
3. ***Intra-articular fibrocartilages, articular discs or menisci, complete or incomplete:*** Help in spreading the synovial fluid throughout the joint cavity, but particularly between the articular surfaces, e.g. temporomandibular joint (Fig. 3.15). The disc divides the joint into two cavities for diverse movements. The disc strengthens the joint.
4. ***Haversian fatty pads (Haversian glands):*** Occupy extra spaces in the joint cavity between the incongruous bony surfaces. All of them are covered with synovial membrane, and perhaps function as swabs to spread the synovial fluid.
5. ***Bursa:*** It is a bag-like space lined by synovial membrane containing synovial fluid. The digital synovial sheath is a synovial fluid-filled bag or sheath in relation to tendons

(Fig. 3.21), joints and bones to prevent friction. The tendons are supplied by blood through vincula brevia and vincula longa (Fig. 3.22). The inflammation of bursa is called bursitis. Bursa reduces friction and permits limited free movements.

Types of bursae

1. ***Subcutaneous bursae:*** These are present between bony prominences and skin, e.g. prepatellar bursa and subcutaneous infrapatellar bursa (Fig. 3.21).
2. ***Articular bursa:*** This bursa functions as a joint, e.g. bursa between dens of axis and transverse ligament of atlas vertebra (Fig. 3.13).
3. ***Subtendinous bursa:*** These are present between bone and tendon, e.g. supraspinatus bursa; between bone and ligament, e.g. bursa deep to tibial collateral ligament; or bursa between the tendons, e.g. anserine bursa.

Blood Supply

The articular and epiphysial branches given off by the neighbouring arteries form a periarticular arterial plexus. Numerous vessels from this plexus pierce the fibrous capsule and form a rich vascular plexus in the deeper parts of synovial membrane. The blood vessels of the synovial membrane terminate around the articular margins in a fringe of looped anastomoses

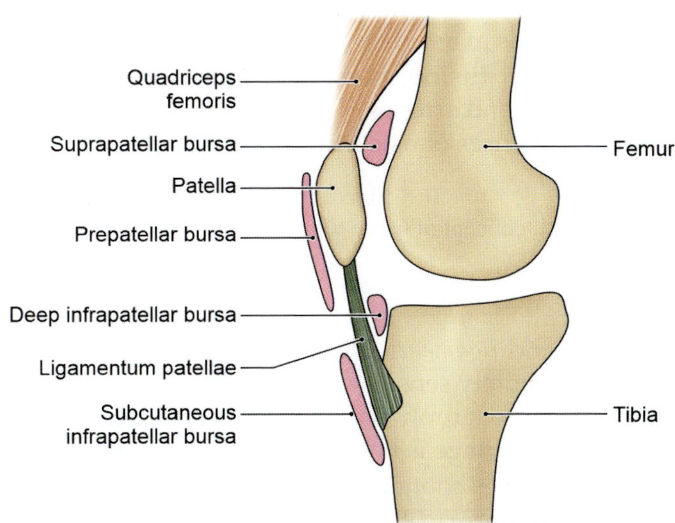

Fig. 3.21: Bursae in relation to knee joint

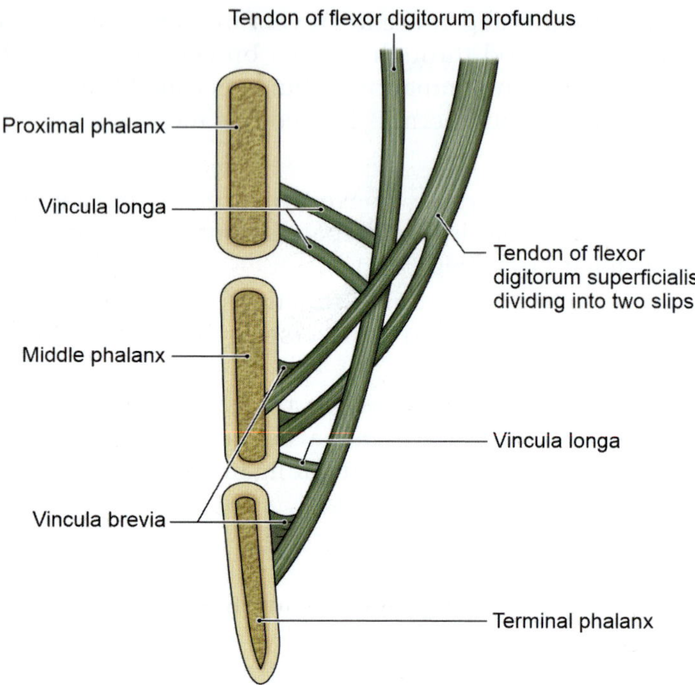

Fig. 3.22: Vincula longa and vincula brevia

termed the circulus vasculosus (*circulus articularis vasculosus*). It supplies capsule, synovial membrane and the epiphysis. The articular cartilage is avascular.

After epiphysial fusion, communications between circulus vasculosus and the end arteries of metaphysis are established, thus minimizing the chances of osteomyelitis in the metaphysis.

> *Competency achievement:* The student should be able to:
> AN 2.6 Explain the concept of nerve supply of joints and Hilton's law

Nerve Supply

1. The *capsule* and *ligaments* possess a rich nerve supply, which makes them acutely sensitive to pain. The synovial membrane has a poor nerve supply and is relatively insensitive to pain. The articular cartilage is non-nervous and totally insensitive.

   Articular nerves contain sensory and autonomic fibres.

   Some of the sensory fibres are proprioceptive in nature; these are sensitive to position and movement, and are concerned with the reflex control of posture and locomotion. Other sensory fibres are sensitive to pain.

Autonomic fibres are vasomotor or vasosensory.

The joint pain is often diffuse, and may be associated with nausea, vomiting, slowing of pulse and fall in blood pressure.

The pain commonly causes reflex contraction of muscles which fix the joint in a position of maximum comfort. Like visceral pain, the joint pain is also referred to uninvolved joints.

2. The principles of distribution of nerves to joints were first described by Hilton (1891). *Hilton's law* states that a motor nerve to the muscle acting on joint tends to give a branch to that joint (capsule) and another branch to the skin covering the joint.

   The concept of innervation of a joint was further elucidated by Gardner (1948) who observed that each nerve innervates a specific region of the capsule, and that the part of the capsule which is rendered taut by a given muscle is innervated by the nerve supplying its antagonists. Thus the pattern of innervation is concerned with the maintenance of an efficient stability at the joint.

Segmental Innervation of Joints of Limbs

Joints of *upper limb* are supplied by spinal segments in sequence. These are shown in Fig. 3.23. Joints of *lower limb* are also supplied by the respective spinal segments shown in Fig. 3.24.

Lymphatic Drainage

Lymphatics form a plexus in the subintima of the synovial membrane, and drain along the blood vessels to the regional deep nodes.

Stability

The various factors maintaining stability at a joint are described here in order of their importance.

1. ***Muscles:*** The tone of different groups of muscles acting on the joint is the most important and indispensable factor in maintaining the stability. Without muscles, the knee and shoulder would be unstable, and arches of the foot would collapse.

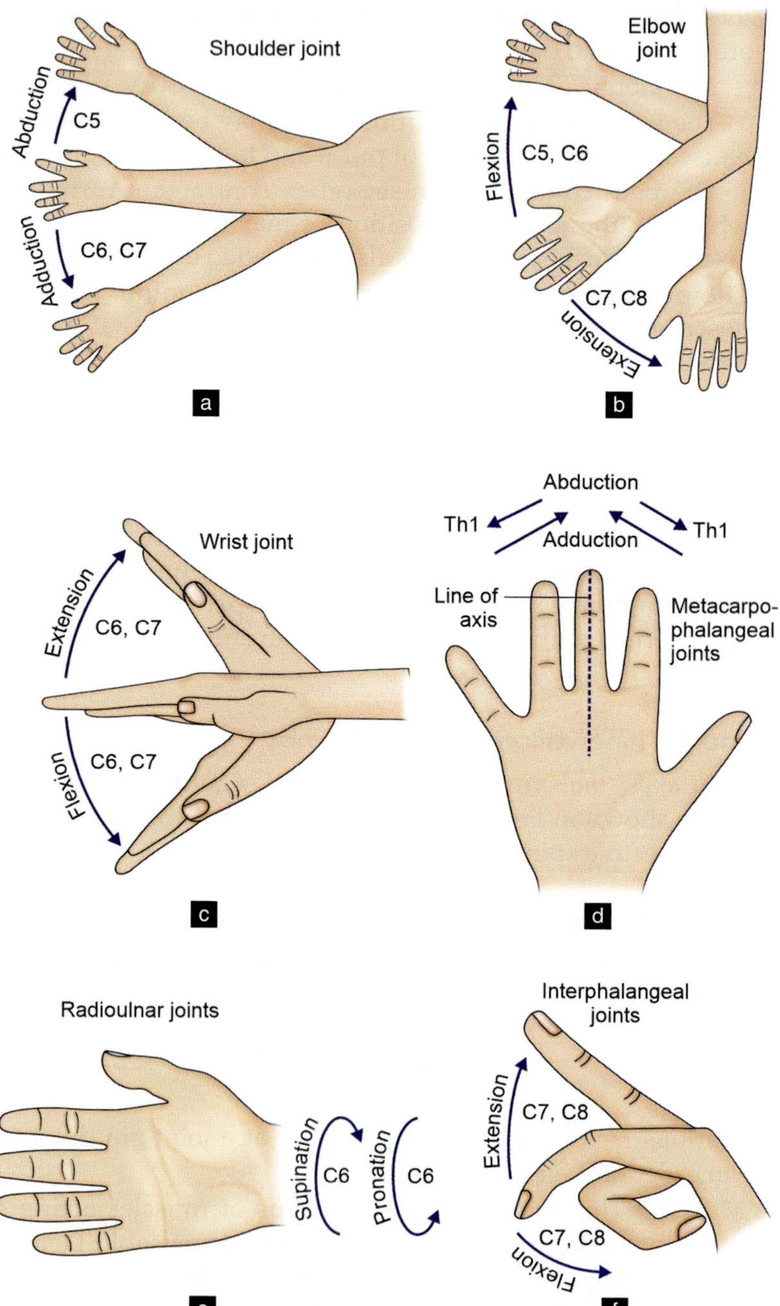

Fig. 3.23a to f: Segmental innervation of joints of upper limb

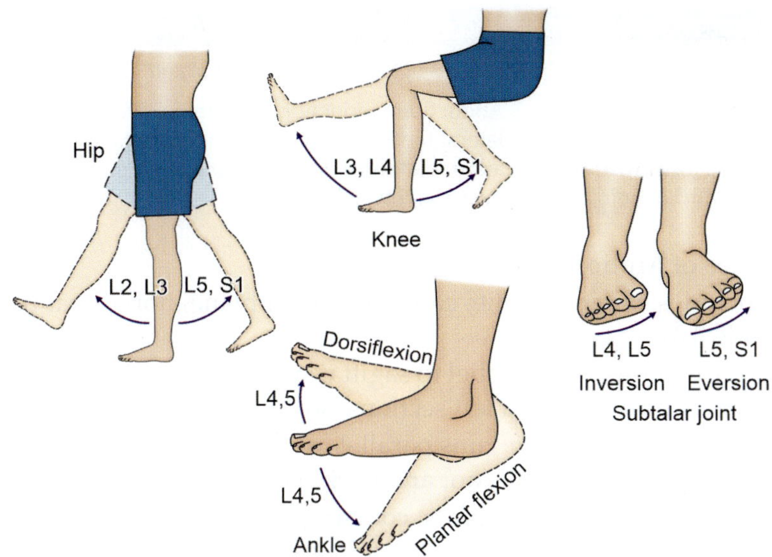

Fig. 3.24: Segmental innervation of joints of lower limb

2. ***Ligaments:*** These are important in preventing any over-movement, and in guarding against sudden accidental stresses. However, they do not help against a continuous strain, because once stretched, they tend to remain elongated. In this respect, the elastic ligaments (ligamenta flava and ligaments of the joints of auditory ossicles) are superior to the common type of white fibrous ligaments.
3. ***Bones:*** Help in maintaining stability only in some type of joints, like the hip and ankle. Otherwise in most of the joints (shoulder, knee, sacroiliac, etc.), their role is negligible.

BIOMECHANICS

Biomechanics: Study of forces and their effects on living system.

It is a discipline that uses principle of physics to quantitatively study flow forces interact within a living body.

Kinematics: Area of biomechanics includes description of motion without regard for forces producing motion.

Kinetics: Area of biomechanics concerned with forces producing motion or maintaining equilibrium.

Osteokinematics: It refers to the rotatory movement of bones in space during physiological joint motion.

Table 3.4: Common movements around different planes		
Sagittal plane	*Frontal plane*	*Horizontal plane*
Flexion, extension dorsiflexion, plantar flexion forward and backward bending	Abduction, adduction lateral flexion, ulnar, and radial deviation, eversion, inversion	Internal (medial) and external (lateral) rotation, axial rotation

Planes of Motion

It includes: Sagittal plane, coronal/frontal plane, horizontal plane (Table 3.4).

Sagittal plane runs parallel to sagittal suture of the skull, dividing the body into right and left sections (*see* Fig. 1.14).

Coronal/frontral plane runs parallel to coronal suture of the skull, dividing the body into front and back sections.

Horizontal (transverse) plane courses parallel to horizontal plane and divides the body into upper and lower sections.

Axis of rotation: Bones rotate about a joint in a plane that is perpendicular to an axis of rotation.

Degrees of freedom are the number of independent movements allowed at a joint. A joint can have up to 3 degrees of angular freedom.

For example, shoulder has 3 degree of freedom, one for each plane.

Sagittal plane (flexion, extension)

Frontal plane (abduction, adduction)

Horizontal plane (internal and external rotation).

Arthrokinematics refers to types of motion that occur between articular surfaces of a joint. The term roll, slide and spin are used to describe the type of motion that the moving part performs.

Roll: Multiple points along one rotating articular surface contact multiple points on another articulating surface (Fig. 3.25).

Slide: A single point on one articulating surface contacts multiple points on another articular surface.

Spin: A single point on one articular surface rotates on single point on another articular surface.

Convex–Concave Rule

When a concave articulating surface is moving on a stable convex surface, sliding and rolling is considered to occur in same direction (Fig. 3.26).

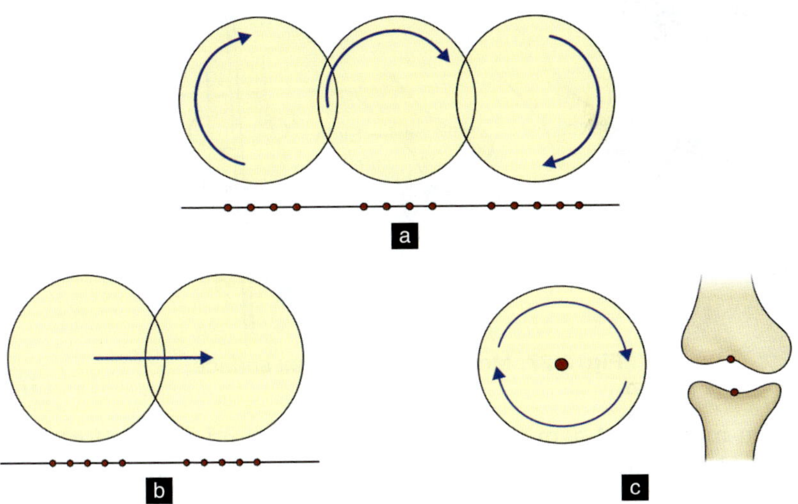

Fig. 3.25: (a) Roll, (b) slide and (c) spin

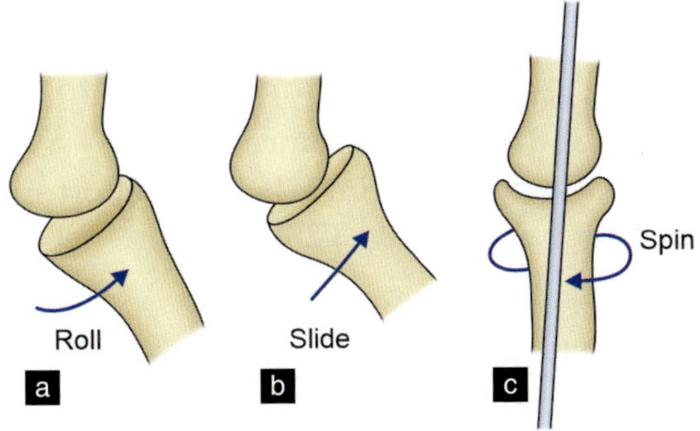

Fig. 3.26: Movement of concave surface

When a convex joint surface moves on a concave surface, the bone typically rolls in one direction and slide in opposite direction (Fig. 3.27a to c).

Levers

A lever is any rigid segment that rotates around a fulcrum.

In a lever system, the forces that are producing the resultant torque is called effort force (EF). Because other force must be creating an opposing torque, it is known as resistance force (RF). Effort force is always the winner in the torque game, and the resistance force is always the loser by producing motion.

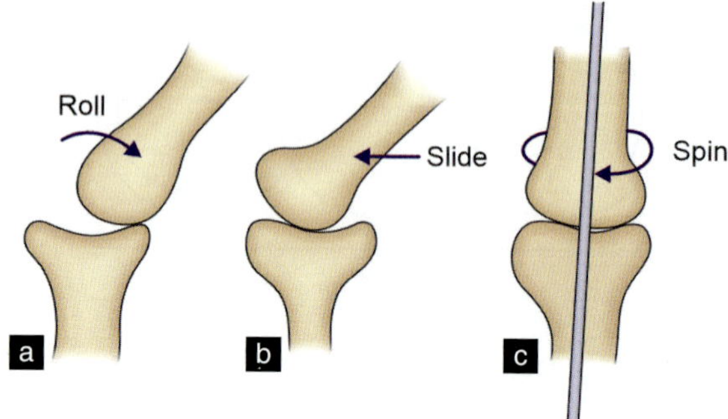

Fig. 3.27: Movements of convex surface

The movement arm for effort force is referred to as effort arm (EA), whereas arm for resistance force is referred to as the resistance arm (RA).

First Class Lever System

In a first class lever system, EA may be greater than RA, smaller than RA or {EA = RA, EA > RA, EA < RA}.

Muscles of neck act as effort (E)

Weight of skull and face as resistance (R)

Atlanto-occipital joint as fulcrum in between effort and resistance.

It is designed for balance (Fig. 3.28).

Second Class Lever System

Effort arm (EA) is always larger than resistance arm (RA).

Tendocalcaneus muscle is effort

Weight of lower limb is resistance in middle

Metatarsophalangeal joint is fulcrum at one end. It is best used for power (Fig. 3.29).

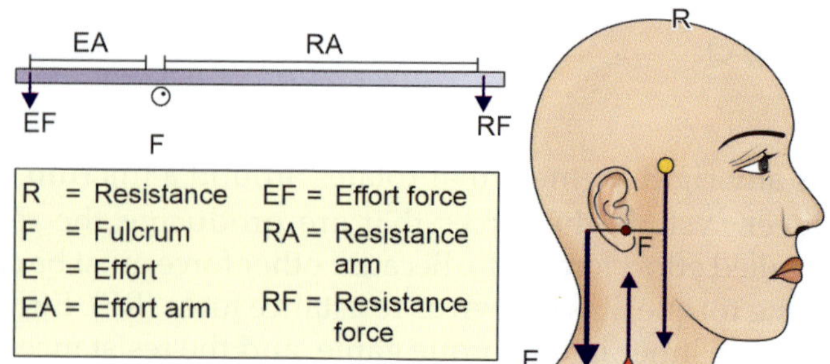

Fig. 3.28: First class lever system

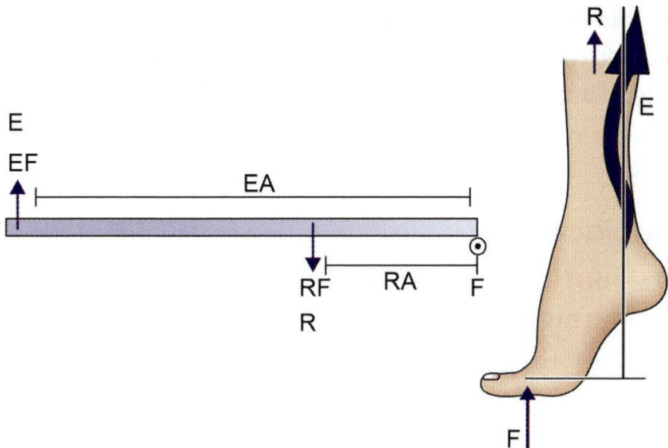

Fig. 3.29: Second class lever system

Third Class Lever System

Effort arm (EA) is always smaller than the resistance arm (RA)

Biceps brachii is effort arm in middle

Forearm weight is resistance

Elbow joint is fulcrum at one end

It is ideally designed for range of motion. Third class lever is the most common type of lever in the body (Fig. 3.30).

Mechanical Advantage

$$\text{M. Ad} = \frac{\text{EA}}{\text{RA}}$$

Mechanical advantage is related to classification of a lever and provides an understanding relationship between the torque of an external force and the torque of muscular force.

In third class lever, the mechanical advantage will always be less than one because effort arm is always smaller than resistance arm. So,

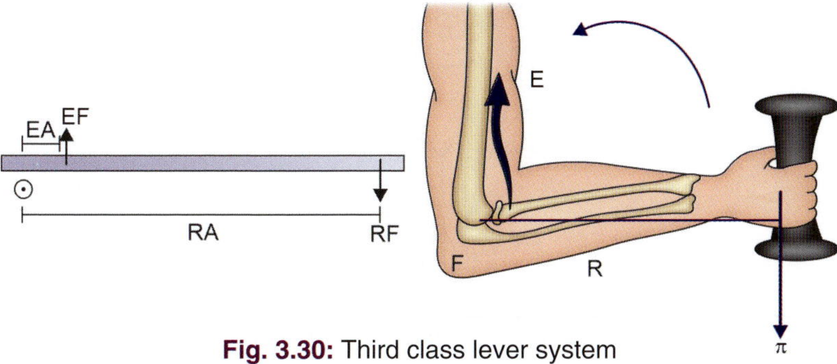

Fig. 3.30: Third class lever system

it works as mechanically inefficient or working at a disadvantage in terms of force output. In order to balance torque equilibrium the muscles must produce force much greater than the opposing external force.

This is also a reason why the muscles in human body are near to the joint axis.

Types of Displacement

Translatory motion (linear displacement) is the movement of a segment in a straight line.

Rotatory motion (angular displacement) is movement of a segment around a fixed axis (centre of rotation; COR) in curved path.

Curvilinear motion is a combination of rotatory and translatory motion, e.g. while taking the glass of water to mouth.

Clinical Anatomy of Joints

- Intervertebral disc forms secondary cartilaginous joint between the bodies of the vertebrae. If the nucleus pulposus part of the disc protrudes backwards, it may press on the spinal nerve leaving out from the intervertebral foramina. The condition is known as *herniation of the disc* or disc prolapse. If disc prolapse occurs in lumbar vertebrae, there is radiating pain in the lower limb, and the condition is called **sciatica** (Fig. 3.31).

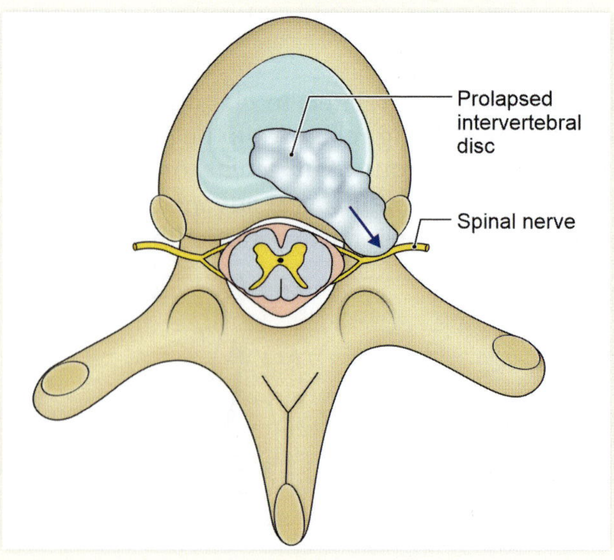

Fig. 3.31: Herniation of the disc

- The joints may get dislocated, i.e. the end of one of the bones gets out of its socket. In subluxation, the end of the bone partially leaves its socket (Fig. 3.32).
- Rheumatic fever causes fleeting pain in the joints, accompanied by streptococcal pharyngitis. It is mostly temporary pain in the joints. The toxins of the bacteria may affect the mitral valve of the heart or the kidneys.
- Rheumatoid arthritis is an inflammatory systemic disease resulting in thickened synovial membranes of small joints of the hands. Due to chronic inflammatory process there is erosion of bones leading to deformity of the fingers (Figs 3.33 and 3.34).

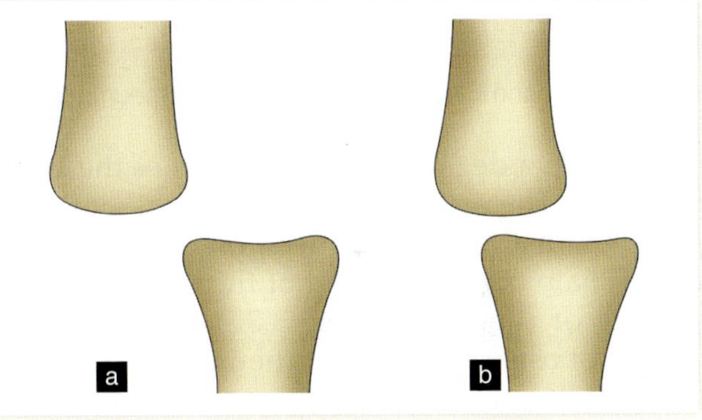

Fig. 3.32: (a) Dislocation, (b) Subluxation

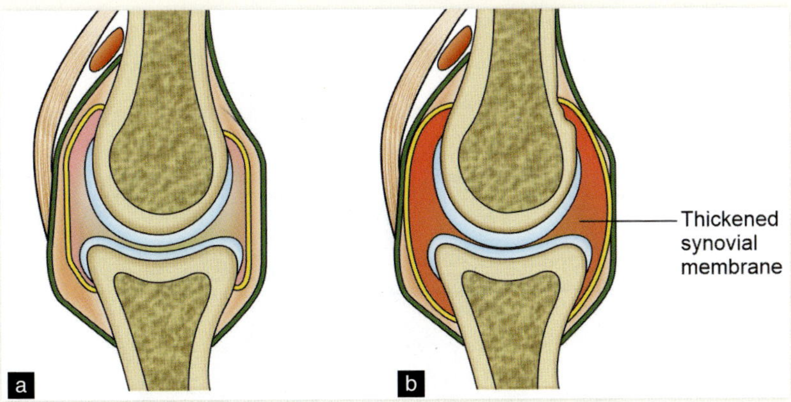

Fig. 3.33: (a) Synovial membrane in a normal joint and (b) thickened in a rheumatoid arthritis patient

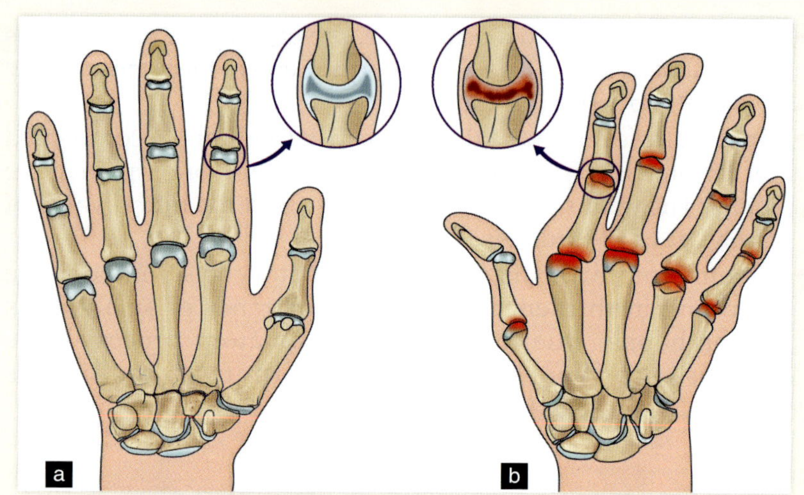

Fig. 3.34: (a) Joints of hand in normal subject and (b) in rheumatoid arthritic hand

- Osteoarthritis is a degenerative condition of the large weight-bearing joints. The articular cartilage wears out, degenerates and there is formation of peripheral osteophytes. The patients feel a lot of pain due to rubbing of the bones together during movements of the joints (Fig. 3.35). Table 3.5 shows the comparison of osteoarthritis and rheumatoid arthritis.
- The degenerative changes or spondylitis may occur in the cervical spine, leading to narrowed intervertebral foramen, causing pressure on the spinal nerve (Fig. 3.36).

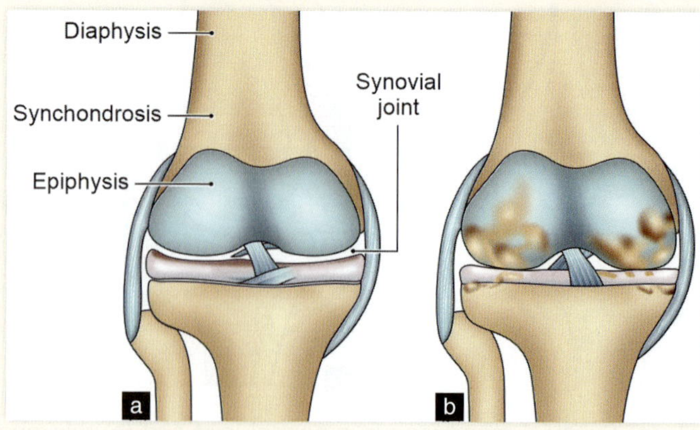

Fig. 3.35: (a) Knee joint of a normal subject and (b) An osteoarthritic patient

Table 3.5: Comparison of osteoarthritis and rheumatoid arthritis			
	Age and joints	*Disorder and initial damage*	*Systemic disease*
Osteoarthritis	Middle age, single large weight bearing joint	Degenerative, articular cartilage damaged	None ESR—normal, Rheumatoid factor absent
Rheumatoid arthritis	Any age, multiple small joints of hands and feet	Inflammatory, synovial membrane inflammed	Systemic disease, ESR—raised, anaemia + rheumatoid factor present

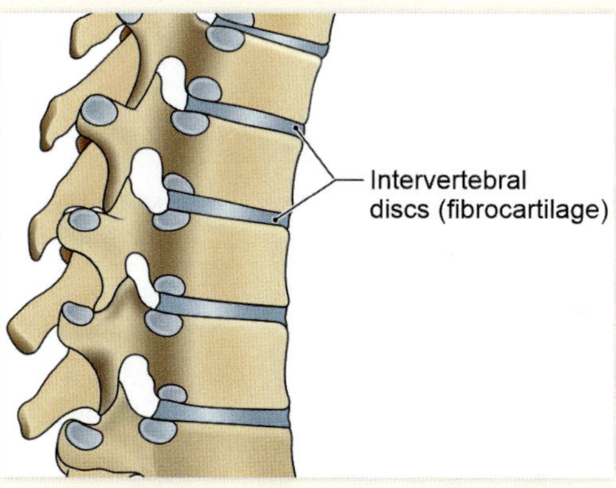

Fig. 3.36: Bony changes in spondylitis

- There may be injury to various structures in the joints. At times the medial meniscus of the knee joint may get injured. In that case it needs to be removed (Fig. 3.37).
- The metaphysis, the end of diaphysis or shaft is the actively growing end of the bone. In some joints, the capsule encloses the metaphysis as well. In such joints, infection from metaphysis would reach the joint cavity and cause septic arthritis (Fig. 3.38).
- There may be fracture into the joint space leading to collection of blood and broken pieces of ends of the bones in the joint cavity.
- If joints have been diseased for a very long time with no hope of recovery, these can be replaced.

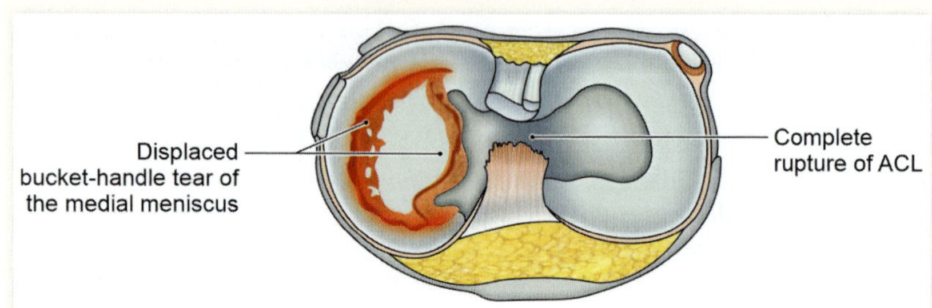

Fig. 3.37: Injury of knee joint involving tear of medial meniscus and rupture of anterior cruciate ligament

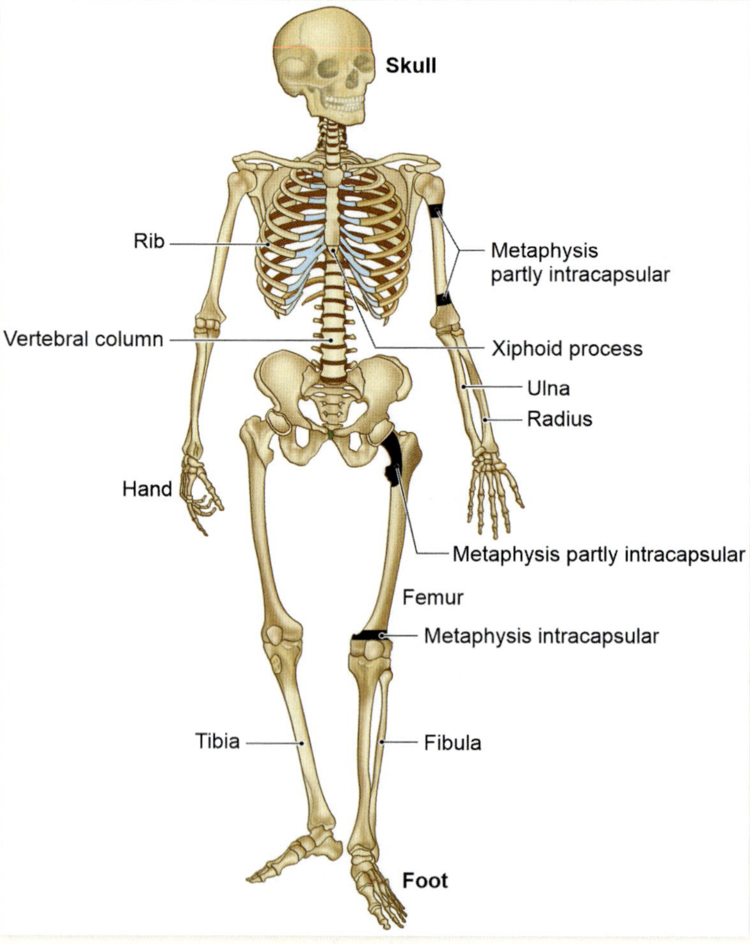

Fig. 3.38: Relations of capsule of joints to their metaphyses

- Stiffness of joints is related to weather. The viscosity of synovial fluid increases with fall in temperature. This accounts for stiffness of the joints in cold weather. Mobility of joint in itself is an important factor in promoting lubrication. Thus the stiffness of joints experienced in the morning gradually passes off as the movements are resumed.
- Neuropathic joint is the result of its complete denervation, so that all reflexes are eliminated and the joint is left unprotected and liable to mechanical damage. A neuropathic joint shows painless swelling, excessive mobility and bony destruction. It is commonly caused by leprosy, tabes dorsalis and syringomyelia.

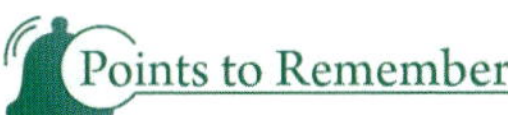

Points to Remember

- Joint is a junction between two or more bones or cartilages.
- Joints are classified as fibrous, cartilaginous and synovial types.
- There are more joints in a child than in an adult. The primary cartilaginous joints at the ends of long bones after fusion disappear in the adult, decreasing the number of joints.
- Joints help in increasing the length of bones, increasing the size of cranial, thoracic and pelvic cavities.
- Joints in thorax help in respiratory movements.
- Joints are vital for locomotion.
- The secondary cartilaginous joints are in midline of the body.
- Joints in ossicles of middle ear are synovial joints.
- Joints chiefly suffer in osteoarthritis and rheumatoid arthritis.
- Joints in the laryngeal cartilages help us in speech.

Multiple Choice Questions

1. Which of the following joint contains an intra-articular disc?

a. Ankle joint
b. Sternoclavicular joint
c. Elbow joint
d. Shoulder joint

2. Which statement about articular cartilage is correct?

a. It is devoid of perichondrium
b. It is devoid of nerves
c. It is covered by synovial membrane
d. It contains lots of capillaries

3. **Synovial membrane lines or encloses all structures *except*:**
   a. Articular cartilage
   b. Inner aspect of the capsule
   c. Intracapsular tendons
   d. Intracapsular parts of the articulating bones
4. **All the statements about synovial membrane are correct *except*:**
   a. It is avascular
   b. It is modification of deep fascia
   c. It secretes synovial fluid
   d. If damaged, it regenerates
5. **Which of the following is a hinge joint?**
   a. Superior radioulnar b. Wrist
   c. Metacarpophalangeal d. Elbow
6. **Which of the following is not the ball and socket joint?**
   a. Incudostapedial b. Shoulder
   c. Talocalcaneonavicular d. Incudomalleolar
7. **Definition of Hilton's law is:**
   a. The nerve supplying a muscle also supplies the overlying skin and underlying joint
   b. Muscles around the joint act on the same joint
   c. The capsule is rich in nerve fibres
   d. The synovial membrane is rich in capillaries
8. **The articular surfaces of articulating bones in synovial joints are covered by:**
   a. Articular cartilage b. Joint capsule
   c. Synovial membrane d. Periosteum
9. **Condylar joints are:**
   a. Uniaxial b. Biaxial
   c. Multiaxial d. Symphysis
10. **Which of the following is not a saddle joint?**
    a. Sternoclavicular
    b. Temporomandibular
    c. Wrist joint
    d. First carpometacarpal
11. **Which is not a fibrous joint?**
    a. Sutures b. Gomphosis
    c. Xiphisternal d. Inferior tibiofibular

12. Following are the features of manubriosternal joint *except*:
a. It is a secondary cartilaginous joint
b. It is a symphysis type of joint
c. It shows synovial cavity in 30% of cases
d. It moves slightly during respiration

13. Which of the following is a primary cartilaginous joint?
a. Ist sternochondral
b. Xiphicostal
c. Intervertebral
d. Sternoclavicular

14. Synostosis is defined as union of bones by:
a. Hyaline cartilage
b. Bone
c. Fibrocartilage
d. Interosseous ligament

15. Name the joint present between epiphysis and diaphysis:
a. Fibrous
b. Primary cartilaginous
c. Secondary cartilaginous
d. Synovial

16. First sternochondral joint is:
a. Synchondrosis
b. Syndesmosis
c. Symphysis
d. None of the above

Answers

1. b	**2.** a	**3.** a	**4.** a	**5.** d	**6.** d	**7.** a	**8.** a
9. b	**10.** c	**11.** c	**12.** c	**13.** a	**14.** b	**15.** b	**16.** a

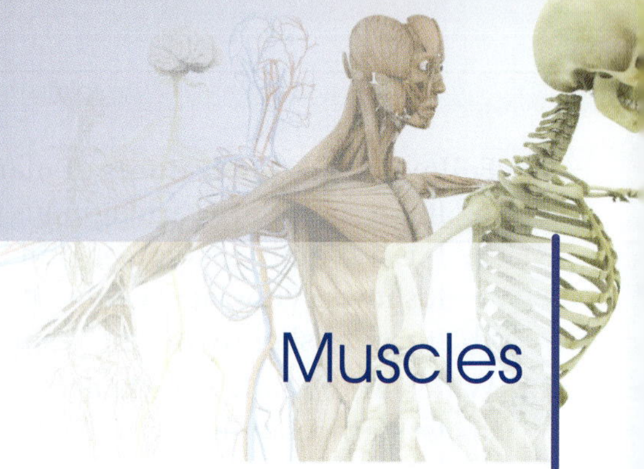

Chapter 4

Muscles

Smile does not cost anything, but it improves your "face value, much better than any cosmetics."

DERIVATION OF NAME

Muscles (L Mus = mouse) are so named because, many of them resemble a mouse, with their tendons representing the tail.

Definition

Muscle is a contractile tissue which brings about movements. Muscles can be regarded as motors of the body.

Types of Muscles

The muscles are of three types, skeletal, smooth and cardiac. The characters of each type are summarized in Table 4.1.

Table 4.1: Types of muscles

Striated/skeletal	*Non-striated/smooth*	*Cardiac*
1. Striated muscles are present in the limbs, body wall, tongue, pharynx and beginning of oesophagus (Fig. 4.1)	Oesophagus (distal part), urogenital tract, urinary bladder, blood vessels, iris of eye, arrector pili muscle of hair (Fig. 4.2)	Wall of heart (Fig. 4.3)
2. Long and cylindrical	Spindle shaped	Short and cylindrical

(Contd.)

Table 4.1: Types of muscles (*Contd.*)		
Striated/skeletal	*Non-striated/smooth*	*Cardiac*
3. Fibres unbranched	Fibres unbranched	Fibres branched
4. Multinucleated	Uninucleated	Uninucleated
5. Bounded by sarcolemma	Bounded by plasma-lemma	Bounded by plasma-lemma
6. Light and dark bands present	Light and dark bands absent	Faint light and dark bands present
7. No intercalated disc	No intercalated discs	Intercalated disc present and a characteristic feature
8. Nerve supply from cranial nervous system	Nerve supply from autonomic nervous system	Nerve supply from autonomic nervous system
9. Blood supply is abundant	Blood supply is scanty	Blood supply is abundant
10. Very rapid contraction	Slow contraction	Rapid contractions
11. They soon get fatigued	They do not get fatigued	They never get fatigued
12. Voluntary	Involuntary	Involuntary

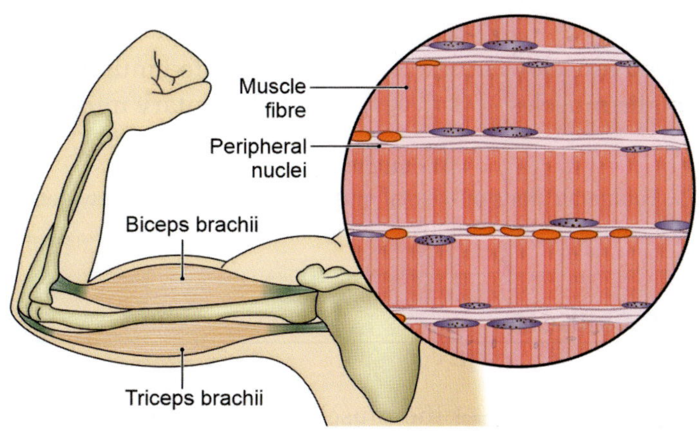

Fig. 4.1: Skeletal muscle

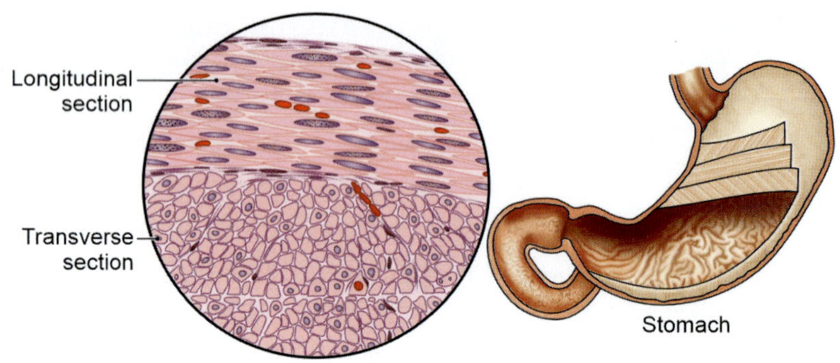

Fig. 4.2: Smooth muscle

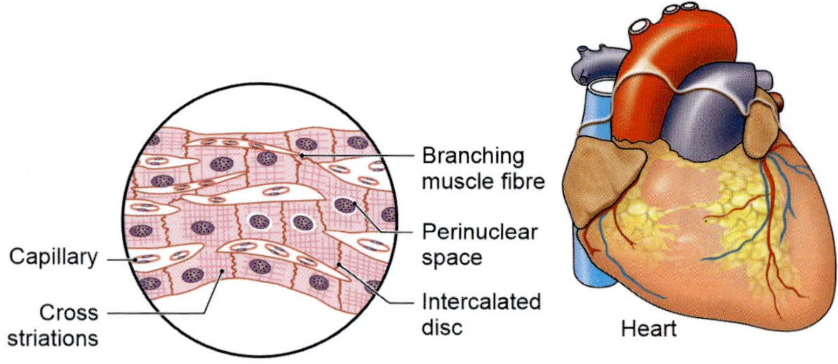

Fig. 4.3: Cardiac muscle

SKELETAL MUSCLES

Synonyms

1. Striped muscles
2. Striated muscles
3. Somatic muscles
4. Voluntary muscles

Competency achievement: The student should be able to:
AN 3.2 Enumerate parts of skeletal muscle and differentiate between tendons and aponeuroses. Give examples

PARTS OF A MUSCLE

A. Two Ends

1. ***Origin*** is one end of the muscle which mostly remains fixed during its contraction.

2. ***Insertion*** is the other end which mostly moves during its contraction. In the ***limb*** muscles, the origin is usually proximal to insertion.

However, the terms origin and insertion, are at times interchangeable, and at other times difficult to define, as in the intercostal muscles. Muscles of pharynx, oesophagus, and the diaphragm act as involuntary muscles.

B. Two Parts

1. ***Fleshy part*** is contractile, and is called the 'belly'.
2. ***Fibrous part*** is noncontractile and inelastic. When cord-like or rope-like, it is called tendon (Fig. 4.4); when flattened, it is called aponeurosis. The tendon receives Golgi tendon nerve endings. It is supplied by capillaries extending from the fleshy part and also from the periosteal arteries of the bone where the tendon terminates or gets inserted.

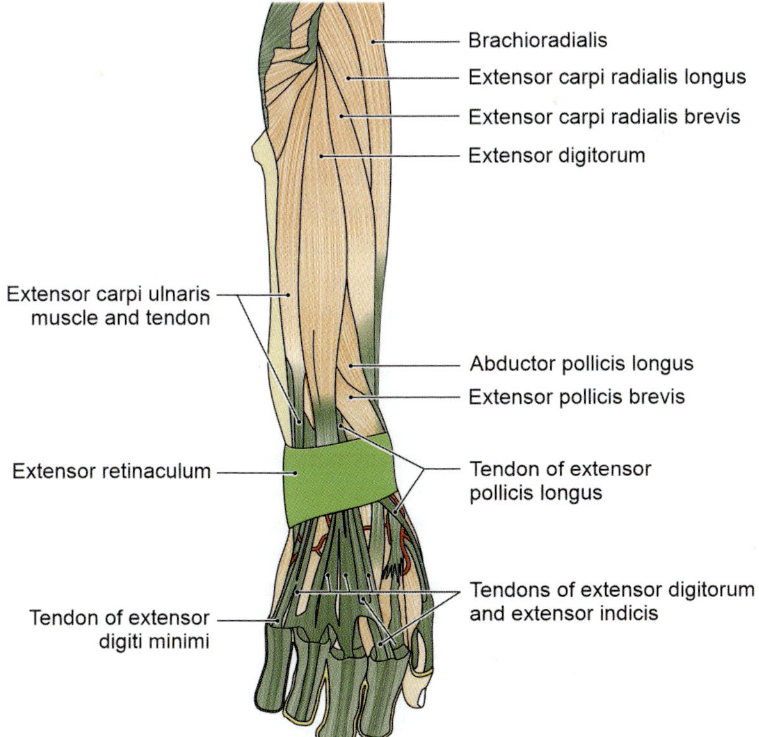

Fig. 4.4: Muscles and tendons of extensor compartment of forearm

STRUCTURE OF STRIATED MUSCLE

A. Contractile Tissue

Each muscle is composed of numerous muscle fibres. Each *muscle fibre* is a multinucleated, cross-striated cylindrical cell (myocyte) 1–300 mm long. It is made up of sarcolemma (cell membrane) enclosing sarcoplasm (cytoplasm).

Embedded in the sarcoplasm there are: (a) Several hundred nuclei arranged at the periphery beneath the sarcolemma (Fig. 4.1) and (b) a number of evenly distributed longitudinal threads called *myofibrils*. Each myofibril shows alternate dark and light bands. Dark bands are known as A bands (anistropic) and the light bands as I bands (isotropic). The bands of adjacent fibrils are aligned transversely so that the muscle fibre appears cross-striated. In the middle of dark band there is a light H band. In the middle of I band there is a dark Z line or Krause's membrane. The segment of myofibril between two Z lines is called sarcomere (Fig. 4.5).

Muscle → fasciculi → fibres → myofibril → myofilaments

B. Supporting Tissue

Supporting tissue helps in organization of the muscle. *Endomysium* surrounds each muscle fibre separately. *Perimysium* surrounds bundles (fasciculi or myonemes) of muscle fibres of various sizes. *Epimysium* surrounds the entire muscle. The connective tissue of the muscle becomes continuous with the tendon (Fig. 4.6).

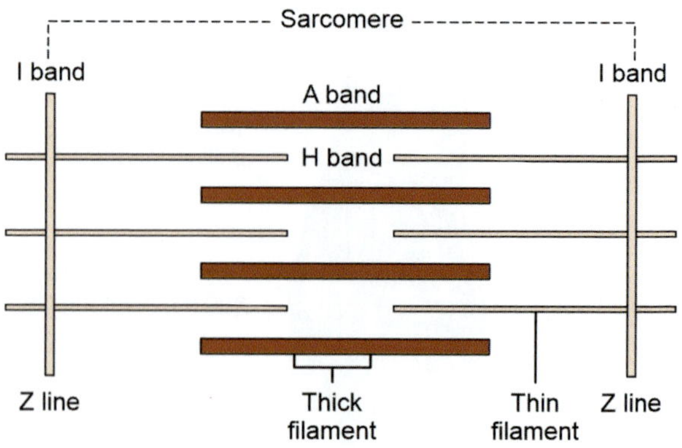

Fig. 4.5: Myofibrils in skeletal muscle

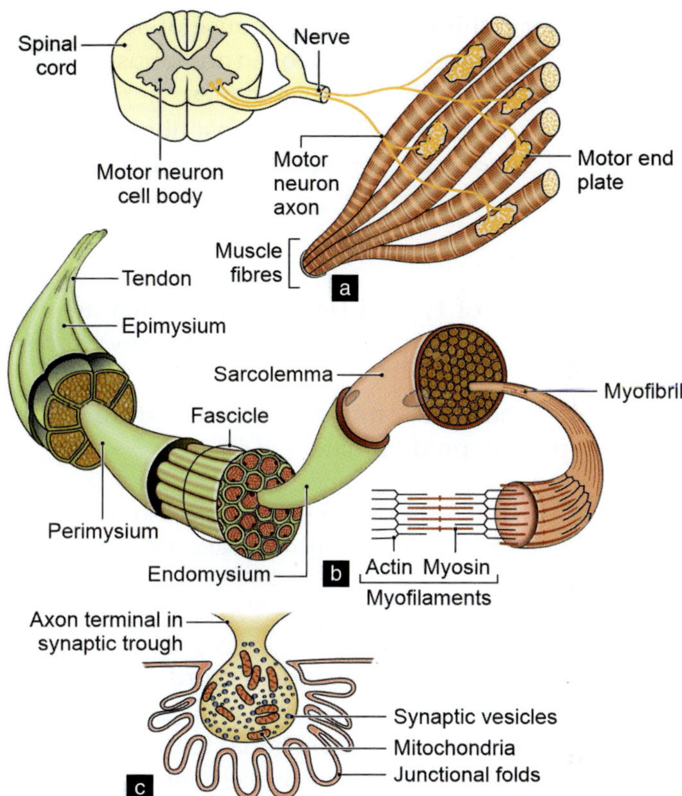

Fig. 4.6: Supporting tissue of a muscle. Nerve supply to muscle fibres also shown (a) nerve supply to muscle fibres; (b) supporting tissue of a muscle; (c) motor end plate

C. Types of Fibres

1. Type I (Slow) Fibres

Show a slow 'tonic' contraction characteristic of postural muscles like gluteus maximus.

These are red in colour because of large amounts of myoglobin. The fibres are rich in mitochondria and oxidative enzymes, but poor in phosphorylases.

Because of a well-developed aerobic metabolism, slow fibres are highly resistant to fatigue.

2. Type II (Fast) Fibres

Show a fast 'phasic' contraction required for large-scale movements of body segments.

These are paler (white) in colour because of small amounts of myoglobin. The fibres are rich in glycogen and phosphorylases, but poor in mitochondria and oxidative enzymes.

Because of a glycolytic respiration, the fast fibres are quite easily fatigued. Table 4.2 shows the comparison betwee type I and type II muscle fibres.

3. Intermediate Fibres

Represent a variant of type II (fast) fibres which are relatively resistant to fatigue, although less than type I (slow) fibres (Burke et al, 1973).

In man, most of the skeletal muscles show a mixture of fibre types, but any one type may predominate.

> *Competency achievement:* The student should be able to:
> AN 3.1 Classify muscle tissue according to structure and action

Fascicular Architecture of Muscles

The arrangement of muscle fibres varies according to the direction, force and range of habitual movement at a particular joint. The force of movement is directly proportional to the number and size of muscle fibres, and the range of movement is proportional to the length of fibres. The muscles can be classified according to the arrangement of their fasciculi into the following groups.

Table 4.2: Comparison between type I and type II muscle fibres

	Red fibres/type I	*Pale fibres/type II*
Diameter	Small	Large
Blood supply	Rich blood supply	Poor blood supply
Nerve supply	Small nerve fibres	Large nerve fibres
Contraction	Slow twitch	Fast switch
Force of contraction	Weak, sustained	Strong, less sustained
Fatigue	Fatigue later	Easily fatigued
Myoglobin	Plenty, gives it red color	Scanty
Mitochondria	Rich	Scanty
ATP and glycogen	Poor	Rich
Oxidative enzymes	Rich	Poor

A. Parallel Fasciculi

When the fasciculi are parallel to the line of pull, the muscle may be:

1. *Quadrilateral* (thyrohyoid) (Fig. 4.7a).
2. *Strap-like* (sternohyoid and sartorius) (Fig. 4.7b).
3. *Strap-like with tendinous intersections* (rectus abdominis) (Fig. 4.7c).
4. *Fusiform* (biceps brachii, digastric, etc.). The range of movement in such muscles is maximum (Fig. 4.7d and e).

B. Oblique Fasciculi

When the fasciculi are oblique to the line of pull, the muscle may be triangular, or pennate (feather-like) in the construction. This arrangement makes the muscle more powerful, although the range of movement is reduced. Oblique arrangements are of the following types:

1. *Triangular*, e.g. temporalis (Fig. 4.7f), adductor longus (Fig. 4.7g).
2. *Unipennate*, e.g. flexor pollicis longus, extensor digitorum longus, peroneus tertius, palmar interossei (Fig. 4.7h).

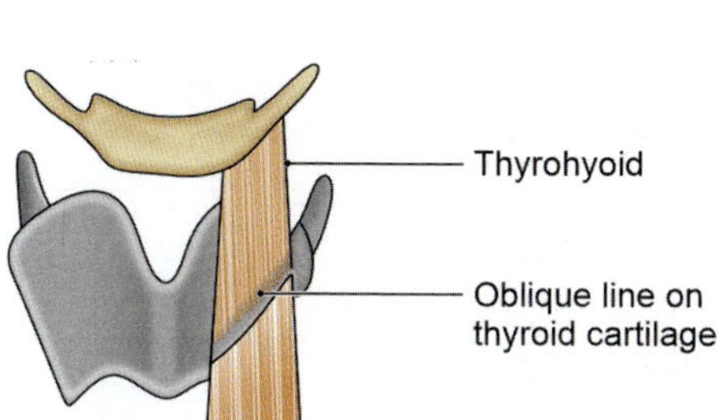

Fig. 4.7a: Quadrilateral muscle

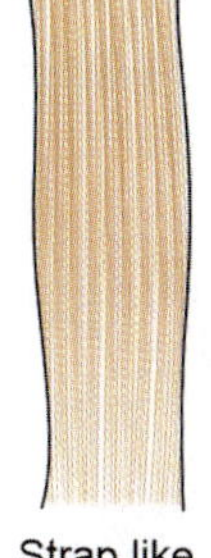

Fig. 4.7b: Sartorius

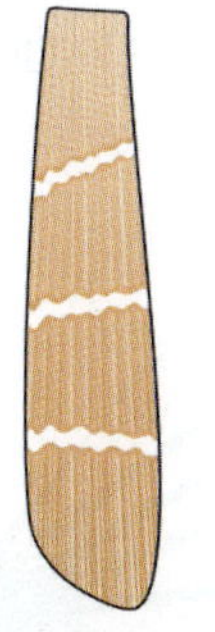

Fig. 4.7c: Rectus abdominis

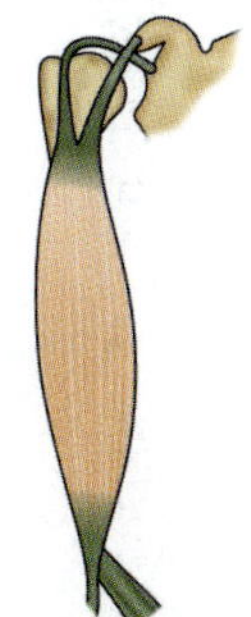

Fig. 4.7d: Biceps brachii

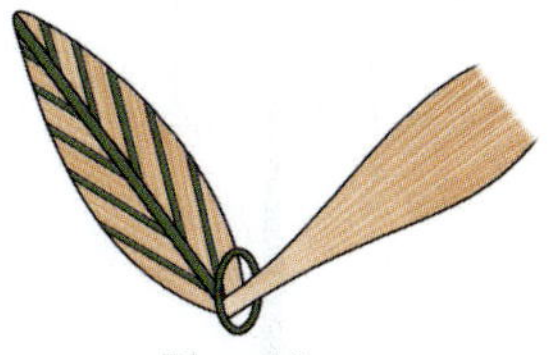

Fig. 4.7e: Digastric muscle

3. *Bipennate*, e.g. rectus femoris, dorsal interossei (Fig. 4.7i), peroneus longus, flexor hallucis longus.
4. *Multipennate*, e.g. subscapularis (Fig. 4.7j), deltoid (acromial fibres).
5. *Circumpennate*, e.g. tibialis anterior.

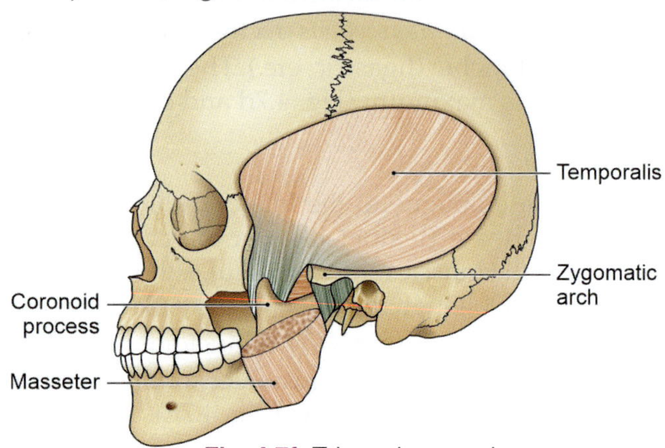

Fig. 4.7f: Triangular muscle

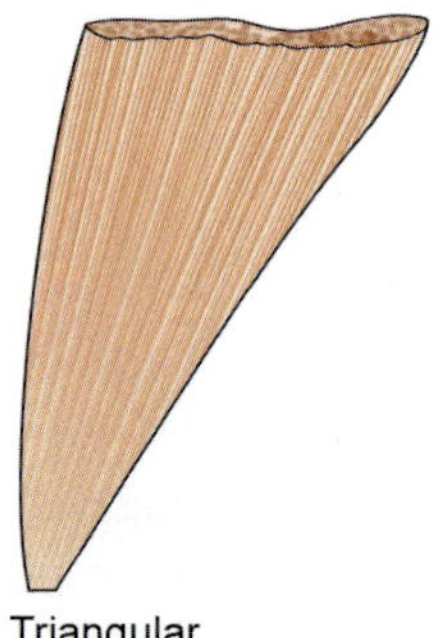

Fig. 4.7g: Adductor longus

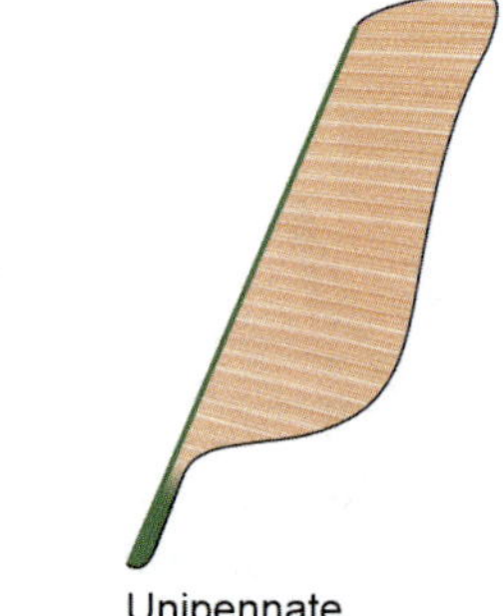

Fig. 4.7h: Flexor pollicis longus

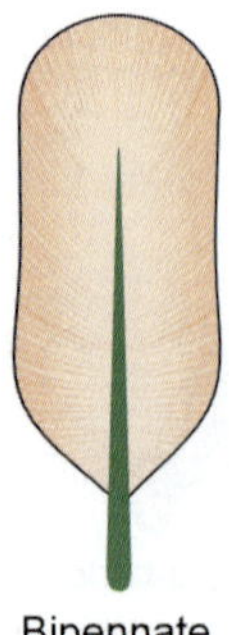

Fig. 4.7i: Rectus femoris

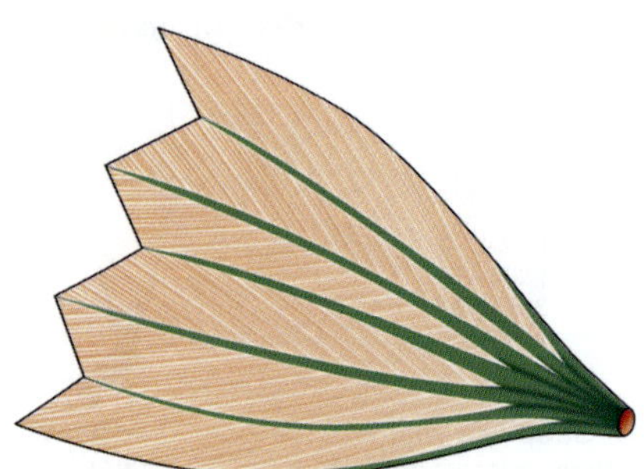

Fig. 4.7j: Subscapularis

C. Spiral or Twisted Fasciculi

Spiral or twisted fibres are found in trapezius, pectoralis major, latissimus dorsi, supinator, etc. (Fig. 4.7k). In certain muscles the fasciculi are crossed. These are called cruciate muscles, e.g. sternocleidomastoid (Fig. 4.7*l*), masseter, and adductor magnus.

NAMING THE MUSCLES

Features Used in Naming Muscles

Following features are used for naming the muscles:

Shape

Deltoid (triangular, Fig. 4.8a)
Quadratus (quadrangular)—quadratus femoris (Fig. 4.8b)
Rhomboid (diamond shaped)—rhomboid major
Teres (round)—teres major (Fig. 4.8d)
Gracilis (slender)—gracilis (Fig. 4.8c)
Lumbrical (worm-like)—lumbricals of palm
Rectus (straight)—rectus abdominis (Fig. 4.7b)

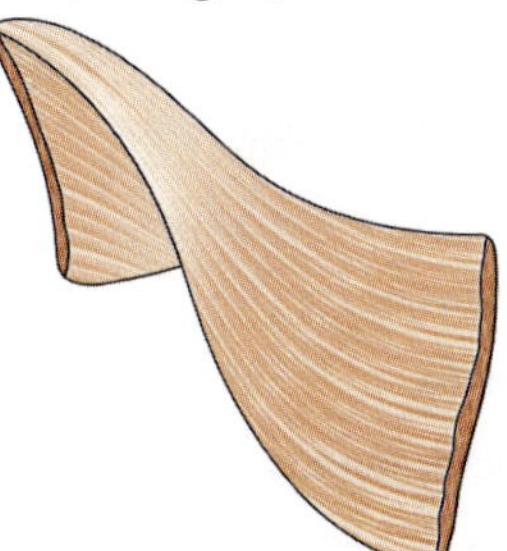

Fig. 4.7k: Spiral

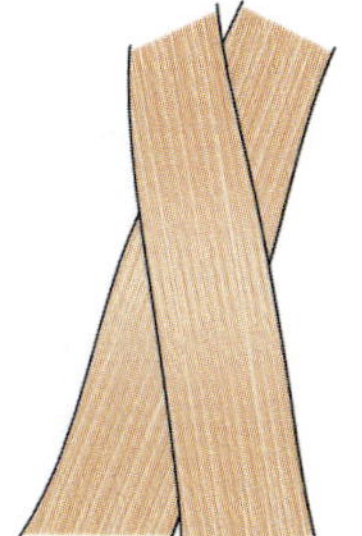

Fig. 4.7*l*: Cruciate

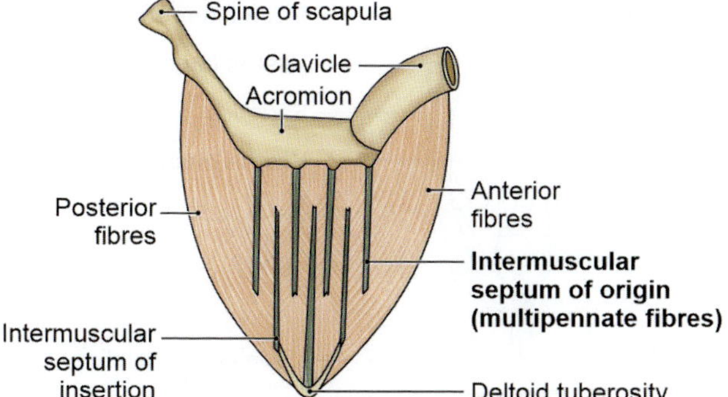

Fig. 4.8a: Multipennate fibres

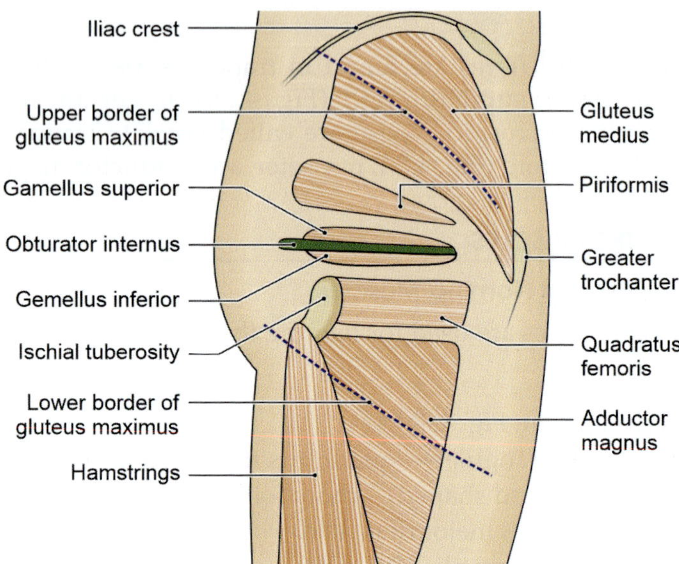

Fig. 4.8b: Quadrangular muscle

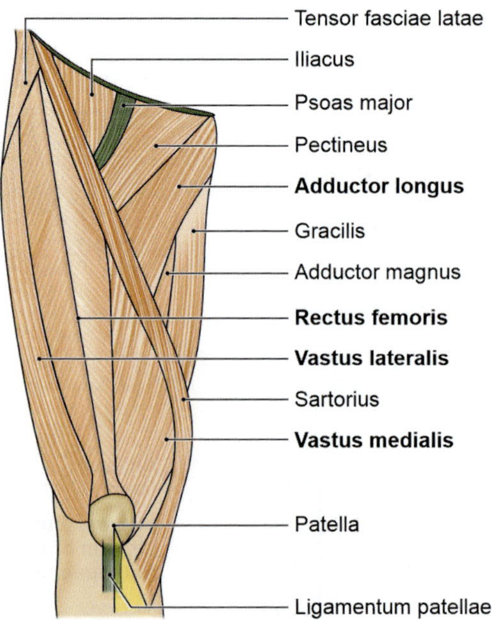

Fig. 4.8c: Nomenclature of muscles

Size

Major (big)—pectoralis major
Minor (small)—pectoralis minor
Longus (long)—adductor longus (Fig. 4.8c)
Brevis (small)—abductor pollicis brevis
Latissimus (broadest)—latissimus dorsi (Fig. 4.8d)
Longissimus (longest)—longissimus thoracis

Number of Heads

Biceps (two heads)—biceps brachii (Fig. 4.8e)
Triceps (three heads)—triceps brachii (Fig. 4.8f)
Quadriceps (four heads)—quadriceps femoris (Fig. 4.8g)
Digastric (two bellies)—anterior and posterior bellies of digastric (Fig. 4.7e).

Attachment

Sternocleidomastoid (from sternum and clavicle to mastoid process, Fig. 4.8h)
Brachialis (from humerus to ulna, Fig. 4.8i).
Coracobrachialis from coracoid process to the arm (brachium).

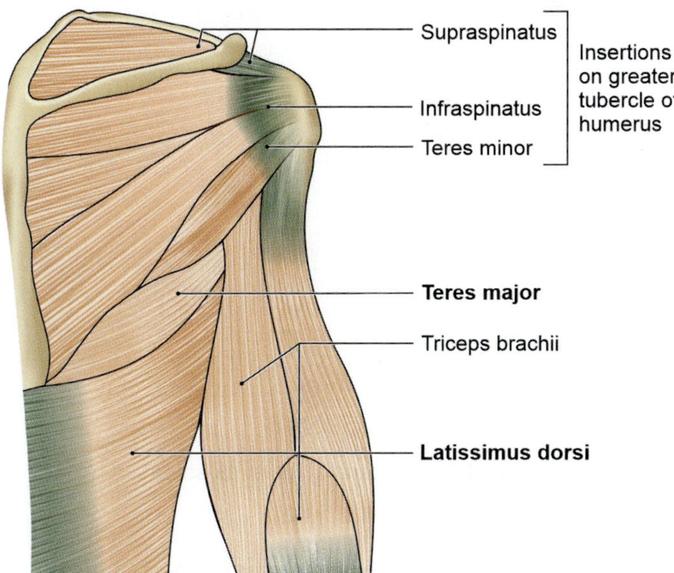

Fig. 4.8d: Nomenclature of muscles

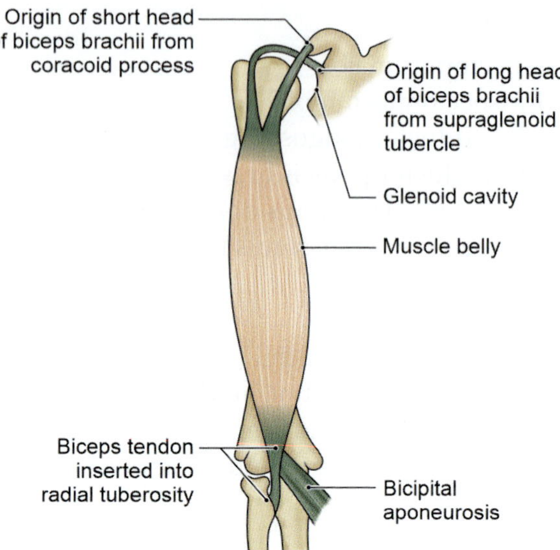

Fig. 4.8e: Nomenclature of muscles

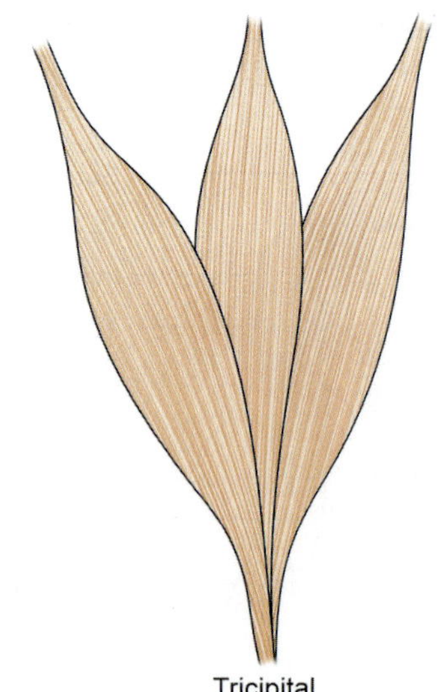

Fig. 4.8f: Nomenclature of muscles

Depth

Superficialis (superficial)—flexor digitorum superficialis [Fig. 4.8j(i)]
Profundus (deep)—flexor digitorum profundus [Fig. 4.8j(ii)]

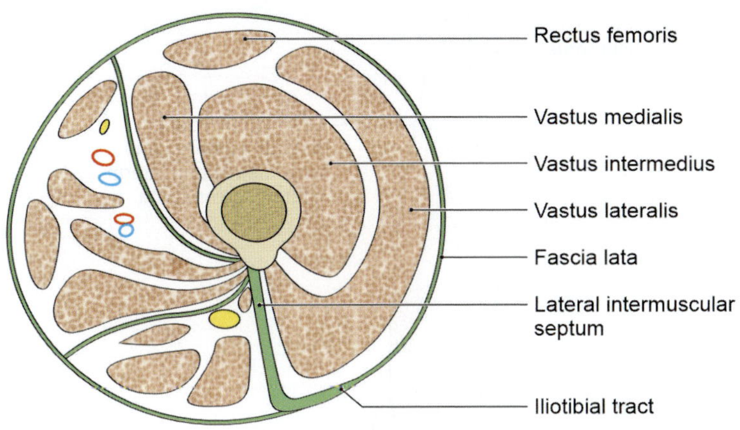

Fig. 4.8g: Nomenclature of muscles

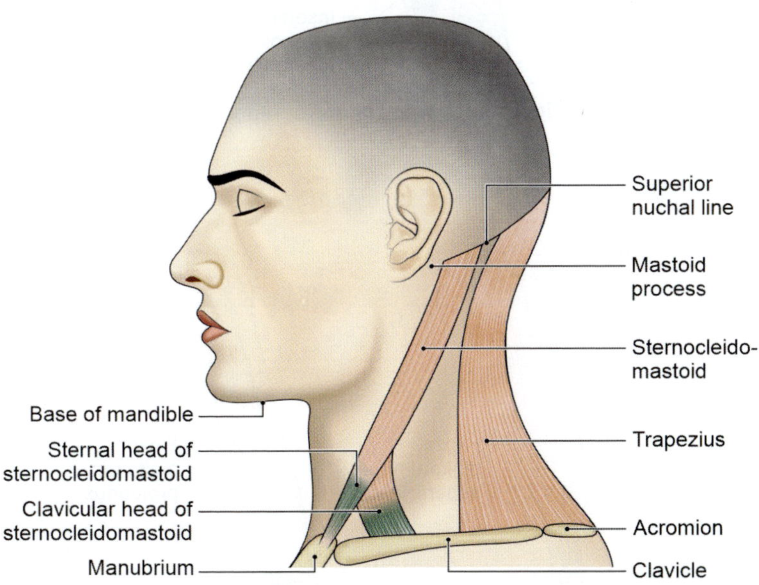

Fig. 4.8h: Nomenclature of muscles

Externus (external)—external oblique of anterior abdominal wall
Internus (internal)—internal oblique of anterior abdominal wall

Position

Anterior (front)—tibialis anterior (Fig. 4.8k)
Posterior (back)—tibialis posterior

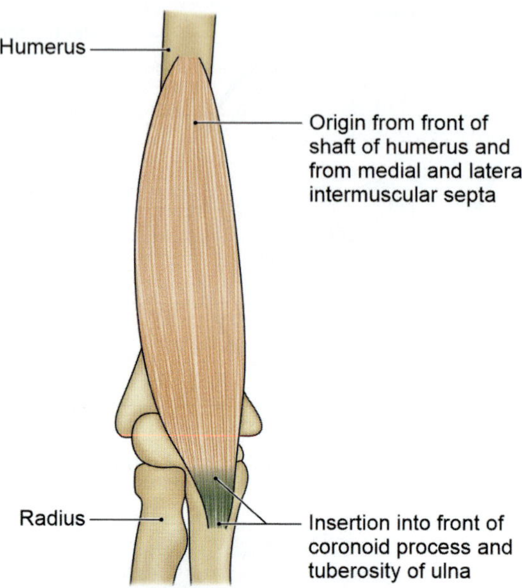

Fig. 4.8i: Nomenclature of muscles

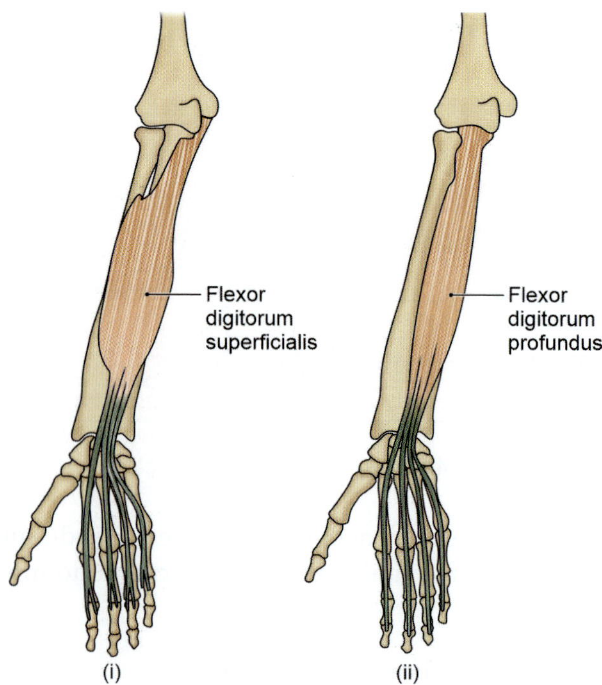

Fig. 4.8j: Nomenclature of muscles

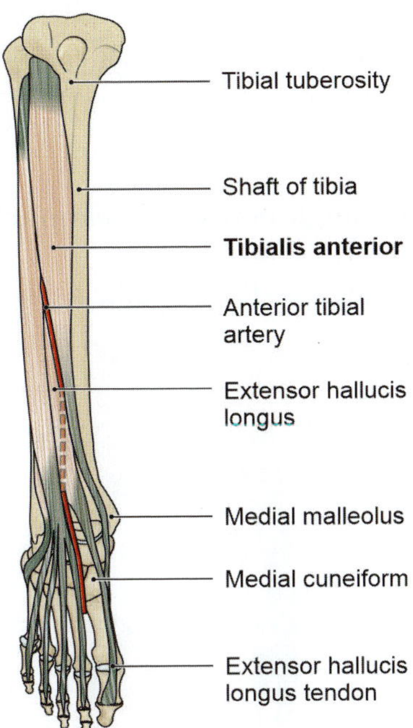

Fig. 4.8k: Muscles of anterior compartment of leg

Lateralis (lateral side)—vastus lateralis (Fig. 4.8c)
Medialis (medial side)—vastus medialis (Fig. 4.8c)
Superior (upper side)—superior rectus of eyeball
Inferior (lower side)—inferior rectus of eyeball
Supra (above)—supraspinatus (Fig. 4.8d)
Infra (lower)—infraspinatus (Fig. 4.8d)
Dorsi (of the back)—latissimus dorsi (Fig. 4.8e)
Brachii (of the arm)—biceps brachii
Femoris (of the thigh)—rectus femoris
Oris (of the mouth)—orbicularis oris
Oculi (of the eye)—orbicularis oculi (Fig. 4.8*l*)

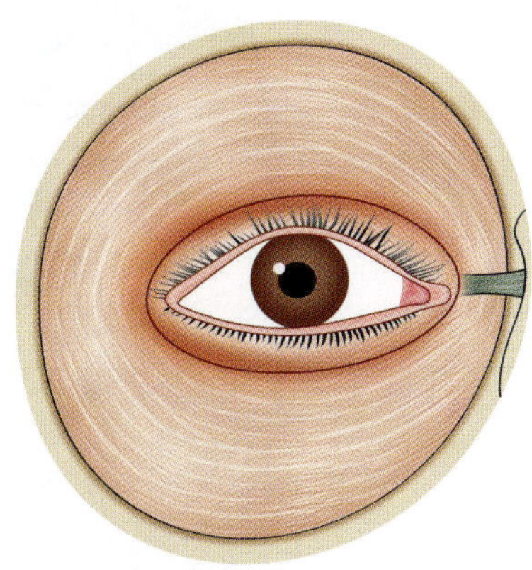

Fig. 4.8*l*: Orbicularis oculi muscle

Structure

Half muscle, half tendon—semitendinosus (Fig. 4.8m)
Serrated edges serratus anterior (Fig. 4.8n)

Action

Extensor (increase the angle between forearm and palm)—extensor pollicis longus (Fig. 4.4)
Flexor (decrease the angle)—flexor pollicis longus

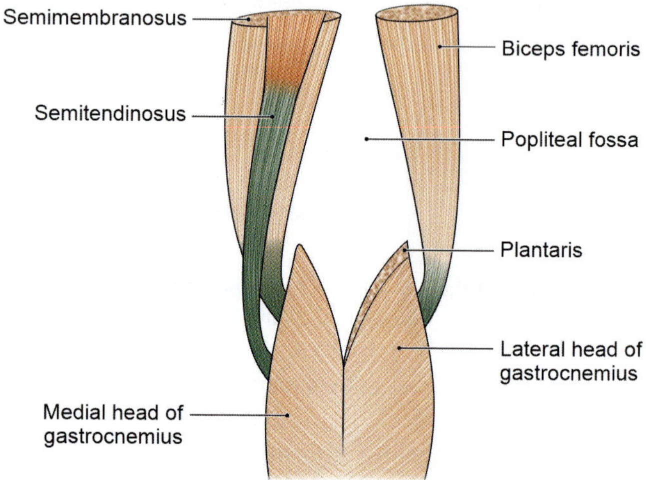

Fig. 4.8m: Muscles forming boundaries for popliteal fossa

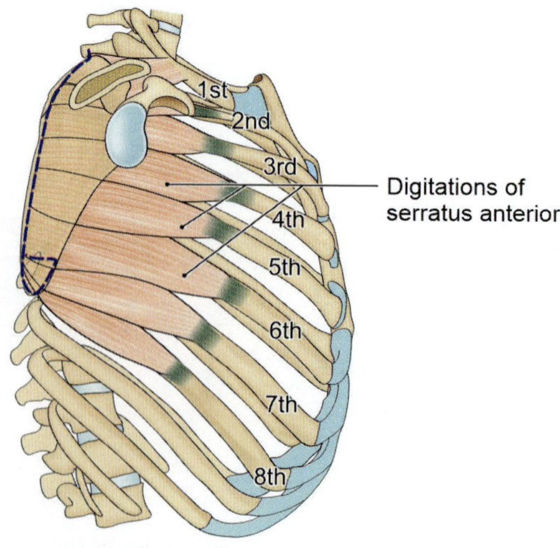

Fig. 4.8n: Serratus anterior muscle

Abductor (take away)—abductor digiti minimi (Fig. 4.8p)
Adductor (take towards midline)—adductor pollicis
Levator (to elevate)—levator scapulae
Depressor (to pull down)—depressor anguli oris (Fig. 4.8o)
Supinator (turning palm anteriorly)—supinator
Pronator (turning palm posteriorly)—pronator teres
Constrictor (to narrow)—constrictor pupillae
Dilator (to dilate)—dilator pupillae
Abduction of digits—dorsal interossei (Fig. 4.8p).

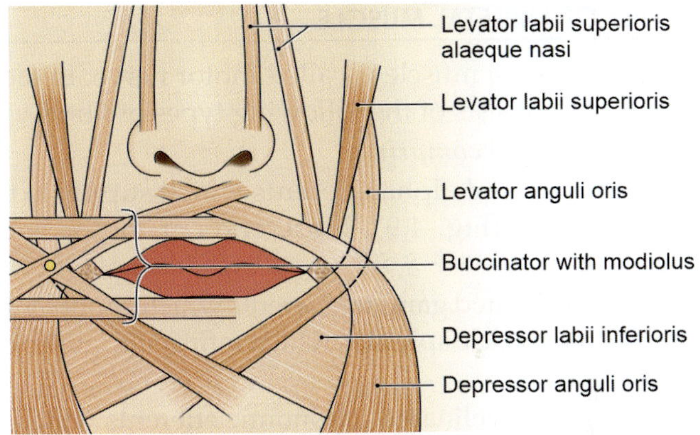

Fig. 4.8o: Muscles of facial expressions

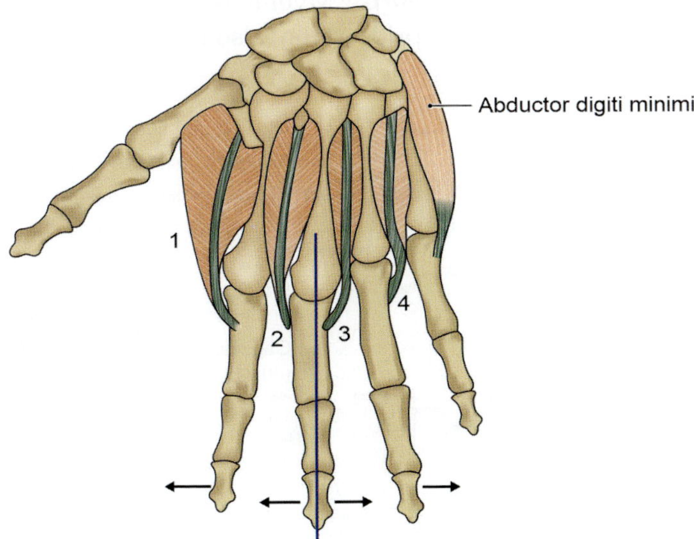

Fig. 4.8p: Dorsal interossei and abductor digiti minimi

Competency achievement: The student should be able to:
AN 3.3 Explain shunt and spurt muscles
AN 7.5 Describe principles of sensory and motor innervation of muscles

Spurt muscle: Its origin is away but the insertion is close to the joint of its action, e.g. brachialis (Fig. 4.8i).

Shunt muscle: Its origin is close to the joint of its action, but insertion is away, e.g. brachioradialis (Fig. 4.4).

NERVE SUPPLY OF SKELETAL MUSCLE

The nerve supplying a muscle is called motor nerve. In fact it is a mixed nerve and consists of the following types of fibres.

1. ***Motor fibres (60%) comprise:***
   a. Large myelinated alpha efferents which supply extrafusal muscle fibres (Fig. 4.9). Fibre ends at motor end plate (Fig. 4.6).
   b. Smaller myelinated gamma efferents which supply intrafusal fibres of the muscle spindles which refine and control muscle contraction.
   c. The fine non-myelinated autonomic efferents which supply smooth muscle fibres of the blood vessels.
2. ***Sensory fibres (40%) comprise:*** Myelinated fibres distributed to muscle spindles for proprioception, also to tendons.

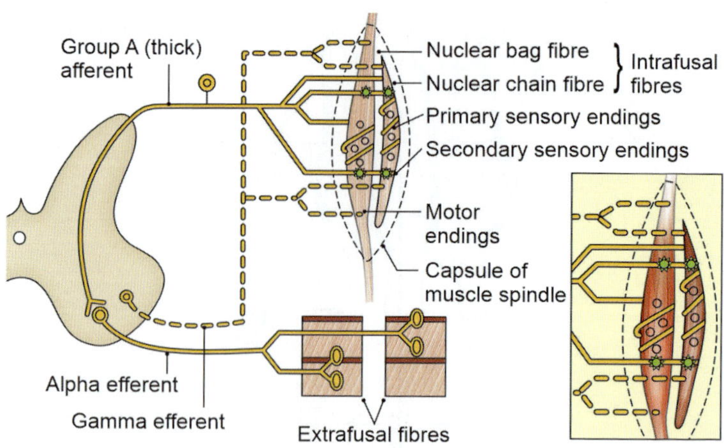

Fig. 4.9: Muscle spindle

4

Muscle spindles are spindle-shaped sensory end organs of the skeletal muscle. Each spindle contains 6–14 intrafusal muscle fibres which are of two types, the larger *nuclear bag fibres*, and the smaller *nuclear chain fibres* (Fig. 4.9). The spindle is innervated by both the sensory and motor nerves. The sensory endings are of two types, the primary sensory endings (annulospiral endings) around the central nuclear region of the intrafusal fibres, and the secondary sensory endings (*flower spray endings*) beyond the nuclear region on either side of these fibres.

The motor nerve supply of the spindle is derived from gamma motor neurons of the spinal cord. Muscle spindles act as stretch receptors. They record and help regulate the degree and rate of contraction of the extrafusal fibres by influencing the alpha neurons, which act on "motor end plates."

Motor point is the site where the motor nerve enters the muscle. It may be one or more than one. Electrical stimulation at the motor point is more effective.

Motor unit is defined as a single alpha motor neuron together with the muscle fibres supplied by it. The size of motor unit depends upon the precision of muscle control. Small motor units (5–10 muscle fibres) are found in muscles of fine movements (extraocular muscles). Large motor units (100–2000 muscle fibres) are found in muscles of gross movements (proximal limb muscles).

Composite/hybrid muscle: Muscle supplied by two different motor nerves with different root values is called a *composite* or *hybrid* muscle, e.g. adductor magnus, flexor digitorum profundus and pectoralis major.

Adductor magnus comprises an adductor part, supplied by obturator nerve (L 2, 3, 4) and an hamstring part supplied by sciatic nerve (L 4, 5, S 1, 2, 3).

Flexor digitorum profundus comprises part destined for index and middle fingers is supplied by median nerve (C 5, 6, 7, 8 T1). The part destined for ring and little fingers gets supplied by ulnar nerve (C 7, 8, T1). Pectoralis major, pectoralis minor are also hybrid muscles.

Vascular pedicle: Vascular pedicle is the pedicle containing one vein and one artery for the supply of skeletal muscle. Accordingly these are classified as:

Type I: Muscle with only one pedicle	e.g. tensor fascia latae
Type II: 1 main and a few small pedicles	gracilis
Type III: 2 main pedicles	gluteus maximus

Type IV: Many pedicles sartorius
Type V: One main and many smaller pedicles latissimus dorsi

Knowledge of vascular pedicles is useful in muscle grafting whenever required.

Nerve Supply of Smooth Muscle

According to nerve supply by autonomic nervous system the smooth muscles are classified into:

Single-unit type: Seen in intestines. The nerve impulse reaches one muscle cell, is transmitted to other cells by the mechanical pull through the fused cell membrane. The nerve supply is sparse.

Multi-unit type: Seen in the muscles of the ductus deferens. Each muscle cell receives a separate nerve fibre. The contraction is simultaneous. The nerve supply is rich.

Nerve Supply of Cardiac Muscle

Heart is supplied by sympathetic and parasympathetic nerve fibres. Sympathetic nerves stimulate both the heart rate and blood pressure and dilate the coronary arteries. The sensory fibres convey painful impulses from heart.

Parasympathetic fibres decrease and normalise the heart rate. Their sensory fibres are involved with visceral reflexes.

Molecular Regulation of Muscle Formation

MYO-D and MYF5, members of the family of myogenic regulatory factors (MRFs), are considered to play an important role in the induction of myogenesis in mesenchymal cells.

Signaling molecules involved in the regulation of beginning of myogenesis and induction of myotomes are:

- *Sonic hedgehog (SHH) protein* secreted from the ventral neural tube and notochord.
- *WNTs and BMP4* secreted from the dorsal neural tube and the overlying ectoderm.

ACTIONS OF MUSCLES

1. Broadly, when a muscle contracts, it shortens by one-third (30%) of its belly-length, and brings about a movement. The range of movement depends on the length of fleshy fibres, and the power or force of movement on the number of fibres.

However, the actual behaviour of muscle contraction is more complex.

i. Length may remain unchanged (*isometric* contraction), e.g. holding the hand in outstretched position. Exercise without movement is isometric contraction.
ii. During contraction the length of the muscle may increase or decrease but the tension is constant (*isotonic* contraction). Exercise with movement is isotonic contraction.
iii. Length may increase, according to the functional demands of the body. It is called *eccentric* contraction, e.g. when the upper limb is lowered to the side of the body.
iv. *Concentric* contraction is when there is increasing tension in the muscle as it contracts and shortens. Most of contractions of muscle are concentric.

In each circumstance the tension generated at the ends may either increase, persist, or decrease, depending upon the number and state of its active motor units and the external conditions like loading. Daily activities involve use of both isotonic and isometric contractions.

2. Each movement at a joint is brought about by a coordinated activity of different groups of muscles. These muscle groups are classified and named according to their function.
   a. ***Prime movers (agonists)*** bring about the desired movement. It is the chief/prime muscle for the movement, e.g. brachialis is prime mover for flexion of elbow joint. When a prime mover helps opposite action by active controlled lengthening against gravity, it is known as action of paradox. For example, putting a glass back on the table is assisted by gravity but controlled by a gradual active lengthening of biceps (paradoxical or eccentric action).
   b. ***Antagonists (opponents)*** oppose the prime movers. They help the prime movers by active controlled relaxation, so that the desired movement is smooth and precise. Thus, the antagonists cooperate rather than oppose the prime movers (Fig. 4.1). This is due to reciprocal innervation of the opposite groups of muscles, regulated by the spinal cord through stretch reflex (Fig. 4.10). It is called Law of Sherrington.
   c. ***Fixators*** are the groups of muscles which stabilize the proximal joints of a limb, so that the desired movement at

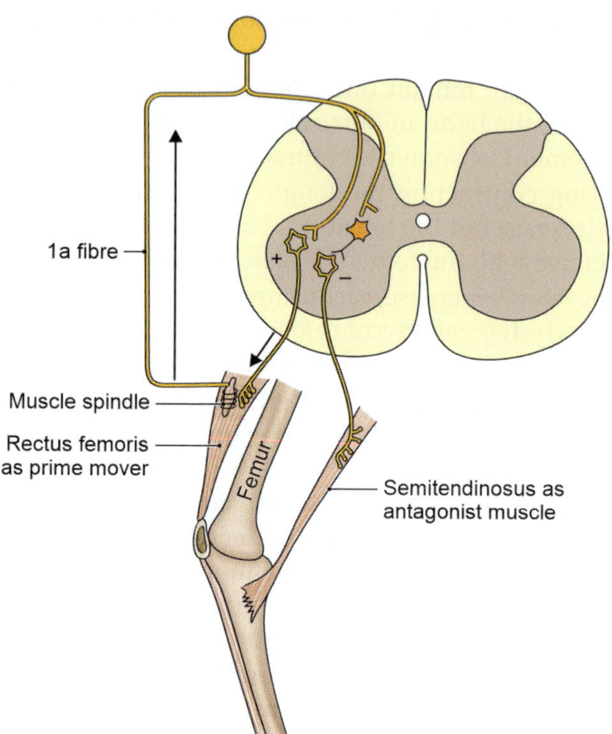

Fig. 4.10: Nerve supply of prime movers and antagonists

the distal joint may occur on a fixed base. Muscles acting on shoulder joint, e.g. trapezius, deltoid fix it for better movement of fingers.

d. ***Synergists:*** Two or more muscles causing one movement are synergist (Fig. 4.11).

When the prime movers cross more than one joint, the undesired actions at the proximal joints are prevented by certain muscles known as synergists. For example, during making a tight fist by long digital flexors the wrist is kept fixed in extension by the synergists (extensors of wrist). Thus, the synergists are special fixators and partial antagonists to the prime movers.

> *Competency achievement:* The student should be able to:
> AN 7.6 Describe concept of loss of innervation of a muscle with its applied anatomy

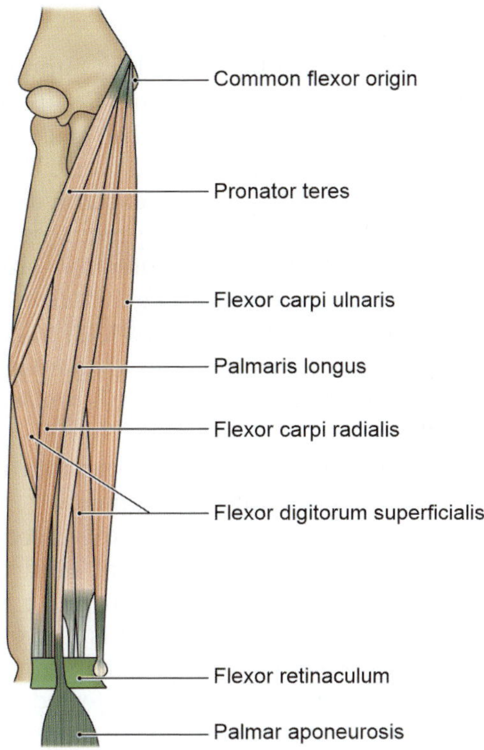

Fig. 4.11: Muscles of front of forearm acting as synergist

Clinical Anatomy of Muscles

- ***Paralysis:*** Loss of motor power (power of movement) is called paralysis. This is due to inability of the muscles to contract, caused either by damage to the motor neural pathways (upper or lower motor neuron), or by the inherent disease of muscles (myopathy). Damage to the upper motor neuron causes *spastic paralysis* with exaggerated tendon jerks. Damage to the lower motor neuron causes *flaccid paralysis* with loss of tendon jerks, e.g. poliomyelitis (Fig. 4.12).
- ***Muscular spasm:*** These are quite painful. Localized muscle spasm is commonly caused by a 'muscle pull'. In order to relieve its

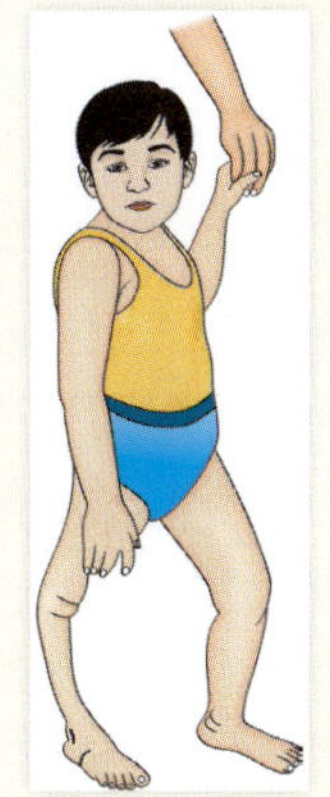

Fig. 4.12: Case of poliomyelitis

pain, the muscle should be relaxed by appropriate treatment. Generalized muscle spasms occur in tetanus and epilepsy.

- ***Disuse atrophy and hypertrophy:*** The muscles which are not used for long times become thin and weak. This is called *disuse atrophy*. Conversely, adequate or excessive use of particular muscles causes their better development, or even *hypertrophy* (Fig. 1.2). Muscular 'wasting' (reduction in size) is a feature of lower motor neuron paralysis and generalized debility.
- ***Regeneration of skeletal muscle:*** Skeletal muscle is capable of limited regeneration. If large regions are damaged, regeneration does not occur and the missing muscle is replaced by connective tissue.
- ***Hyperplasia:*** Increase in number of smooth muscle fibres. It always occurs in uterus during pregnancy.
- ***Myasthenia gravis*** is an autoimmune disease of unknown origin. Antibodies are produced that bind to acetylcholine receptor and block it. The nerve impulse transmission to muscle fibres is therefore blocked. This leads to extensive and progressive muscle weakness although the muscles are normal. Extraocular and eyelid muscles are affected first, followed by those of the neck and limbs. It affects more women than men and usually those between age of 20 and 40 years (Fig. 4.13).

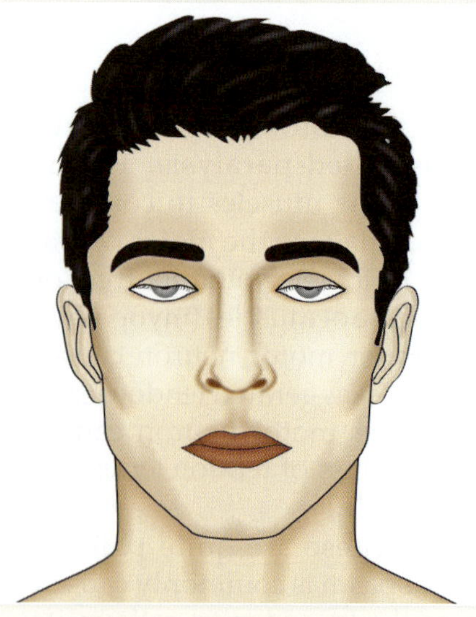

Fig. 4.13: Myasthenia gravis

- ***Polymyositis*** is a disease of muscle characterized by inflammation of the muscle fibres. It starts when white blood cells (immune cells of inflammation) spontaneously invade the muscle. Muscles close to trunk or torso are mostly affected by polymyositis that results in severe weakness. Polymyositis associated with skin rash is referred to as "dermamyositis".
- ***Fibrillation*** is the abnormal contraction of cardiac muscle. The cardiac chambers do not contract as a whole resulting in the disruption of pumping action. In atrial fibrillation, there is rapid and uncoordinated contraction of atria, ineffective pumping and abnormal contraction of the AV node. Ventricular fibrillation is characterized by very rapid and disorganized contraction of ventricle. This leads to disruption of ventricular function.
- ***Angina pectoris*** is episode of chest pain due to temporary ischaemia of cardiac muscle. It is usually relieved by rest and nitrites.
- ***Myocardial ischaemia:*** Persistent ischaemia due to blockage of more than one arteries or a main artery results in necrosis (death) of the cardiac muscle (Fig. 4.14). Pain, not relieved by rest, gets referred to left arm, chest, and neighbouring areas.

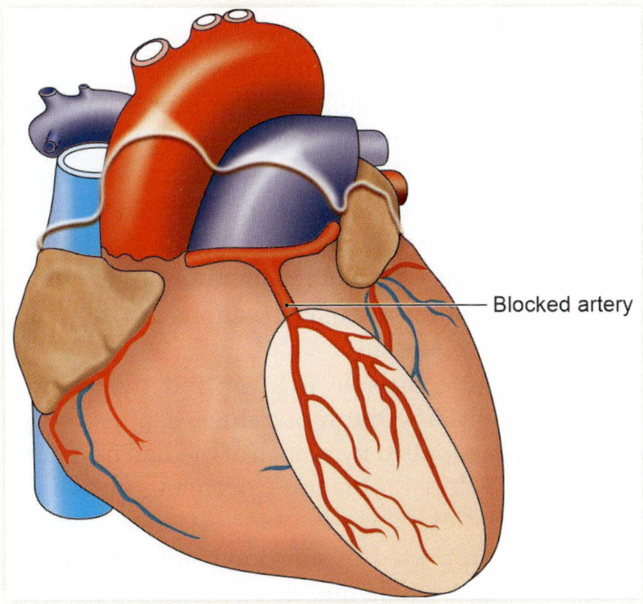

Fig. 4.14: Myocardial infarction

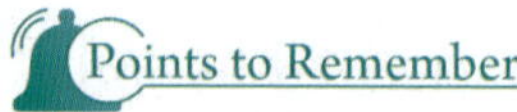

Points to Remember

- Cardiac muscles are least in amount, smooth are intermediate and the skeletal are maximum in amount and weight.
- Some muscles are vestigial, e.g. muscles of auricle, palmaris brevis of palm.
- Some tendons and ligaments are separated/divorced parts of the muscles, e.g.

Palmar aponeurosis	– part of palmaris longus
Plantar aponeurosis	– part of plantaris
Tibial collateral ligament	– part of adductor magnus
Sacrotuberous ligament	– degenerated tendon of long head of biceps femoris
Sacrospinous ligament	– degenerated part of coccygeus muscle
Long plantar ligament	– part of peroneus longus

- Sartorius is the longest muscle with parallel fibres.
- The tendocalcaneus is the longest tendon.
- Soleus is called peripheral heart as it contains many venous sinuses.
- Gluteus maximus is the largest muscle.
- Red muscle fibres are used in marathons.
- Richest nerve supply is to extraocular muscles as these have small motor units. One nerve fibre supplies 5–10 muscle fibres.
- Smooth/visceral muscles have maximum regeneration capacity, skeletal muscles repair sparsely due to multiplication of satellite cells. Cardiac muscle does not regenerate.
- Muscles used for intramuscular injections are deltoid, gluteus medius and vastus lateralis.
- Hybrid/composite muscle is supplied by two different motor nerves with different root values, e.g. flexor digitorum profundus partly supplied by branch of median nerve and partly by ulnar nerve. Adductor magnus, pectineus and digastric are other hybrid muscles.
- Muscle fibre is supported by endomysium, muscle fasciculus by perimysium and whole muscle by epimysium.
- Contractile unit of the muscle is a sarcomere.

Multiple Choice Questions

1. All the following are non-striated muscles *except*:
a. Palmaris brevis
b. Muscle of iris
c. Dartos muscle of scrotum
d. Arrector pilorum

2. Skeletal and smooth muscles are mixed in all *except* one muscle:
a. Anal sphincter
b. Upper eyelid
c. Middle region of oesophagus
d. Tongue

3. Myocyte with multiple nuclei are:
a. Smooth
b. Cardiac
c. Skeletal
d. All of the above

4. Connective tissue sheath around each muscle fibre of skeletal muscle is:
a. Epimysium
b. Perimysium
c. Endomysium
d. Sarcolemma

5. Sarcomere is the part of myofibril between which two adjacent lines:
a. A band
b. Z lines
c. H band
d. I band

6. All the following are characteristics of cardiac muscle *except*:
a. Striations
b. Multinucleated
c. Intercalated disc
d. Involuntary

7. Which of the following structure has maximum blood supply:
a. Bones
b. Cartilages
c. Tendons
d. Ligaments

8. Tendinous intersections are present in one of the following muscles:
a. Rectus femoris
b. Rectus abdominis
c. Biceps brachii
d. Biceps femoris

9. Which one is an unipennate muscle?
a. Deltoid
b. Gluteus medius
c. Flexor pollicis longus
d. Rectus femoris

10. Which muscle does not have spirally arranged fibres?
a. Pectoralis major
b. Latissimus dorsi
c. Sternocleidomastoid
d. Serratus anterior

11. What is the role of triceps brachii during flexion of elbow joint?
a. Synergist
b. Antagonist
c. Prime mover
d. Fixator

12. Which muscle has the longest muscle fibres?

a. Deltoid
b. Soleus
c. Gluteus maximus
d. Sartorius

13. Which fibres of deltoid are multipennate?

a. Clavicular
b. Acromial
c. Spine of scapula
d. All the fibres

14. Muscle cancelling unwanted movements produced by prime movers are called:

a. Synergists
b. Antagonists
c. Fixators
d. Prime movers

15. A "motor unit" is:

a. Spinal segment with all the muscles it supplies
b. A gamma neurons with all the muscle spindles it innervates
c. An alpha motor neuron with all the muscle fibres it innervates
d. A nerve with all the muscles it innervates

Answers

1. a	**2.** d	**3.** c	**4.** c	**5.** b	**6.** b	**7.** a	**8.** b
9. c	**10.** d	**11.** b	**12.** d	**13.** b	**14.** a	**15.** c	

Chapter 5

Circulatory System

"Health is the greatest possession, contentment is the greatest treasure, confidence is the greatest friend". ***—Lao Tzu***

Blood vessels form the transport system of the body, through which the nutrients are conveyed to places where these are utilized, and the metabolites (waste products) are conveyed to appropriate places from where these are expelled.

The conveying medium is a liquid tissue, the blood, which flows in tubular channels called *blood vessels*. The circulation is maintained by the central pumping organ called the heart.

COMPONENTS

1. ***Heart:*** It is a four-chambered muscular organ which pumps blood to various parts of the body (Fig. 5.1). Each half of the heart has a receiving chamber called *atrium*, and a pumping chamber called *ventricle*. It is the first organ of the body which starts functioning.
2. ***Arteries:*** These are distributing channels which carry blood away from the heart. Aorta is the largest artery (Fig. 5.1).
   a. These branch like trees on their way to different parts of the body. These contain oxygenated blood except pulmonary trunk and its two branches, the pulmonary arteries, which carry deoxygenated blood. During foetal life the umbilical arteries contain deoxygenated blood.
   b. The large arteries are rich in elastic tissue, but as branching progresses there is an ever-increasing amount of smooth muscle in their walls.

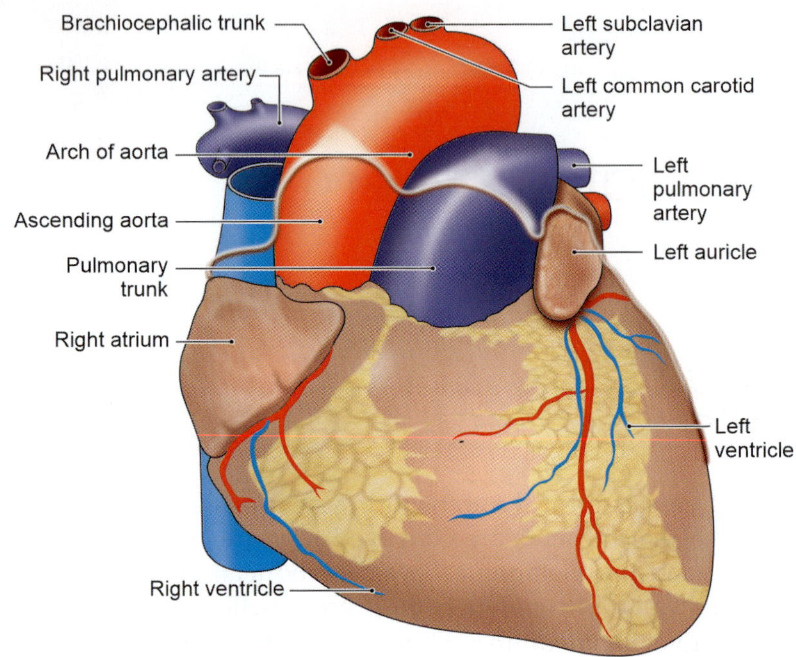

Fig. 5.1: Heart with main blood vessels

c. The minute branches which are just visible to naked eye are called *arterioles* (Fig. 5.2). These give maximum peripheral resistance.

d. *Angeion* is a Greek word, meaning a vessel (blood vessel or lymph vessel). Its word derivatives are angiology, angiography, haemangioma, and thromboangiitis obliterans.

3. ***Veins:*** These are draining channels which carry deoxygenated blood from different parts of the body back to the heart.
   a. Like rivers, the veins are formed by tributaries.
   b. The small veins (venules) join together to form larger veins (Fig. 5.2). These in turn unite to form great veins called *venae cavae*. Inferior vena cava is the largest vein. The four pulmonary veins carry oxygenated blood. In foetal life the umbilical vein carries oxygenated blood.

Capillaries: These are networks of microscopic vessels which connect arterioles with the venules (Fig. 5.2).

- These come in intimate contact with the tissues for a free exchange of nutrients and metabolites across their walls between the blood and the tissue fluid.

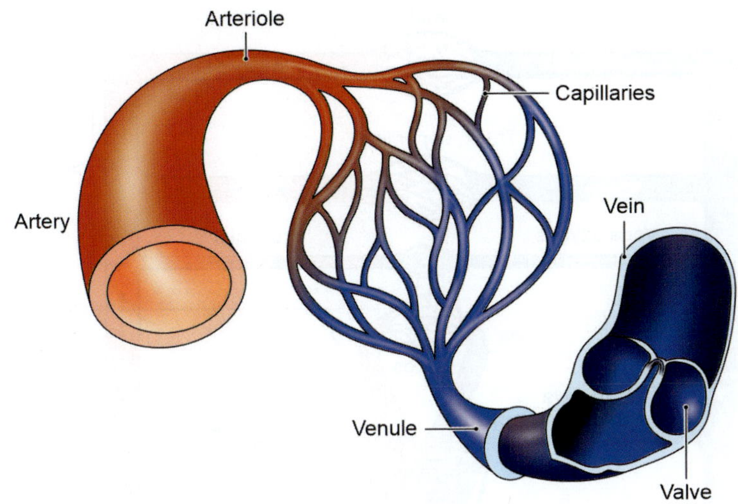

Fig. 5.2: Arteriole, capillaries and venule

- The metabolites are partly drained by the capillaries and partly by lymphatics.
- Capillaries are replaced by sinusoids in certain organs, like liver and spleen.

Functionally, the blood vessels can be classified into the following five groups.

a. *Distributing vessels*, including arteries (Fig. 5.2)
b. *Resistance vessels*, including arterioles and precapillary sphincters
c. *Exchange vessels*, including capillaries, sinusoids, and postcapillary venules
d. *Reservoir (capacitance) vessels*, including larger venules and veins; and
e. *Shunts*, including various types of anastomoses.

> *Competency achievement:* The student should be able to:
> AN 5.2 Differentiate between pulmonary and systemic circulation

Types of Circulation of Blood

Total amount of blood in adult is 4.5–5 litres.

Systemic (greater) circulation: The blood flows from the left ventricle, through various parts of the body, to the right atrium, i.e. from the left to the right side of the heart (Fig. 5.3).

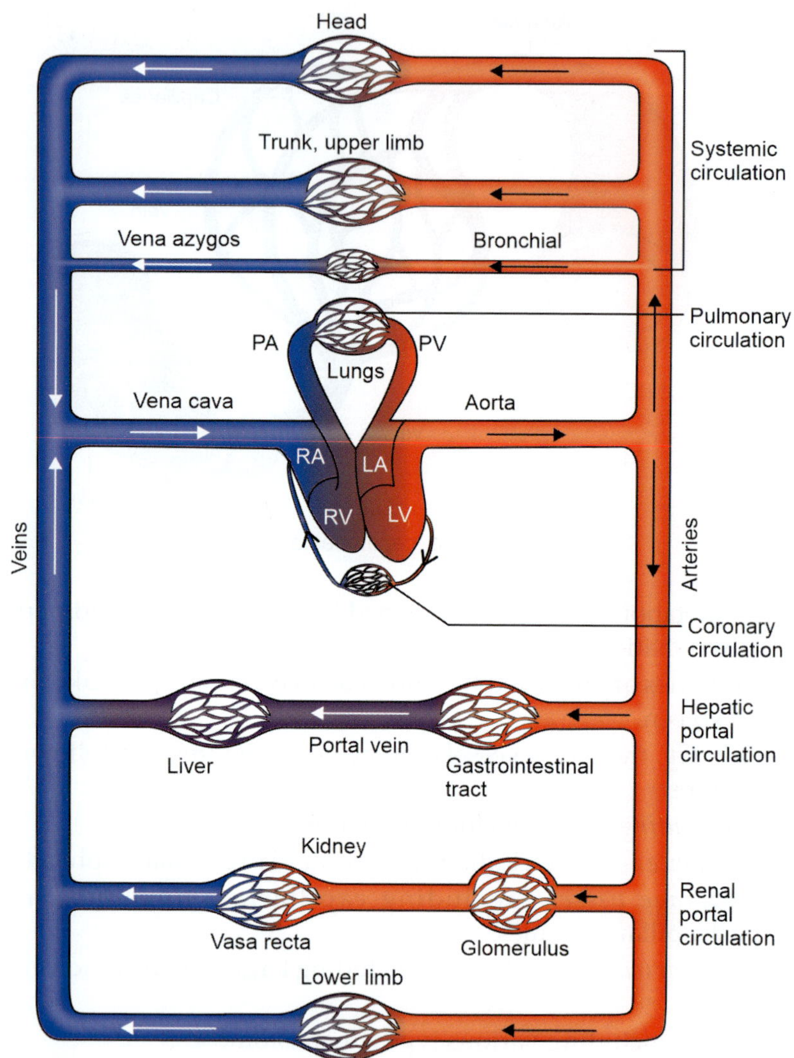

Fig. 5.3: Types of circulation

Pulmonary (lesser) circulation: The blood flows from the right ventricle, through the lungs, to the left atrium, i.e. from the right to the left side of the heart.

Table 5.1 shows the comparison between systemic circulation and pulmonary circulation.

Portal circulation: It is a part of systemic circulation, which has the following characteristics.

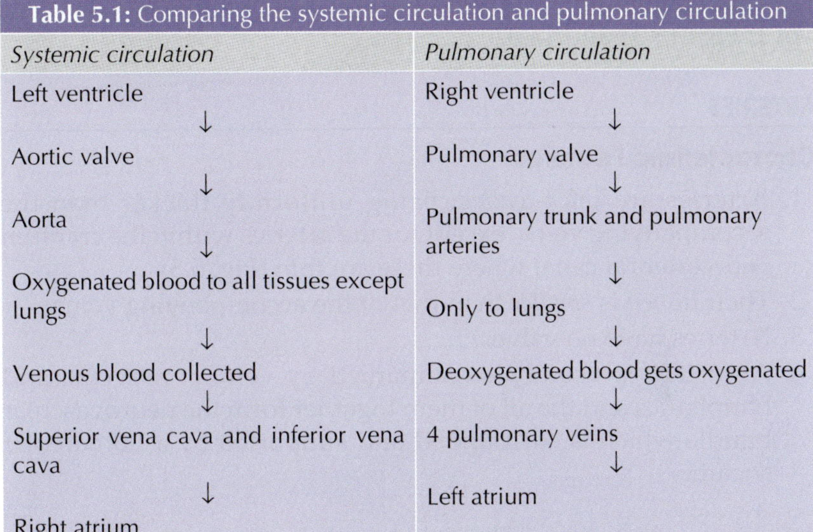

Table 5.1: Comparing the systemic circulation and pulmonary circulation

Systemic circulation	*Pulmonary circulation*
Left ventricle	Right ventricle
↓	↓
Aortic valve	Pulmonary valve
↓	↓
Aorta	Pulmonary trunk and pulmonary arteries
↓	↓
Oxygenated blood to all tissues except lungs	Only to lungs
↓	↓
Venous blood collected	Deoxygenated blood gets oxygenated
↓	↓
Superior vena cava and inferior vena cava	4 pulmonary veins
↓	↓
Right atrium	Left atrium

a. The blood passes through two sets of capillaries before draining into a systemic vein (Fig. 5.3).
b. The vein draining the first capillary network is known as portal vein which branches like an artery to form the second set of capillaries or sinusoids. *Examples:* Hepatic portal circulation, hypothalamo-hypophyseal portal circulation (Fig. 5.4) and renal portal circulation (Fig. 5.3).

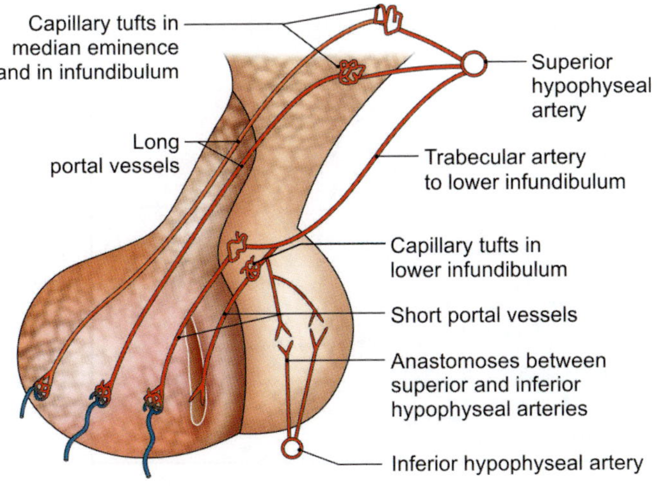

Fig. 5.4: Hypothalamo-hypophyseal circulation

Foetal circulation; see 9th edition, *BD Chaurasia's Human Anatomy*, Vol 1, Figs 18.31 and 18.32.

ARTERIES

Characteristic Features

1. Arteries are *thick-walled*, being uniformly thicker than the accompanying veins, except for the arteries within the cranium and vertebral canal where these are thin (Fig. 5.5).
2. Their *lumen* is *smaller* than that of the accompanying veins.
3. Arteries have no valves.
4. An artery is usually accompanied by vein(s), nerve(s), and lymphatics and the all of them together form the neurovascular bundle which is surrounded and supported by a fibroareolar sheath.

Competency achievement: The student should be able to:
AN 5.4 Explain functional differences between elastic, muscular arteries and arterioles

Types of Arteries and Structure

1. *Large arteries of elastic type*, e.g. aorta and its main branches (brachiocephalic, common carotid, subclavian, common iliac and the pulmonary trunk (Fig. 5.1)).
2. *Medium and small arteries of muscular type*, e.g. ulnar, radial, femoral and popliteal, etc. (Fig. 5.6)

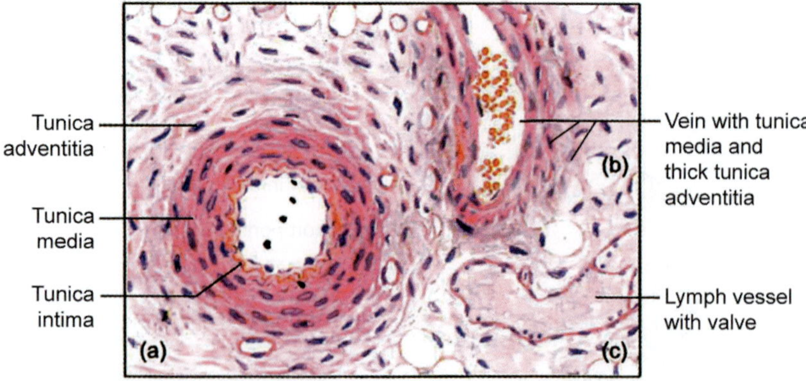

Fig. 5.5: Microscopic structure of (a) an artery, (b) vein and (c) lymph vessel

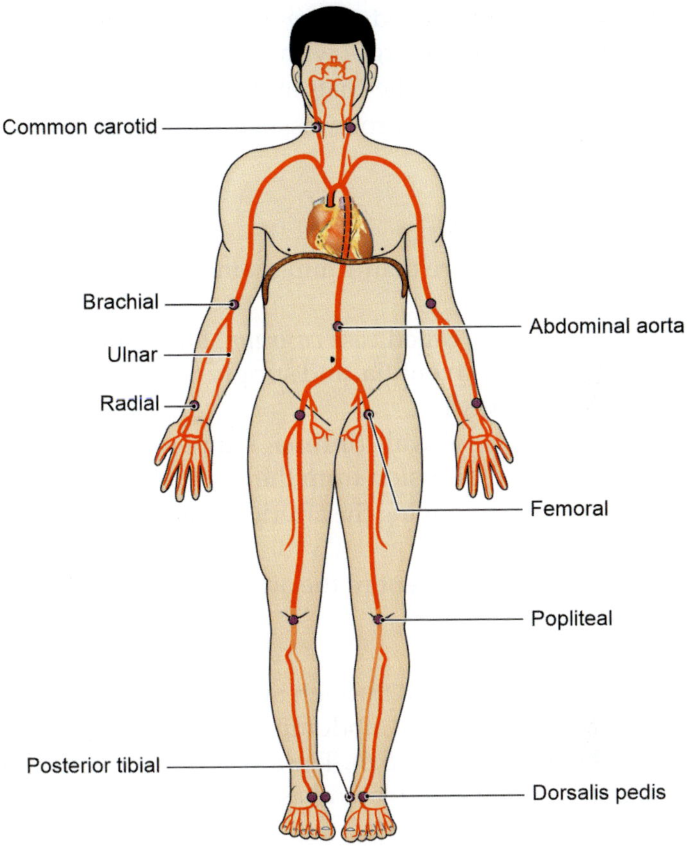

Fig. 5.6: Main arteries and various palpable arteries (with dots)

3. *Smallest arteries of muscular type* are called arterioles. They measure 50–100 micron in diameter. Arterioles divide into terminal arterioles with a diameter of 15–20 micron, and having one or two layers of smooth muscle in their walls. The side branches from *terminal arterioles* are called *metarterioles* which measure 10–15 micron at their origin and about 5 micron at their termination. The terminal narrow end of metarteriole is surrounded by a *precapillary sphincter* which regulates blood flow into the capillary bed. It is important to know that the muscular arterioles are responsible for generating peripheral resistance, and thereby for regulating the diastolic blood pressure.

Microscopically, all arteries are made up of three coats.

a. The inner coat is called *tunica intima* (Fig. 5.5).
b. The middle coat is called *tunica media*.

c. The outer coat is called *tunica adventitia*. It is made up of collagen fibres and merges with the perivascular sheath.

The relative thickness of the coats and the relative proportion of the muscular, elastic and fibrous tissues vary in different types of arteries (Table 5.2).

Blood Supply of Arteries

The large arteries (of more than 1 mm diameter) are supplied with blood vessels.

The nutrient vessels, called *vasa vasorum*, form a dense capillary network in the tunica adventitia, and supply the adventitia and the outer part of tunica media.

The rest of the vessel wall (intima + inner part of media) is nourished directly by diffusion from the luminal blood.

Minute veins accompanying the arteries drain the blood from the outer part of arterial wall.

Lymphatics are also present in the adventitia.

Palpable Arteries

Some arteries can be palpated through the skin. These are: Common carotid, facial, brachial, radial, abdominal aorta, femoral, posterior tibial and dorsalis pedis (Fig. 5.6). The most commonly felt pulse is the radial pulse on the anterolateral aspect of wrist. Carotid pulse next to trachea is also easily felt.

Table 5.2: Types of arteries

Layers	*Elastic artery*	*Muscular artery*	*Arteriole*
Tunica intima	Endothelium + subendothelial tissue and ill-defined internal elastic lamina	Endothelium + subendothelial tissue and prominent internal elastic lamina	Endothelium + subendothelial tissue and internal elastic lamina poorly developed
Tunica media	40–80 fenestrated elastic fibres, thin external elastic lamina	20–40 layers of smooth muscle cells, prominent external elastic lamina	Only 1–4 layers of smooth muscle cells
Tunica adventitia	Fibroelastic layer and prominent vasavasorum	Fibroelastic layer, vasa-vasorum not prominent	Loose connective tissue only

Nerve Supply of Arteries

The nerves supplying an artery are called *nervi vascularis*.

The nerves are mostly thinly myelinated sympathetic fibres which are vasoconstrictor in function. A few fibres are myelinated, and are believed to be sensory to the outer and inner coats of the arteries.

Vasodilator innervation is restricted to the following sites.

a. The skeletal muscle vessels are dilated by cholinergic *sympathetic nerves*.
b. The exocrine gland vessels are dilated on parasympathetic stimulation.
c. The cutaneous vessels are dilated locally to produce the flare (redness) after an injury. The vasodilatation is produced by the afferent impulses in the cutaneous nerves which pass antidromically in their collaterals to the blood vessels (*axon reflex*).

> *Competency achievement:* The student should be able to:
> AN 5.3 List general differences between arteries and veins

VEINS

Characteristic Features

1. Veins are *thin-walled*, being thinner than the arteries (Fig. 5.7).
2. Their *lumen* is *larger* than that of the accompanying arteries.

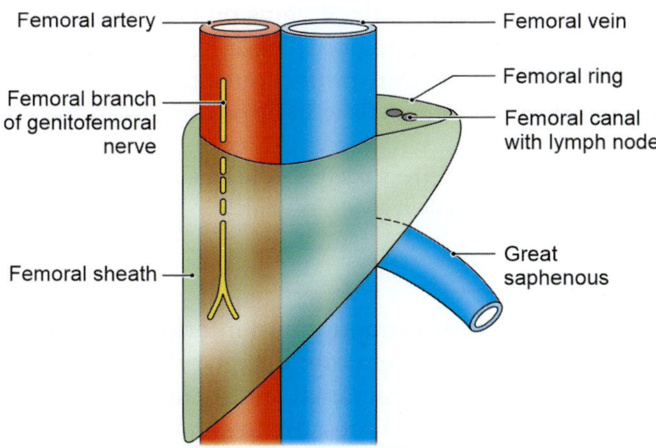

Fig. 5.7: Femoral sheath with its contents

3. Veins have valves which maintain the unidirectional flow of blood, even against gravity (Fig. 5.8).

   Since the venous pressure is low (7 mm Hg), the valves are of utmost value in the venous return. However, the valves are absent:

   a. In the veins of less than 2 mm diameter.
   b. In the venae cavae.
   c. In the hepatic, renal, uterine, ovarian (not testicular), cerebral, spinal, pulmonary, and umbilical veins.

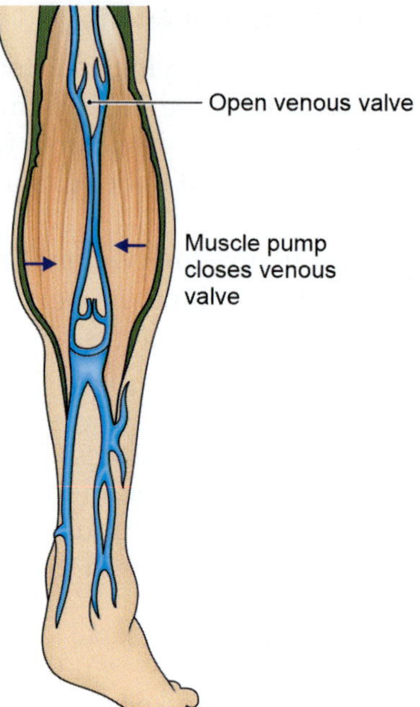

Fig. 5.8: Venous valves for unidirectional flow of venous blood

4. The muscular and elastic tissue content of the venous walls is much less than that of the arteries. This is directly related to the low venous pressure.
5. Large veins have *dead space* around them for their dilatation during increased venous return; e.g. femoral canal medial to femoral vein. The dead space commonly contains the regional lymph nodes (Fig. 5.7 and Table 5.3).
6. Venae comitantes are a pair of veins on each side of the artery in the forearm and leg region. These help in return of blood towards the heart by transmitted pulsation of the artery. The blood in artery and veins flow in opposite direction.

> *Competency achievement:* The student should be able to:
> AN 5.5 Describe portal system giving examples

Venous System

1. Caval system includes superior and inferior caval veins. Veins associated with the system are: Emissary veins of the cranial cavity, these connect intracranial and extracranial veins. These help to lower intracranial pressure in some situations. Also the infection from outside may reach the cranial cavity.

5

2. Portal system is made up of two sets of capillaries, e.g. hepatic portal: Capillaries join to form veins which form portal vein. It divides into branches which form veins/sinusoids. Hypophyseal portal system seen in anterior pituitary gland is an example of this system, other example is portal vein in gastrointestinal system.

Structure of Veins

Veins are made up of usual three coats which are found in the arteries. But the coats are ill-defined, and the muscle and elastic tissue content is poor (Fig. 5.5).

In poorly developed tunica media, the amount of collagen fibres is more than the elastic and muscle fibres. The adventitia is thickest and best developed. The smooth muscle is altogether absent:

a. In the veins of maternal part of placenta
b. In the cranial venous sinuses and pial veins
c. In the retinal veins
d. In the veins of cancellous bone
e. In the venous spaces of the corpora cavernosa and corpus spongiosum of penis.

After studying both the arteries and veins, a comparison is drawn between them.

Table 5.3 shows the comparison of various types of veins.

Table 5.4 shows the comparison of arteries and veins.

Blood and Nerve Supply of Veins

The larger veins, like the arteries, are supplied with nutrient vessels called *vasa vasorum*. But in the veins, the vessels may penetrate up

Table 5.3: Types of veins

Layers	*Large veins*	*Medium sized veins*	*Venules*
Tunica intima	Endothelium, basal lamina, subendothelial tissue, valves may be seen	Same as in large vein	Endothelium, basal lamina and pericytes
Tunica media	Smooth muscles and connective tissue	Smooth muscles and connective tissue	A few smooth muscles and loose connective tissue
Tunica adventitia	Smooth muscle fibres seen as longitudinal bundles	Comprises fibroblasts and collagen bundles	A few fibroblasts and thin layer of collagen fibres

Table 5.4: Comparison of arteries and veins

Arteries (Fig. 5.9)	*Veins* (Fig. 5.10)
1. Arteries carry oxygenated blood, away from the heart except pulmonary trunk and pulmonary arteries	Veins carry deoxygenated blood, towards the heart except four pulmonary veins
2. These are mostly deeply situated in the body	These are superficial and deep in location
3. These are thick-walled, highly muscular except arteries of cranium and vertebral column	These are thin-walled
4. These possess narrow lumen	These possess wide lumen
5. Valves are absent	Valves are present which provide unidirectional flow of blood
6. These are reddish in colour	These are bluish in colour
7. These show spurty flow of blood giving pulse	These show sluggish flow of blood
8. Blood in arteries moves with pressure	Blood in veins moves under very low pressure
9. Arteries get empty at the time of death	Veins get filled up at time of death
10. If arterial wall is injured, the blood comes out like a 'fountain' in a large area all around the artery	If venous wall is injured, blood comes out, collects in a pool in a small area around vein

to the intima, probably because of the low venous pressure and the low oxygen tension (Figs 5.9 and 5.10).

Nerves are also distributed to the veins in the same manner as to the arteries, but are fewer in number.

Factors Helping in Venous Return

1. Overflow from the capillaries, pushed from behind by the arteries (*vis-a-tergo*).
2. *Negative intrathoracic pressure* sucks the blood into the heart from all over the body.
3. *Gravity* helps venous return in the upper part of the body.

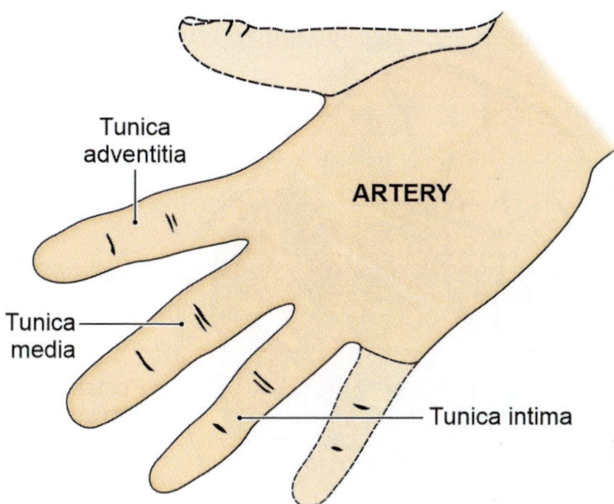

Fig. 5.9: Artery with thick tunica media

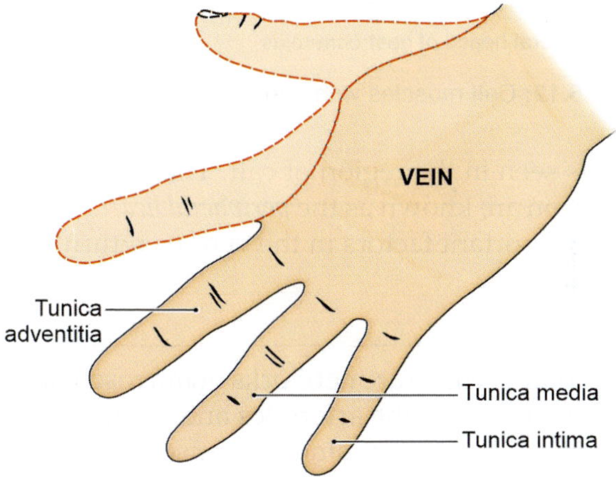

Fig. 5.10: Vein with thick tunica adventitia

4. *Arterial pulsations* press on the venae comitantes intermittently and drive the venous blood towards the heart (Fig. 5.11).
5. *Venous valves* prevent any regurgitation (backflow) of the luminal blood (Figs 5.2 and 5.8).
6. Muscular contractions press on the veins and form a very effective mechanism of venous return. This becomes still more effective within the tight sleeve of the deep

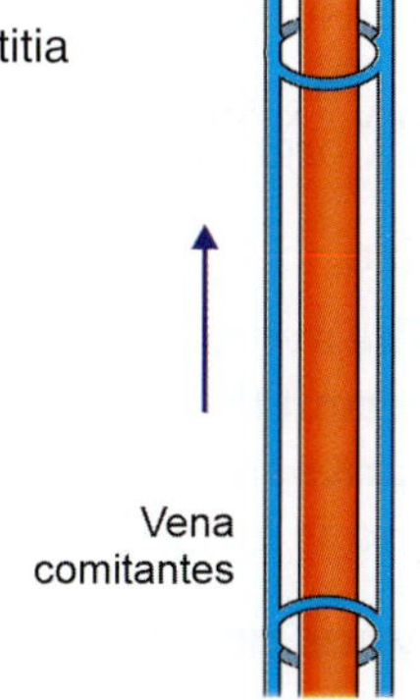

Fig. 5.11: Artery with venae comitantes

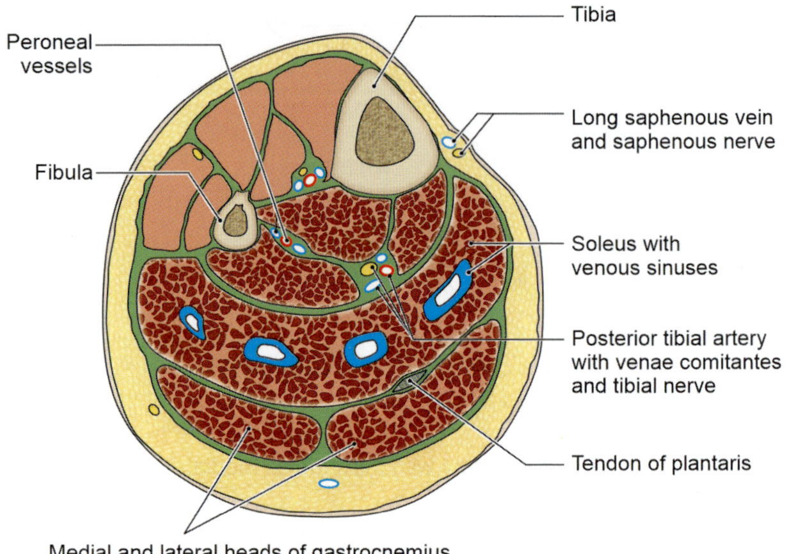

Fig. 5.12: Calf muscles with tight sleeve of deep fascia

fascia, as is seen in the region of calf. The calf muscles (soleus) for this reason are known as the *peripheral heart*. Thus the *muscle pumps* are important factors in the venous return (Fig. 5.12).

CAPILLARIES

Capillaries (capillus = hair) are networks of microscopic endothelial tubes interposed between the arterioles and venules (Fig. 5.2). The true capillaries (without any smooth muscle cell) begin after a transition zone of 50–100 microns beyond the precapillary sphincters.

The capillaries are replaced by cavernous (dilated) spaces in the sex organs, splenic pulp and placenta.

Size

The average diameter of a capillary is 6–8 microns, just sufficient to permit the red blood cells to pass through in 'single file'. But the size varies from organ to organ. It is smallest in the brain and intestines, and is largest (20 microns) in the skin and bone marrow.

Types and Structure

The capillaries are classified as continuous and fenestrated according to the type of junctions between the endothelial cells.

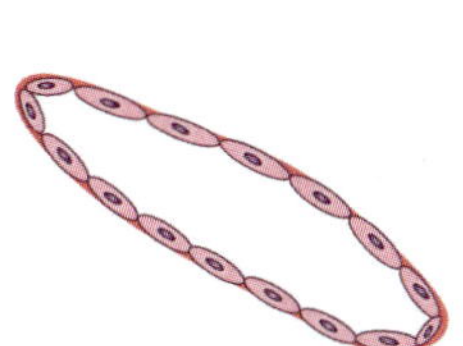

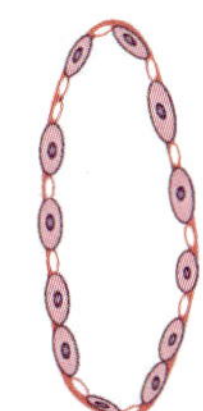

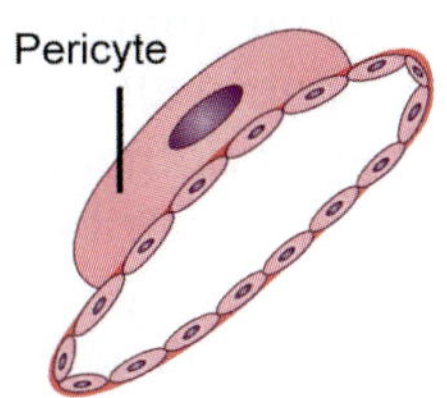

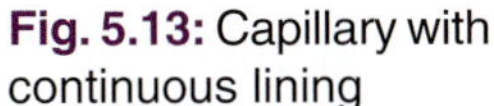

Fig. 5.13: Capillary with continuous lining

Fig. 5.14: Capillary with fenestration

Fig. 5.15: Capillary with pericyte

1. ***Continuous capillaries*** are found in the skin, connective tissue, skeletal and smooth muscles, lung and brain. These allow passage across their walls of small molecules (up to 10 microns size) (Fig. 5.13).
2. ***Fenestrated capillaries*** are found in the renal glomeruli/ intestinal mucosa, endocrine glands and pancreas. These allow passage across their walls of larger molecules (up to 20–100 microns size) (Fig. 5.14).

The capillary bed and postcapillary venules form an enormous area for the exchange of nutrients, gases, metabolites and water, between the blood and interstitial fluid. Capillaries also allow migration of leucocytes out of the vessels.

Total end to end length of the vascular network in an adult is twice the circumference of earth.

Pericytes: These are present on outer suface of capillaries and smallest venules, where there is no adventitia and muscle. Its procesess are wrapped around the endothelium.

Pericytes reveal contractile property

Act as stem cell

Help in repair process and give rise to new blood vessels (Fig. 5.15).

SINUSOIDS

Sinusoids, replace capillaries in certain organs, like liver, spleen, bone marrow, suprarenal glands, parathyroid glands, carotid body, etc.

Characteristics

Sinusoids are large, irregular, vascular spaces which are closely surrounded by the parenchyma of the organ. These differ from capillaries in the following respects:

1. Their lumen is *wider* (up to 30 micron) and irregular.
2. Their walls are *thinner* and may be incomplete. They are lined by endothelium in which the phagocytic cells (*macrophages*) are often distributed. The adventitial support is absent.
3. These may connect arteriole with venule (spleen, bone marrow), or venule with venule (liver).

Cavernous tissue: These are seen in penis and clitoris. Arterioles and venules open into these spaces. These spaces are blood filled spaces are lined by endothelium. Spaces are surrounded by trabeculae which contain smooth muscle fibres.

ANGIOSOME

Angiosome: It is 3D block of tissue supplied by an artery and vein. It is composed of skin, fascia, muscle, and bone. These form 3D jigsaw puzzle. Some have chiefly cutaneous component and some 3D muscle component.

Neighbouring angiosome are linked by "choke" vessels. If one angiosome is blocked, its territory can be rescued from adjacent choke vessel.

NERVE SUPPLY

Efferent autonomic fibres supply tunica adventitia.

Nervi vasorum are unmyelinated and varicose in nature.

Sympathetic cholinergic fibres inhibit smooth muscle contraction and cause vasodilatation.

Neurotransmitters reach muscle from tunica adventitia.

Hormone nitric oxide (NO) and endothelin reach muscle from tunica intima.

Competency achievement: The student should be able to:
AN 5.6 Describe the concept of anastomoses and collateral circulation with significance of end-arteries
AN 5.7 Explain function of meta-arterioles, precapillary sphincters, arterio-venous anastomoses

ANASTOMOSES

Definition

A precapillary or postcapillary communication between the neighbouring vessels is called anastomoses. Circulation through the anastomosis is called *collateral circulation*.

Types

A. ***Arterial anastomoses*** is the communication between the arteries, or branches of arteries. It may be actual or potential.

1. In *actual arterial anastomosis* the arteries meet end to end. For example, palmar arches (Fig. 5.16), plantar arch, circle of Willis, intestinal arcades, labial branches of facial arteries.
2. In *potential arterial anastomoses* the communication takes place between the terminal arterioles. Such communications can dilate only gradually for collateral circulation. Therefore, on sudden occlusion of a main artery, the anastomoses may fail to compensate the loss. The examples are seen in the coronary arteries (Fig. 5.17). The coronary arteries get filled during diastole of the heart.

B. ***Venous anastomoses*** is the communication between the veins or tributaries of veins. For example, the dorsal venous arches of the hand and foot (Fig. 5.18).

C. ***Arteriovenous anastomosis (shunt)*** is the communication between an artery and a vein. It serves the function during phasic activity of the organ. When the organ is active, these shunts are closed and the blood circulates through the capillaries (Fig. 5.19).

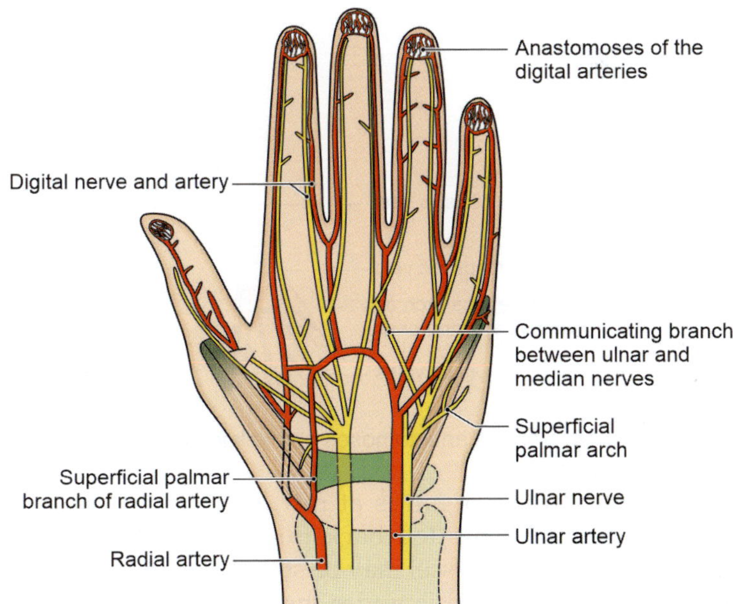

Fig. 5.16: Actual arterial anastomoses

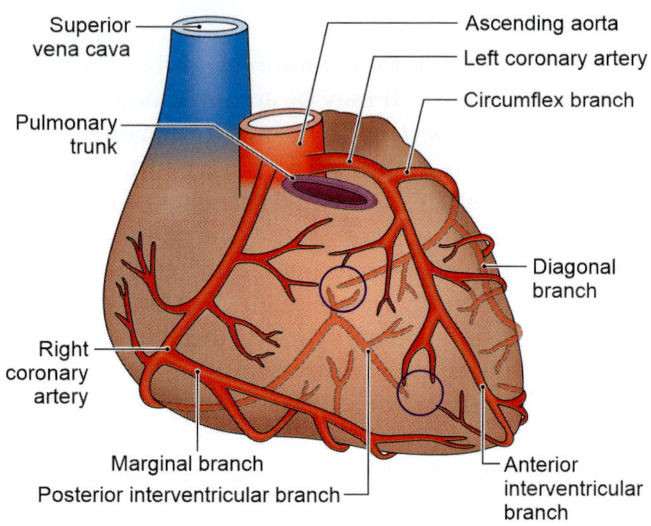

Fig. 5.17: Potential arterial anastomoses shown as circles

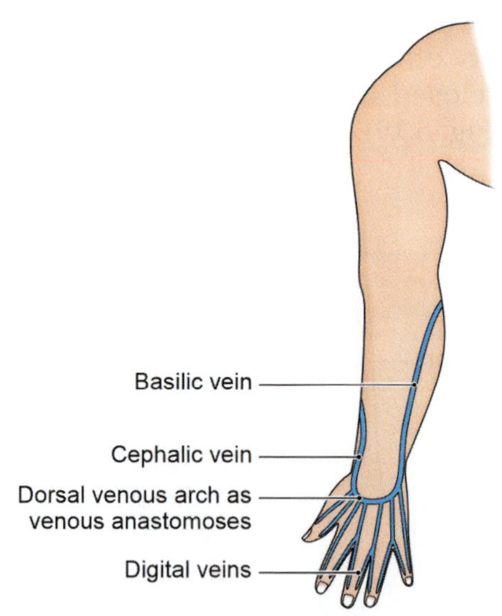

Fig. 5.18: Venous anastomoses on back left upper limb

However, when the organ is at rest, the blood bypasses the capillary bed and is shunted back through the arteriovenous anastomosis. The shunt vessel may be straight or coiled, possesses a thick muscular coat, and is under the influence of sympathetic system (Fig. 5.20).

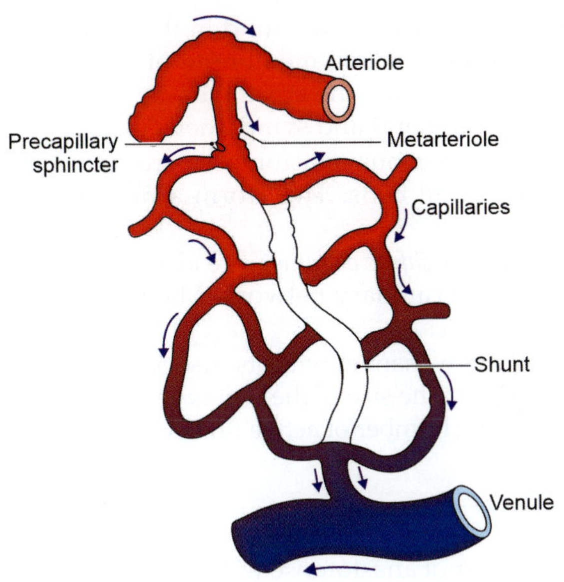

Fig. 5.19: Arteriovenous shunt during active phase of organ

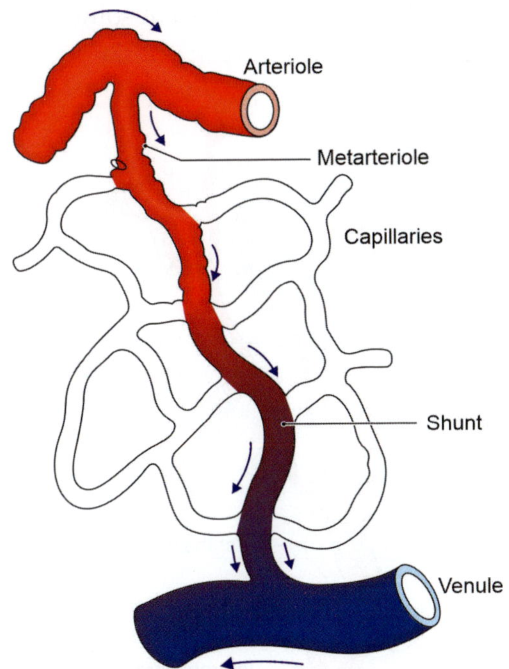

Fig. 5.20: Arteriovenous shunt during the resting phase of the organ

Shunts of *simple* structure are found in the skin of nose, lips and external ear; in the mucous membrane of nose and alimentary canal, the coccygeal body, the erectile tissue of sexual organs, the tongue, the thyroid gland and sympathetic ganglia.

Specialized arteriovenous anastomoses are found in the skin of digital pads and nail beds. They form a number of small units called glomera.

Preferential 'thoroughfare channels' are also a kind of shunts. They course through the capillary network. Many true capillaries arise as their side branches.

One thoroughfare channel with its associated capillaries forms a *microcirculatory unit*. The size of the unit is variable from 1–2 to 20–30 true capillaries. The number of active units varies from time to time.

END ARTERIES

Definition

Arteries which do not anastomose with their neighbours are called *end arteries*. Examples:

1. Central artery of retina (Fig. 5.21) and labyrinthine artery of internal ear are the best examples of absolute end arteries.

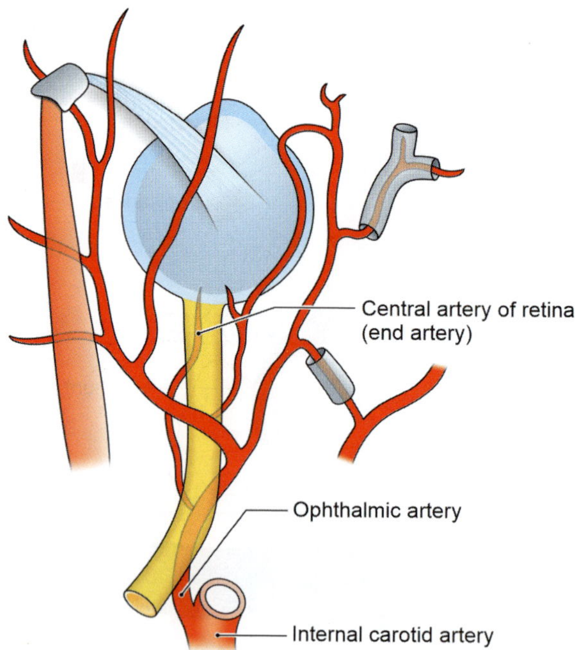

Fig. 5.21: End artery of retina

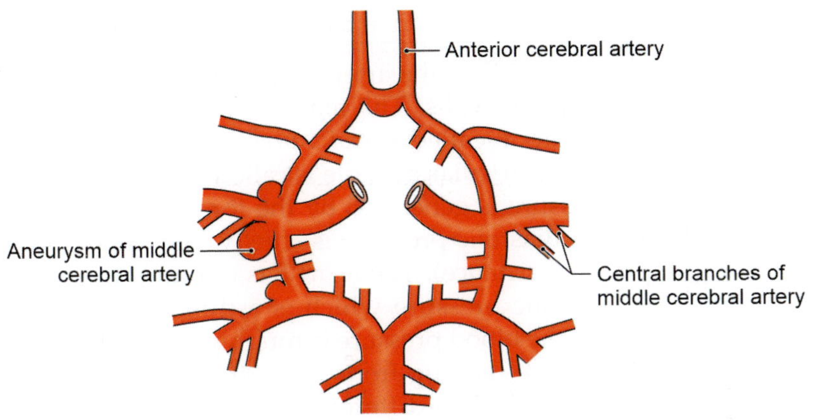

Fig. 5.22: Central branches of cerebral artery. Aneurysms in the cerebral arteries

2. Central branches of cerebral arteries (Fig. 5.22) and vasa recta of mesenteric arteries are anatomical end arteries.
3. Arteries of spleen, kidney, lungs and metaphyses of long bones.

Functional end arteries, e.g. coronary arteries. These are not true end arteries. Their anastomoses cannot meet demand of the myocardium.

Anastomoses are between of right and left coronary arteries including many anastomoses between the branches of these coronary arteries.

Importance

Occlusion of an end-artery causes serious nutritional disturbances resulting in death of the tissue supplied by it. For example, occlusion of central artery of retina results in blindness.

Molecular regulation of angiogenesis and vasculogenesis: Molecular regularization of vasculogenesis is by fibroblast growth factor 2 (FGF 2) and vasculoendothelial growth factor (VEGF). Sprouting of new vessels from existing one is by VEGF and maturation and modeling of vasculature is by platelet-derived growth factor (PDGF) and transforming growth factor-β (TGF-β).

Competency achievement: The student should be able to:
AN 5.8 Define thrombosis, infarction and aneurysm

Clinical Anatomy of Circulatory System

- ***The blood pressure*** (BP) is the arterial pressure exerted by the blood on the arterial walls. The maximum pressure during ventricular systole is called *systolic pressure*; the minimum pressure during ventricular diastole is called *diastolic pressure*. The systolic pressure is generated by the force of contraction of the heart; the diastolic pressure is chiefly due to arteriolar tone (peripheral resistance). The heart has to pump the blood against the diastolic pressure which is a direct load on the heart. Normally, the blood pressure is roughly 120/80 mm Hg, the systolic pressure ranging from 110–130, and the diastolic pressure from 70–80. The difference between systolic and diastolic pressure is called *'pulse pressure'*. BP is universally measured by auscultating the brachial artery at the elbow joint (Fig. 5.23).
- ***Haemorrhage*** (bleeding) is the obvious result of rupture of the blood vessels. Arterial haemorrhage causes spurting of blood, venous haemorrhage causes pooling of blood (Fig. 5.24).
- ***Vascular catastrophies*** are of three types:
  a. *Thrombosis:* Intravascular clot blocking the vessel.
  b. *Embolism:* Movement of the clot to block some other artery.
  c. *Haemorrhage:* Rupture of the vessel.

  All of them result in a loss of blood supply to the area of distribution of the vessel involved, unless it is compensated by collateral circulation.

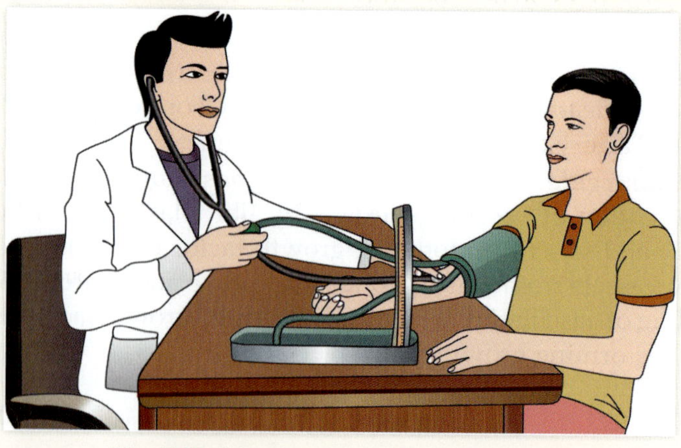

Fig. 5.23: Measurement of blood pressure

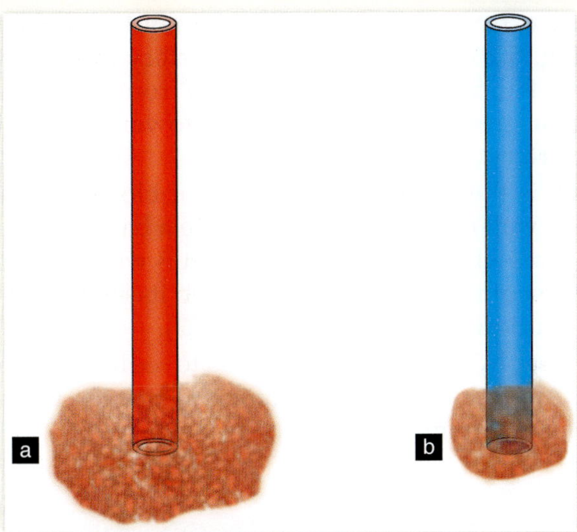

Fig. 5.24: Bleeding from (a) an artery and (b) a vein

- ***Arteriosclerosis:*** In old age the arteries become stiff. This phenomenon is called arteriosclerosis. This causes a variable reduction in the blood supply to the tissues and a rise in systolic pressure.
- ***Arteritis and phlebitis:*** Inflammation of an artery is known as arteritis, and inflammation of a vein as phlebitis.
- ***Atheroma*** are patchy changes developed in the tunica intima of arteries due to accumulation of cholesterol and other lipid compounds. Arteries most commonly narrowed are those in the heart, brain, small intestine, kidneys and lower limbs. The changes are called atheromatous plaque (Fig. 5.25).

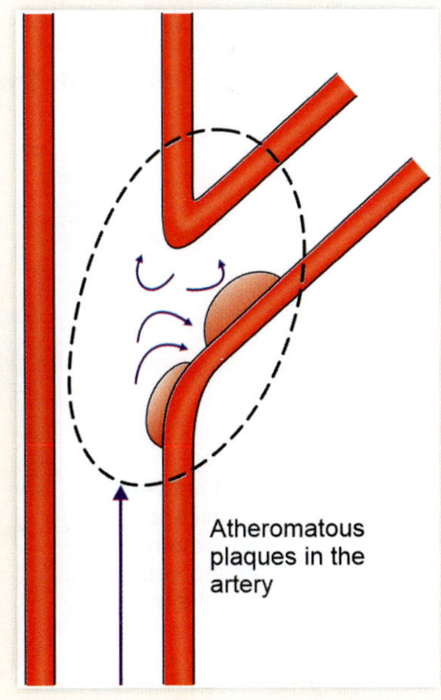

Fig. 5.25: Atheromatous changes in the artery

- ***Coronary arteries blockage:*** These may be opened up by stents (Fig. 5.26). Blocked coronary artery may be replaced by a graft (Fig. 5.27). The graft is taken from the longest vein, the long or great saphenous vein of lower limb or internal thoracic artery.
- ***Aneurysm*** is the swelling or dilation of blood vessels where part of the wall of an artery inflates like a balloon. The wall of the blood vessel at the site of aneurysm is weaker and thinner than the rest of the blood vessels. Due to its likelihood to burst it poses a serious risk to health (Fig. 5.22).

Angiography is an imaging method to see lumen of coronary arteries. Angiography of the coronary arteries is known as coronary angiogram.

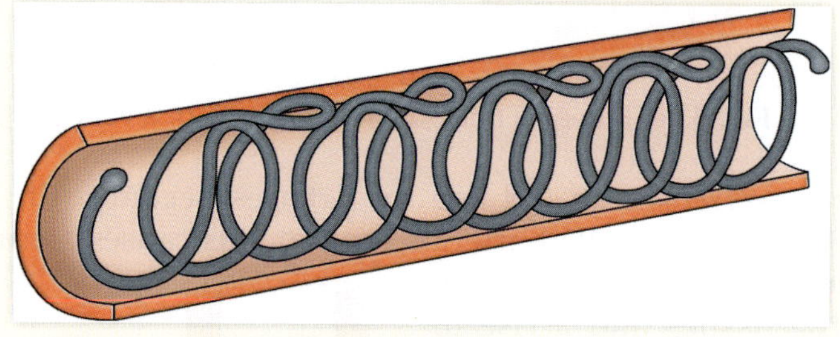

Fig. 5.26: Stent within an artery

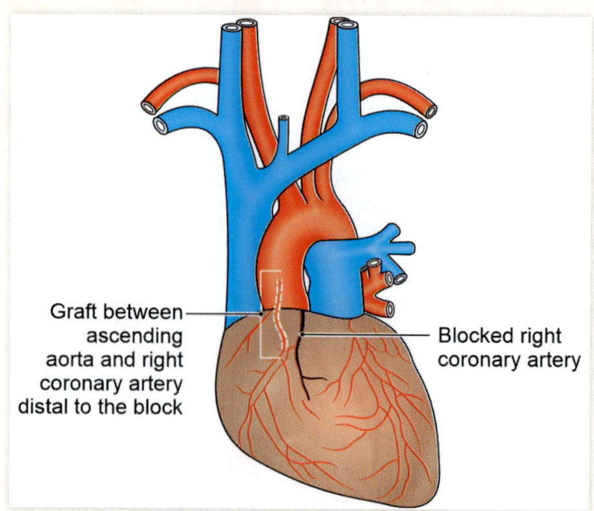

Fig. 5.27: Graft for bypassing the blocked coronary artery

- ***Buerger's disease (thromboangiitis obliterans):*** This is a very painful condition. There is inflammation of small peripheral arteries of the legs. The victim is a young person and a heavy smoker.
- ***Raynaud's phenomenon:*** In this condition there is spasmodic attack of pallor of the fingers due to constriction of small arteries and arterioles in response to cold.
- ***Acute phlebothrombosis:*** The veins of the lower limbs are affected. Due to lack of movement of the legs there is thrombus formation with mild inflammation. This thrombus may get dislodged and flow in the blood and may block any other artery. This condition is called *embolism*.
- ***Varicose veins:*** When the vein wall is subjected to increased pressure over long time there is atrophy of muscle and elastic tissue with fibrous replacement. This leads to stretching of the vein with tortuosity and localized bulging (Fig. 5.28). Venous congestion of the feet is relieved by putting feet on the stool, that is higher than the trunk, helping in venous return and

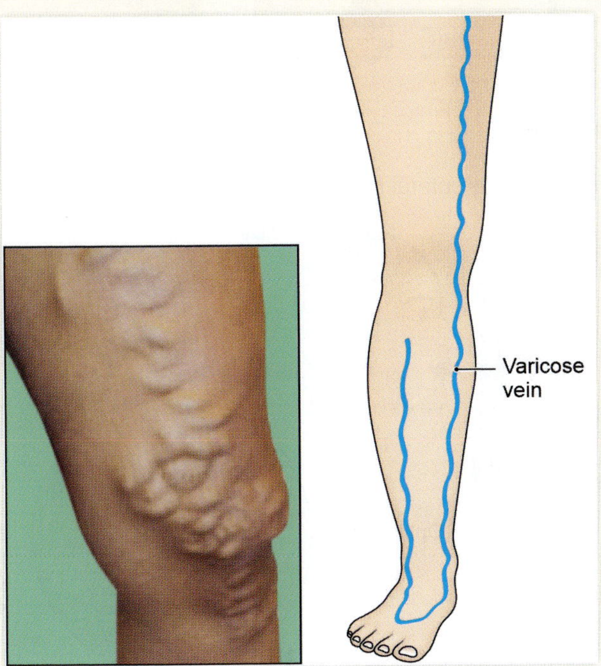

Fig. 5.28: Varicose veins in lower limb

relief in tiredness. Varicose veins may occur at the lower end of oesophagus or in the anal canal.

- At times parenteral nutrition can be given through the right subclavian vein (Fig. 5.29).
- Blood vessels can be examined in the retina by ophthalmoscope, especially in cases of diabetes and hypertension (Fig. 5.30).

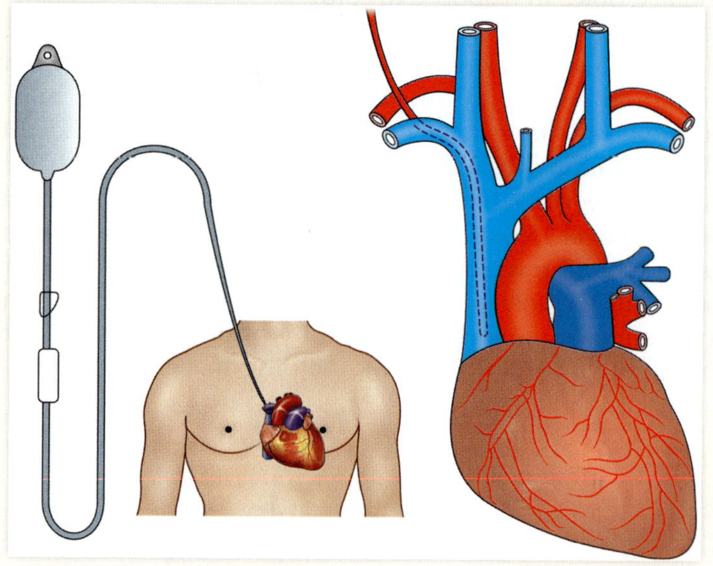

Fig. 5.29: Parenteral nutrition through right subclavian vein

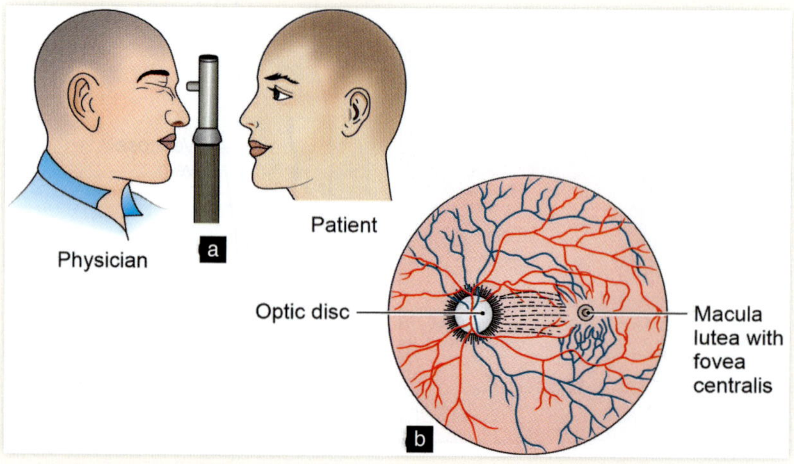

Fig. 5.30: Ophthalmoscopic examination (a) to view the retina (b)

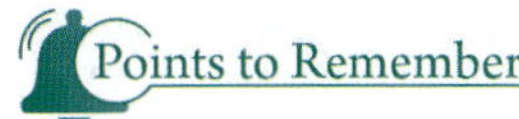

Points to Remember

- Systemic circulation starts from left ventricle, goes to most of the tissues of the body and returns to right atrium of heart.
- Pulmonary circulation starts from right ventricle, goes to lungs and returns to left atrium of heart.
- Portal circulation passes through two sets of capillaries. It starts like a vein, but ends like an artery. This circulation carries nutritive substances, hormone releasing factors, etc.
- Vessel wall comprises inner tunica intima, middle tunica media and outermost tunica adventitia. Arteries have thickest tunica media. Veins have thickest tunica adventitia.
- Veins have thinner walls, larger lumen and usually have blood cells in their lumen as compared to their parallel arteries.
- Some arteries in the body are superficial and are palpated to count heart rate. These are radial, common carotid, facial and superficial temporal, etc.
- Arteries of head and neck are used by anaesthetists to count/ monitor the pulse rate. These are called anaesthetist's arteries.
- There is dead/empty space next to a large vein, in which the vein can dilate whenever there is increased venous return.
- Normal functioning valves are responsible for unidirectional flow of blood especially in lower limb.
- End artery is an artery which does not anastomose with any other artery.
- Hypertension or high blood pressure must be controlled, or it may lead to haemorrhage, or aneurysm of the arteries.

Multiple Choice Questions

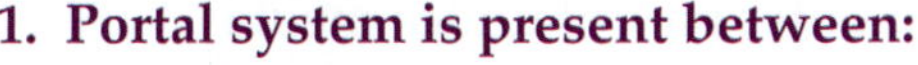

1. Portal system is present between:
   a. Two veins
   b. Two arteries
   c. Vein and artery
   d. Two capillary plexuses

2. One of the following organs does not have sinusoids:
   a. Parotid gland
   b. Spleen
   c. Liver
   d. Bone marrow

3. **Functional end arteries are terminal branches of the arteries which:**
   a. Show extensive anastomoses
   b. Show insufficient anastomoses
   c. Do not anastomose
   d. Show anastomoses
4. **Which vessels show valves?**
   a. Capillaries
   b. Arteries
   c. Veins of neck
   d. Veins of lower limb
5. **Fenestrated capillaries are present in all organs *except*:**
   a. Thyroid gland
   b. Pancreas
   c. Kidney
   d. Brain
6. **Which is the thickest layer in veins?**
   a. Tunica intima
   b. Tunica media
   c. Tunica adventitia
   d. All tunics are of same thickness
7. **Which is the thickest layer in the arteries?**
   a. Tunica intima
   b. Tunica media
   c. Tunica adventitia
   d. All layers of equal thickness
8. **Arterioles have a diameter of:**
   a. 50–100 microns
   b. 200–500 microns
   c. 500–1000 microns
   d. 10–20 microns
9. **Vasa vasorum of an artery are nutrient vessels to:**
   a. All layers of the arterial wall
   b. Tunica adventitia and tunica media
   c. Tunica media and tunica intima
   d. Tunica adventitia and outer part of tunica media
10. **All features of vein are correct *except*:**
    a. Their lumen is larger
    b. These have valves
    c. These are thin walled
    d. Muscle tissue and elastic tissue is more in veins
11. **Anaemia is diagnosed by:**
    a. Decreased number of RBC

b. Increased number of RBC
c. Decreased number of WBC
d. Increased number of WBC

12. Artery is differentiated by following features *except*:
a. Thicker wall
b. Smaller lumen
c. More smooth muscle fibres
d. Thin tunica media

13. End arteries are present in:
a. Skeletal muscle b. Bone
c. Retina d. Middle ear

14. What type of artery is muscular artery?
a. Distribution b. Exchange
c. Resistance d. Reservoir

15. Which of the following is resistance vessel?
a. Arteriole b. Venule
c. Sinusoid d. Vein

16. Cell lining of tunica intima is:
a. Cuboidal b. Columnar
c. Squamous d. Stratified cuboidal

Answers

1. d **2.** a **3.** b **4.** d **5.** d **6.** c **7.** b **8.** a
9. d **10.** d **11.** a **12.** d **13.** c **14.** a **15.** a **16.** c

Chapter 6

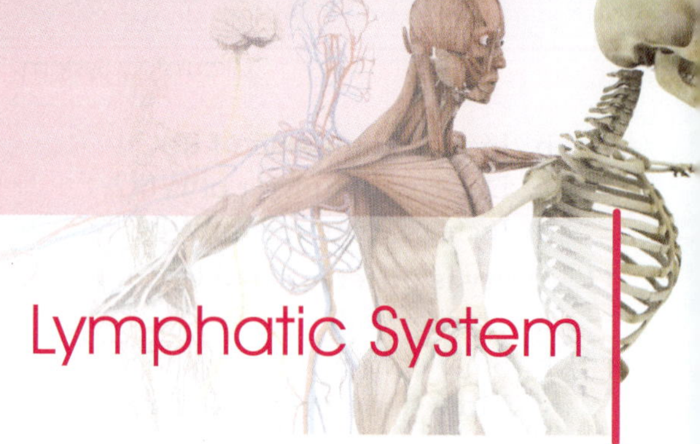

Lymphatic System

"Lives of great men all remind us, we can make our lives subline. And departing leave behind us, foot prints on the sands of time." **—William Wordsworth**

Lymphatic system is essentially a drainage system which is accessory to the venous system (Fig. 6.1).

Most of the tissue fluid formed at the arterial end of capillaries is absorbed back into the blood by the venous ends of the capillaries and the postcapillary venules. The rest of the tissue fluid (10–20%) is absorbed by the lymphatics which begin blindly in the tissue spaces.

It is important to know that the larger particles (proteins and particulate matter) can be removed from the tissue fluid only by the

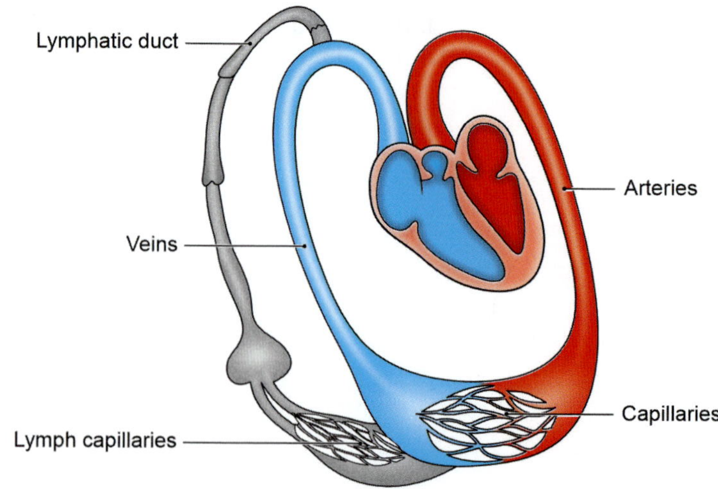

Fig. 6.1: Beginning and termination of lymph vessels

lymphatics. Therefore, the lymphatic system may be regarded as 'drainage system of coarse type' and the venous system as 'drainage system of fine type'.

Certain parts of the lymphatic system (lymphoreticular organs), however, are chiefly involved in phagocytosis, raising immune responses, and contributing to cell populations of the blood and lymph.

The tissue fluid flowing in the lymphatics is called lymph. It passes through filters (lymph nodes) placed in the course of lymphatics, and finally drains into the venous blood.

Lymph from most of the tissues is clear and colourless, but the lymph from small intestine is milky-white due to absorption of fat. The intestinal milky lymph is called chyle, and lymph vessels, the *lacteals*.

Competency achievement: The student should be able to:
AN 6.1 List the components and functions of the lymphatic system
AN 6.2 Describe structure of lymph capillaries and mechanism of lymph circulation

COMPONENTS

The lymphatic system comprises:

1. Lymph capillaries and lymph vessels
2. Central lymphoid tissues
3. Peripheral lymphoid organs
4. Circulating lymphocytes
5. Epithelio-lymphoid system
6. Mononuclear phagocyte system

1. Lymph Capillaries and Lymph Vessels

The lymph capillaries begin blindly in the tissue spaces and form intricate networks. Their calibre is greater and less regular than that of blood capillaries, and their endothelial wall is permeable to substances of much greater molecular size.

Lymph capillaries are absent from the cellular structures like brain, spinal cord, splenic pulp, bone marrow, articular cartilage, epidermis, hair, nail and cornea.

Lymph capillaries have been compared to blood capillaries in Table 6.1.

Table 6.1: Comparison of lymph and blood capillaries	
Lymph capillaries	*Blood capillaries*
1. Colourless, difficult to observe	Reddish, easy to observe
2. Blind (closed at the tip)	Joined to arterioles at one end and to venules at another end
3. Wider than blood capillaries	Narrower than lymph capillaries
4. Wall consists of thin endothelium and poorly developed basement membrane	Wall consist of normal endothelium and basement membrane
5. Contain colourless lymph	Contain red blood
6. Have relatively low pressure	Have relatively high pressure
7. Absorb tissue fluid from intercellular spaces	Add tissue fluid to intercellular spaces

Lymph capillaries start from portal radicle around hepatic lobule. These join together and drain into thoracic duct which ends in the large vein near the heart (Fig. 6.2).

The lymph capillaries join to form lymphatics, which are superficial and deep lymphatics. The superficial lymphatics accompany veins, while the deep lymphatics accompany arteries.

The lymph passes through filters or barriers of the regional lymph nodes which trap the particulate matter.

The filtered lymph passes through larger lymphatics and is eventually collected into two large trunks, the *thoracic duct* and *right*

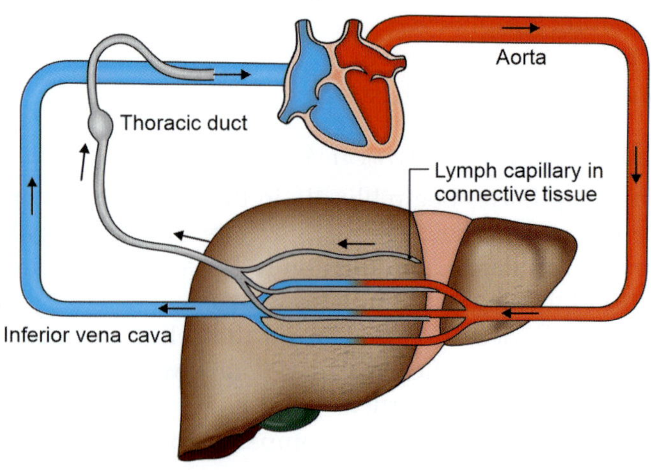

Fig. 6.2: Lymph vessels from the liver

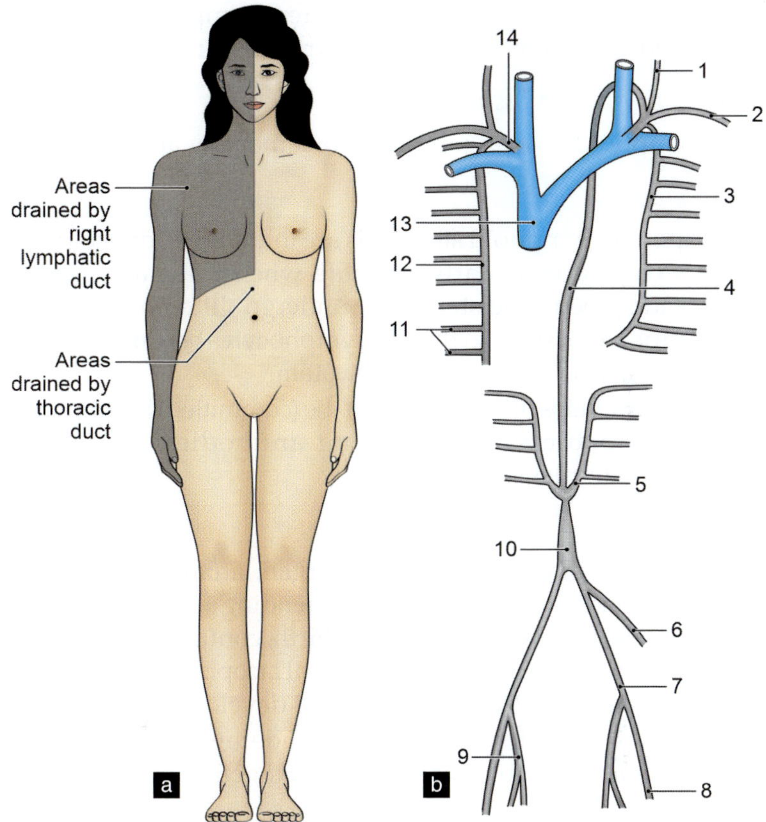

Fig. 6.3: (a) Areas drained by thoracic duct and (b) right lymphatic duct

1. Jugular lymph trunk
2. Subclavian lymph trunk
3. Broncho-mediastinal lymph trunk
4. Thoracic duct
5. Descending thoracic lymph trunk
6. Intestinal lymph trunk
7. Left lumbar lymph trunk
8. External iliac lymph trunk
9. Internal iliac lymph trunk
10. Cisterna chyli
11. Intercostal lymph vessels
12. Right broncho-mediastinal lymph trunk
13. Superior vena cava
14. Right lymphatic duct

lymphatic duct, which pour their lymph into the brachiocephalic veins (Fig. 6.3). Thoracic duct drains both lower limbs, abdomen, left half of thorax, head and neck and left upper limb. Right lymphatic duct drains right half of thorax, head and neck and right upper limb.

The lymphatics anastomose freely with their neighbours of the same side as well as of the *opposite side*. Larger lymphatics are supplied with their vasa vasorum and are accompanied by a plexus of fine blood vessels which form red streaks seen in lymphangitis.

2. Central Lymphoid Tissues

Central lymphoid tissues comprise bone marrow and thymus.

Bone Marrow

All 'pluripotent' lymphoid stem cells are initially produced by bone marrow, except during early fetal life when these are produced by liver and spleen. The stem cells undergo differentiation in the central lymphoid tissues, so that the lymphocytes become competent defensive elements of the immune system.

Bone marrow helps differentiation of the (committed) B-lymphocytes which are capable of synthesizing antibodies after getting transformed into plasma cells.

Thymus

The thymus is an important lymphoid organ, situated in the anterior and superior mediastina of the thorax, extending above into the lower part of the neck. It is well developed at birth, continues to grow up to puberty, and thereafter undergoes gradual atrophy and replacement by fat. It is the only lymphoid organ well developed at birth.

The thymus is a bilobed structure, made up of two pyramidal lobes of unequal size which are connected together by areolar tissue (Fig. 6.4).

Functions

1. The thymus controls lymphopoiesis, and maintains an effective pool of circulating lymphocytes, competent to react to innumerable antigenic stimuli.

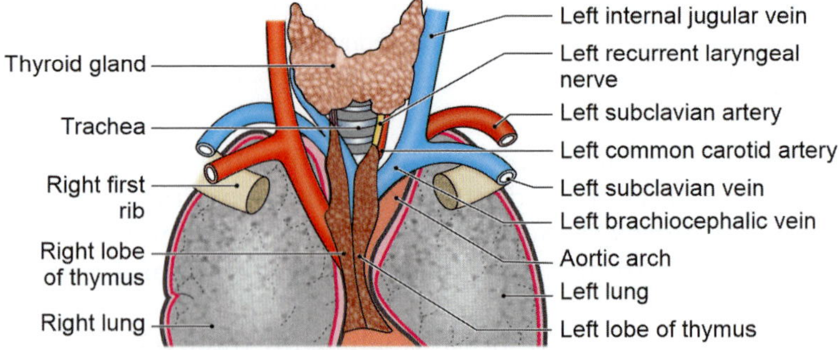

Fig. 6.4: Thymus in a child

2. It controls development of the peripheral lymphoid tissues of the body during the neonatal period. By puberty, the main lymphoid tissues are fully developed.
3. The cortical lymphocytes of the thymus arise from stem cells of bone marrow origin. Most (95%) of the lymphocytes (T lymphocytes) produced are autoallergic (act against the host or 'self antigens'), short-lived (3–5 days) and never move out of the organ. They are destroyed and their remnants are seen in Hassall's corpuscles. The remaining 5% of the T lymphocytes are longer living and join the circulating pool of lymphocytes where they act as immunologically competent but uncommitted cells. On the other hand, the other circulating lymphocytes (from lymph nodes, spleen, etc.) are committed only when exposed to a particular antigen. The process of involution are all intrinsically controlled.
4. The medullary epithelial cells of the thymus are thought to secrete:
   a. *Lymphopoietin*, which stimulates lymphocyte production, both in the cortex of the thymus and in peripheral lymphoid organs.
   b. The *competence-inducing* factor, which may be responsible for making new lymphocytes competent to react to antigenic stimuli.
5. Normally, there are no germinal centres in the thymic cortex. Such centres appear in autoimmune diseases. This may indicate a defect in the normal function of the thymus.

3. Peripheral Lymphoid Organs

Peripheral lymphoid organs comprise lymph nodes, spleen. Any part of this may become overactive on appropriate stimulation.

The progenies of B- and T-lymphocytes reach these organs where the cells may proliferate and mature into competent cells. The mature lymphocytes join the circulating pool of lymphocytes.

Lymphatic Follicle (Nodule)

Collections of lymphocytes occur at many places in the body. Everywhere there is a basic pattern, the *lymphatic follicle*. The follicle is a spherical collection of lymphocytes with a pale centre known as *germinal centre*, where the lymphocytes are more loosely packed.

The central cells are larger in size, stain less deeply, and divide more rapidly, than the peripheral cells.

LYMPH NODES

Lymph nodes are small nodules of lymphoid tissue found in the course of smaller lymphatics.

The lymph passes through one or more lymph nodes before reaching the larger lymph trunks.

The nodes are oval or reniform in shape, 1–25 mm long, and light brown, black (pulmonary), or creamy white (intestinal) in colour.

Usually they occur in groups (cervical, axillary, inguinal, mesenteric, mediastinal, etc.), but at times there may be a solitary lymph node.

Superficial nodes are arranged along the veins, and the deep nodes along the arteries.

Cervical lymph nodes form a ring at the junction of head and neck and vertical chains in the neck (Fig. 6.5). These drain whole of head and neck. On right side jugular lymph trunk drains into right lymphatic duct, while on left side it drains into thoracic duct. Lymph vessels of abdominal wall above a line passing horizontally through umbilicus drain into respective sides of axillary lymph nodes. Lymph vessels below this line drain into

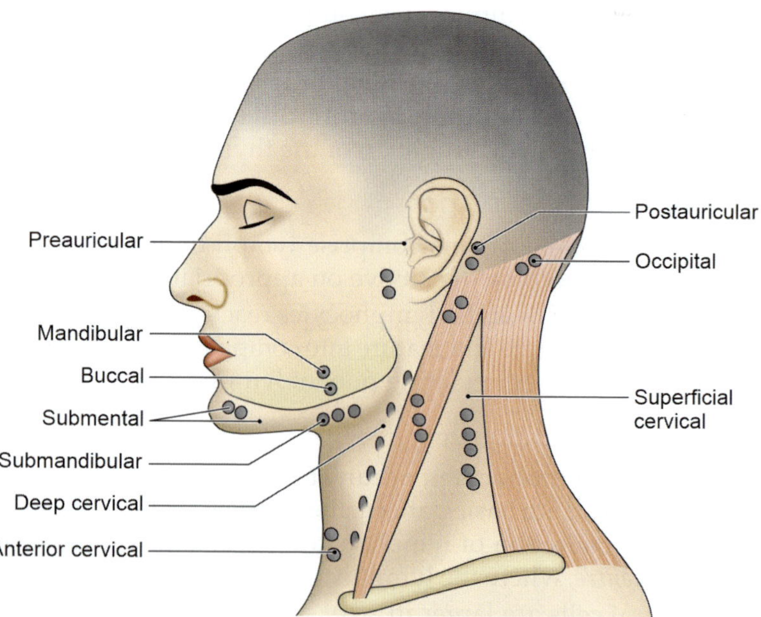

Fig. 6.5: Some lymph nodes of the neck

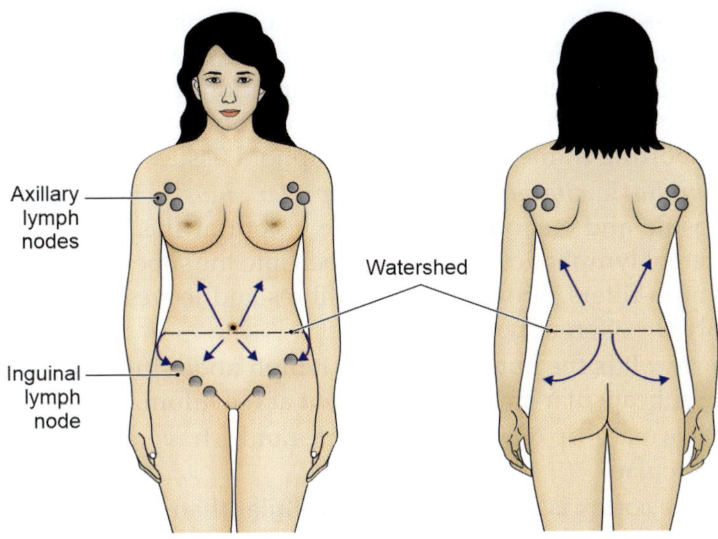

Fig. 6.6: Areas drained by axillary and inguinal lymph nodes

inguinal group of lymph nodes. This line is called "watershed" (Fig. 6.6).

Each lymph node has a slight depression on one side, called hilum. The artery enters the node, and the vein with efferent lymphatic comes out of it, at the hilum.

The afferent lymphatics enter the node at different parts of its periphery.

Structurally, a lymph node is made up of the following parts (Fig. 6.7).

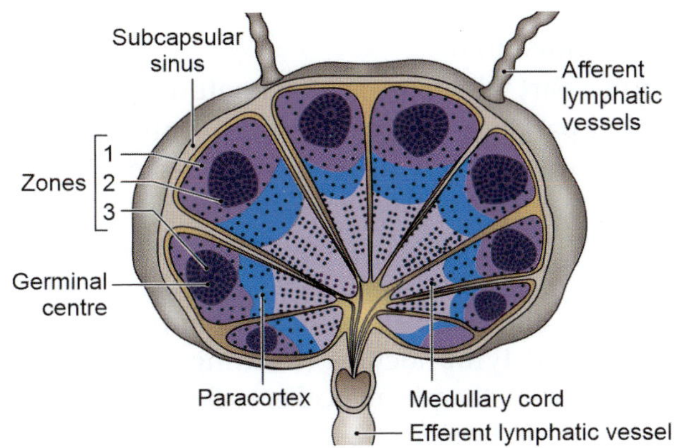

Fig. 6.7: Structure of a lymph node

a. ***Fibrous and reticular framework:*** The lymph node is covered by a capsule. From the deep surface of the capsule a number of trabeculae extend radially into the interior of the node, where they are continuous with the fine reticulum which forms the supporting framework for the lymphoid tissue.

b. ***Lymphatic channels:*** The *subcapsular sinus* lies beneath the capsule and surrounds the node except at the hilum. Many afferent lymphatics of the node open into the subcapsular sinus. Lymph filters through reticulin fibres and leaves the node by only *one* efferent lymphatic vessel.

c. ***Cortex:*** It is the outer part of the lymph node situated beneath the subcapsular sinus, being absent at the hilum.

   It is made up of lymphatic follicles and is traversed by fibrous trabeculae.

   The cortex is far more densely cellular than the medulla.

   It is divided into:

   Zone 1: Containing loosely packed small lymphocytes, macrophages and occasional plasma cells at the periphery of the follicle and extending into the medullary cords.

   Zone 2: Containing more densely packed small lymphocytes and macrophages, and limited to cortical and paracortical (inner cortex) areas.

   Zone 3: Including the germinal centre which contains large lymphocytes and macrophages.

   The maturing lymphocytes pass from zone 3 to zone 2 to zone 1 and to the subcapsular sinus (Fig. 6.7).

   According to the distribution of B- and T-lymphocytes, the cortex is divided into:

   1. An outer part which contains immature B-lymphocytes.
   2. An inner part, between the germinal centre and the medulla, which contains T-lymphocytes. This part is known as *paracortex* or *thymus dependent zone*.

      The mature B-lymphocytes (plasma cells) are found in the medulla.

d. ***Medulla:*** It is the central part of the lymph node, containing loosely packed lymphocytes (forming irregular branching medullary cords), the plasma cells, and macrophages.

e. ***Blood channels:*** The artery enters at the hilum and divides into straight branches which run in the trabeculae. In the cortex

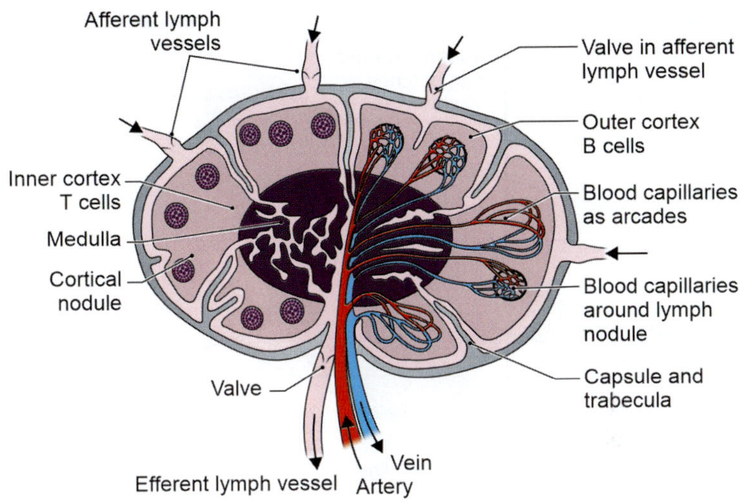

Fig. 6.8: Artery, vein and lymph vessels of the lymph node

the arteries further divide to form arcades of arterioles and capillaries with many anastomosing loops (Fig. 6.8).

The capillaries give rise to venules and veins, which run back to the hilum. The capillaries are more profuse around the follicles, and the postcapillary venules are more abundant in the paracortical zones for lymphatic migration.

Haemal Nodes and Spleen

These are small lymphatic bodies resembling lymph nodes in their structure, which are found in the course of blood vessels.

The afferent and efferent lymphatics are absent. Their sinuses are filled with blood rather than lymph.

These are found in some animals in relation to their abdominal and thoracic viscera.

Haemal nodes may represent an intermediate stage between a lymph node and the spleen. In man, the spleen is a large haemal node.

Spleen

Spleen is the largest lymphoid organ and is covered by a dense connective tissue *capsule* (Fig. 6.9). *Trabeculae* extend inwards from capsule. Cellular material of spleen is divided into *white pulp* and

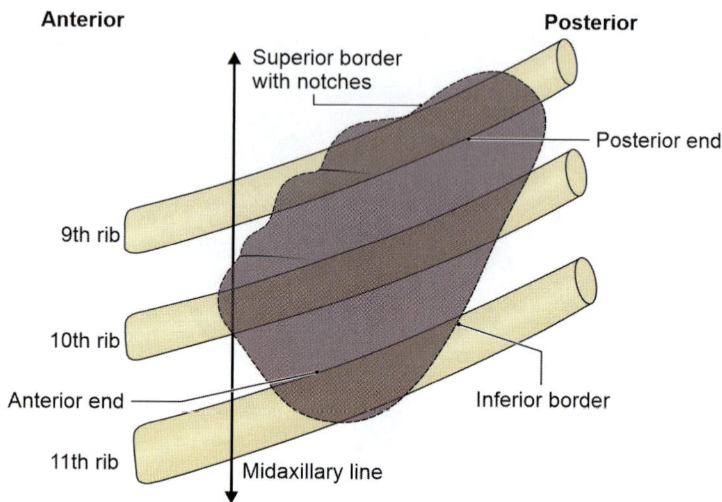

Fig. 6.9: Spleen with its extent, ends and borders (previous view)

red pulp. Red pulp consists of blood filled venous sinuses and white pulp comprises lymphatic tissue, consisting of lymphocytes and macrophages. (*Reference: Gray's Anatomy*, 42nd edition, spleen lies along 10th–12th ribs.)

Spleen is part of the lymphatic system and its functions are:

1. ***Phagocytosis:*** Leukocytes, platelets are phagocytosed in spleen. Old and abnormal RBCs are destroyed in spleen and break down products (bilirubin and iron) are passed to the liver.
2. ***Storage of blood:*** Spleen contains up to 350 ml blood. In shock, sympathetic stimulation can return a large part of this volume to circulation.
3. ***Immunity:*** Spleen contains B- and T-lymphocytes which are important in immune response to infections.
4. ***Erythropoiesis:*** RBC production occurs in spleen and liver in fetal life.
5. Storage of platelets.

4. Circulating Pool of Lymphocytes

The pool contains mature progenies of B- and T-lymphocytes which may be called upon during antigenic emergencies (Roitt, 1977).

Table 6.2 shows the differences between T- and B-lymphocytes.

Table 6.3 shows the approximate percentage of lymphocytes in lymphoid organs.

Table 6.2: Differences between T- and B-lymphocytes		
	T-lymphocytes	*B-lymphocytes*
Origin	Bone marrow → Thymus → lymphoid tissue	Bone marrow → Bursa-equivalent → lymphoid tissue
Life span	Months to years	Less than one month
Location Lymph nodes Spleen Peyer's patches	 Perifollicular Perifollicular Perifollicular	 Germinal centre Germinal centre Central follicles
Number in blood	80%	20%
Function	i. Cell-mediated immunity via Tc cells (cytotoxic) ii. Immunoregulation of T and B-lymphocytes via TH cells (helper) iii. Memory T cells	i. Humoral immunity IgG (most abundant). It is via immunoglobulins produced by plasma cells ii. Formed by enlargement and modification of B-lymphocytes iii. Memory B cells

Table 6.3: Approximate percentage of lymphocytes in lymphoid organs		
Lymphoid organ	*T-lymphocytes*	*B-lymphocytes*
Thymus	100%	0%
Lymph node	60%	40%
Spleen	45%	55%
Bone marrow	10%	90%
Blood	80%	20%

5. Epithelio-lymphoid System

Epithelio-lymphoid system comprises Mucosa Associated Lymphoid Tissue (MALT) in digestive system and Bronchus Associated Lymphoid Tissue (BALT) in respiratory system.

In the region of posterior one-third of tongue, oropharynx, nasopharynx, there is a ring of lymphoid tissue under the mucous membrane. Its components are lingual tonsil, palatine tonsils, tubal tonsils and nasopharyngeal tonsil. This ring is called Waldeyer's ring

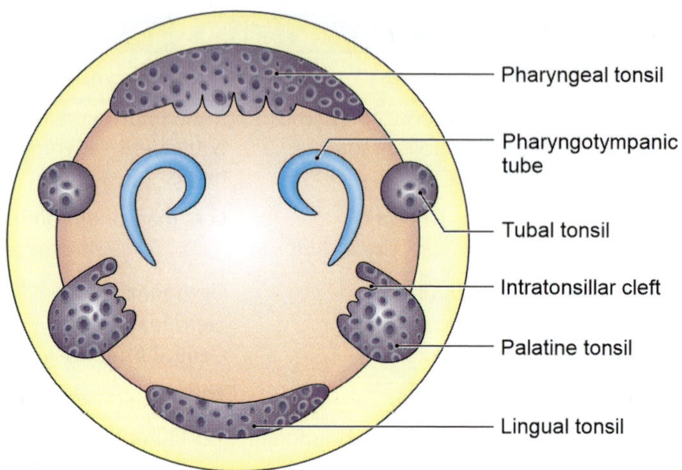

Fig. 6.10: Components of Waldeyer's ring

(Fig. 6.10). Peyer's patches of ileum of small intestine and lymphoid tissue of vermiform appendix belong to MALT.

6. Mononuclear Phagocyte System or Macrophage System (Reticuloendothelial System)

This system is not closely related to lymphatic system because the two are independent structurally and functionally. The macrophage system is made up of highly phagocytic cells which are widely distributed in the body. These cells include:

a. Macrophages of connective tissue, reticular tissue and lungs
b. Monocytes of blood
c. Kupffer's cells of liver
d. Meningocytes of meninges
e. Microglial cells of nervous tissue
f. Foreign body giant cells.

The endothelial cells, fibroblasts, and most leucocytes are not included in this system because of their poor power of phagocytosis.

Functions

1. The system forms first line of defence of the body against micro-organisms, because of the amoeboid and phagocytic properties of its cells.

2. The macrophages of lymphoid tissue are now considered to be intimately concerned with mounting specific immune responses by the neighbouring cells.
3. Many of the prominent sites of RES are also important sites of haemopoiesis.
4. Absorbs fat from intestines to be transported to blood.

Growth Pattern of Lymphoid Tissue

Lymphoid tissue of the body is prominent at birth, and grows rapidly during childhood. There are about 600 lymph nodes in an adult.

The growth ceases at about the time of puberty, and is followed by partial atrophy in the later years.

This growth pattern is shared by lymph nodes, thymus, tonsils, lymphoid tissue of the intestines, and the follicles of spleen.

However, the lymph nodes may enlarge again in response to inflammation (lymphadenitis) or tumour formation (Hodgkin's disease, lymphosarcoma, etc.).

Lymph nodes are commonly enlarged by metastases (spread) of malignant growths (carcinoma).

Functions of Lymphoid System

1. Lymph capillaries absorb and remove the large protein molecules and other particulate matter from the tissue spaces. Thus the cellular debris and foreign particles (dust particles inhaled into the lungs, bacteria and other micro-organisms) are conveyed to the regional lymph nodes. Lymphatics (lacteals) help in transportation of fat from the gut.
2. Lymph nodes serve a number of functions.
    a. They act as filters for the lymph which percolates slowly through the intricate network of its spaces. Thus the foreign particles are prevented from entering the blood stream.
    b. The foreign particles are engulfed by the macrophages in the sinuses.
    c. Antigens are also trapped by the phagocytes.
    d. The mature B-lymphocytes (plasma cells capable of producing antibodies) and mature T-lymphocytes are produced in the node.
    e. Both the cellular and humoral immune responses are mounted against the antigen-laden phagocytes.

f. The circulating lymphocytes can pass back into the lymphatic channels within the node.
g. Humoral antibodies are freely produced by the lymph nodes.

3. Production (proliferation) and maturation of B- and T-lymphocytes is the main function of lymphoid tissue.

> *Competency achievement:* The student should be able to:
> AN 6.3 Explain the concept of lymphoedema and spread of tumors via lymphatics and venous system

Clinical Anatomy of Lymphatic System

- Lymphatics are primarily meant for coarse drainage, from the tissue spaces to the regional lymph nodes.
- Here the foreign and noxious material is filtered off by the phagocytic activity of the macrophage cells. The cell debris is finally disposed by the appropriate immune responses within the node. Thus the lymphatic system forms the *first line of defence of the body*.

While draining from an infected area, the lymphatics and lymph nodes carrying infected debris may become inflammed, resulting in *lymphangitis* (Fig. 6.11) and *lymphadenitis*. In acute cases the lymphatics are marked on the skin as painful red lines leading to the painful and tender swollen lymph nodes which may suppurate. Chronic infections (tuberculosis, syphilis, etc.) cause chronic lymphadenitis.

Lymphoma is a malignant cancer comprising abnormal lymphocytes or stem lymphocytic cells.

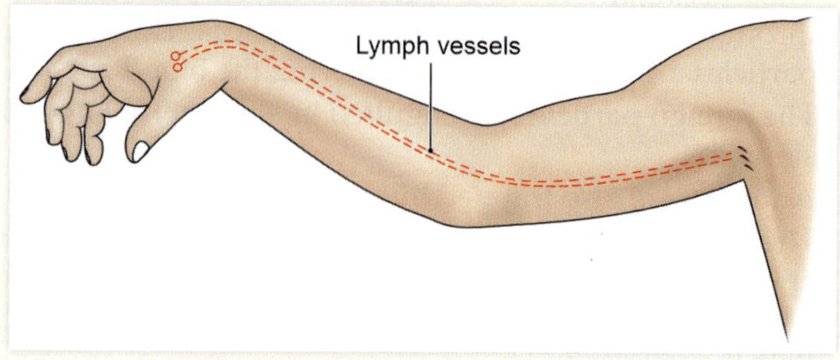

Fig. 6.11: Lymphangitis in upper limb

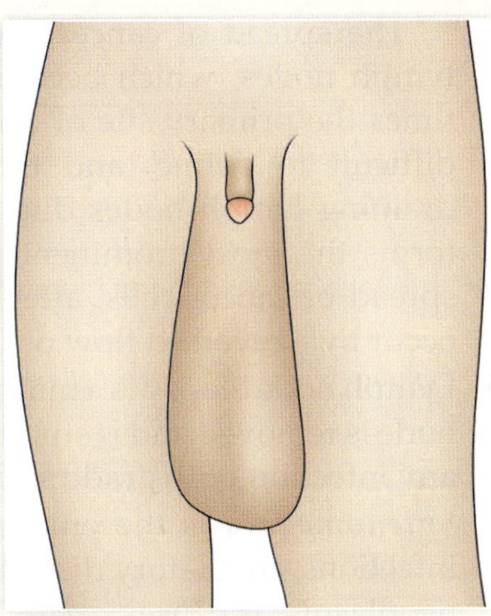

Fig. 6.12: Elephantiasis causing enlarged scrotum

- The filarial parasite lives in the lymphatics, which may become blocked, giving rise to solid oedema (elephantiasis) in the peripheral area of drainage. *Elephantiasis* is characterized by enormous enlargement of the limb or scrotum (Fig. 6.12) due to the thickened skin. The microfilariae enter the blood stream only during night and, therefore, the blood for examination must be collected during night.

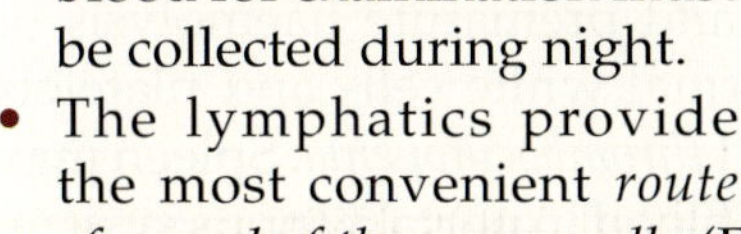

- The lymphatics provide the most convenient *route of spread of the cancer cells* (Fig. 6.13). Therefore, the lymphatic drainage of those organs which are commonly involved in cancer should be studied in greater details. The reasons for detailed study are as follows:
  a. It is helpful in the diagnosis of the primary site of the cancer.
  b. It helps in predicting the prognosis and in classifying the stage of cancer.
  c. It helps the surgeon in doing the block dissections during operative removal of the cancer.

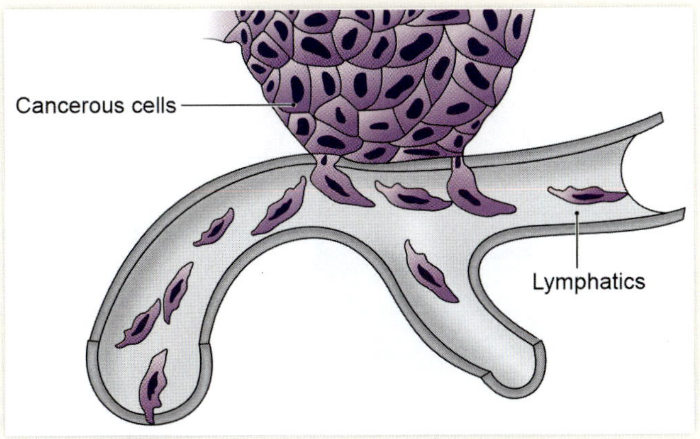

Fig. 6.13: Spread of cancer cells via the lymphatics

The spread of cancer causes enlargement of the regional lymph nodes, which become fixed and stony hard. Many a times the primary site of cancer is quite insignificant or even difficult to define, and the enormous enlargement of the draining lymph nodes due to secondary malignant deposits forms the most prominent part of the disease. A retrograde spread of cancer cells, after the blockage of lymphatics, may occur by a reversed flow of the lymph.

- Lymph node biopsy is a minor surgical procedure where lymph node is removed and is studied microscopically. It is done to see any infection or to grade stage of cancer.
- ***Splenomegaly*** is the enlargement of spleen mainly due to infections, circulatory disorders, blood diseases and malignant neoplasms. It causes excessive and premature haemolysis of red cells or phagocytosis of normal white cells and platelets leading to *anaemia, leukopenia* and *thrombocytopenia*. Spleen may also enlarge due to congestion of blood in portal venous system, in *right-sided heart failure* and in fibrosis caused due to *cirrhosis of liver*. Splenomegaly also occurs to meet the extra work load for removing damaged and abnormal blood cells. Commonest cause of splenomegaly is *malaria* (Fig. 6.14).

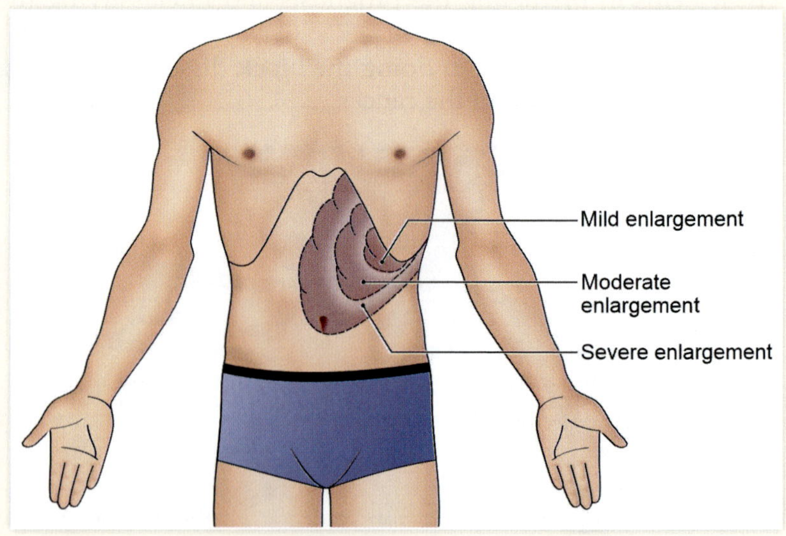

Fig. 6.14: Stages of enlargement of spleen

- Enlargement of thymus may cause *myasthenia gravis*, which produces extreme weakness of the skeletal muscles. It may be treated by removal of enlarged thymus, or by drug treatment.

Disorders of Immune System

Disorders of immune system covers:

1. Allergic reactions
2. Autoimmune disease in which body's immune system fails to recognise normal body cells and attacks the cells.
3. Immunodeficiency diseases, e.g. AIDS where the body's immune system becomes weak and is not able to protect itself, leading to diseases.

Let us discuss them in detail:

1. ***Allergic reactions:*** These can be simple reactions like papules, itching, burning of skin or these can be a major allergic reactions like reaction to intravenous drugs.
2. ***Autoimmune disease:*** It may appear as lupus erythematosus (LE). LE is of two types, discoid LE (DLE) and systemic LE (SLE). In both these cases the body's immune system attacks its own connective tissue.

   DLE affects the skin which becomes thickened with reddish patches on the face, forehead and cheeks.

   In SLE there is butterfly-shaped rash on the face. The joints of the upper limb are also affected.
3. ***Acquired Immunodeficiency Disease Syndrome (AIDS):*** AIDS is caused by HIV human immunodeficiency virus. This is a retrovirus where RNA is enveloped in a protein envelope. The mode of action of this virus is to attack T4 helper cells. These helper cells are vital to immune response and their inefficiency compromises the immune response. It results in minor infections taking on serious form.

   A person can be HIV positive for many years without showing symptoms of AIDS. AIDS is the last stage of HIV disease. Many opportunistic infections like TB invade AIDS patients and cause serious illness which can be fatal. They may also get AIDS, dementia, kaposis sarcoma.

   HIV is transmitted by needle sharing, multiple sexual contacts, multiple sex partners or from mother to the foetus. Public awareness and safe sex has reduced the cases of HIV/AIDS.

Points to Remember

- Lymph mostly consists of macromolecules not able to course through the blood capillaries. Lymph carries absorbed products of fats to the blood circulation.
- Lymph vessels also carry cancer cells from the original site of disease to nearby or distant regions.
- Lymph nodes/palatine tonsil/thymus, etc. are maximum in size till puberty. Then these start involuting/decreasing in size.
- Lymph nodes increase in size (lymphadenitis) during chronic infections like tuberculosis, syphilis, lymphomas.
- Lymphatic system forms the first line of defence of the body.
- Umbilical plane is the line of watershed of lymphatics.

Multiple Choice Questions

1. **Components of lymphatic system are all *except*:**
   a. Lymph vessels
   b. Central lymphoid tissues
   c. Peripheral lymphoid organs
   d. Circulating red blood cells
2. **Lymphoid tissue enlarges in all conditions/stages *except*:**
   a. Childhood
   b. At and after puberty
   c. Lymphadenitis
   d. Metastases of carcinoma
3. **Splenomegaly commonly occurs in:**
   a. Malaria
   b. Cirrhosis of liver
   c. Anaemia
   d. Elephantiasis
4. **Lymph node enlargement draining an organ is useful in all *except*:**
   a. Diagnosis of primary site of the carcinoma
   b. Classifying the stage of carcinoma
   c. Surgeon in doing block dissection
   d. Splenomegaly
5. **Thoracic duct drains the following areas *except*:**
   a. Left upper limb
   b. Left lower limb
   c. Right lower limb
   d. Right upper limb
6. **Which lymphoid tissue contains red pulp and white pulp?**
   a. Lymph node
   b. Palatine tonsil
   c. Spleen
   d. Thymus

7. Lymph capillaries are absent in all *except*:

a. Cornea
b. Epidermis
c. Spinal cord
d. Dermis

8. Thymus has the following features *except*:

a. Lies in superior and anterior mediastinum
b. T-lymphocytes are cytotoxic, helper and memory cells
c. Secretes thymosin
d. Filters blood to get rid of antigens

9. One of the following lymphoid tissues has both afferent and efferent lymphatics:

a. Thymus
b. Spleen
c. Tonsil
d. Lymph node

Answers

1. d **2.** b **3.** a **4.** d **5.** d **6.** c **7.** d **8.** d
9. d

Chapter 7

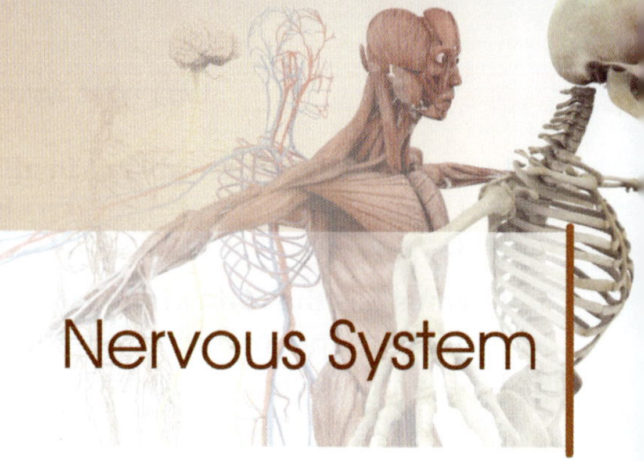

Nervous System

"We only use 5% of our intelligence, while Albert Einstein used up to 15–20%. There is such a gap between what we do and what we can do."

—William James

Nervous system is the chief controlling and coordinating system of the body. It controls and regulates all activities of the body, whether voluntary or involuntary, and adjusts the individual (organism) to the given surroundings.

This is based on the special properties of sensitivity, conductivity and responsiveness of the nervous system.

The protoplasmic extensions of the nerve cells form the neural pathways called nerves. The nerves resemble the electricity wires. Like the electric current flowing through the wires, the impulses (sensory and motor) are conducted through the nerves.

The sensory impulses are transmitted by the sensory (afferent) nerves from the periphery (skin, mucous membranes, muscles, tendons, joints, and special sense organs) to the central nervous system (CNS).

The motor impulses are transmitted by the motor (efferent) nerves from the central nervous system to the periphery (muscles and glands) (Fig. 7.1).

Thus the CNS is kept continuously informed about the surroundings (environment) through various sensory impulses, both general and special.

The CNS in turn brings about necessary adjustment of the body by sending appropriate orders which are passed on as motor impulses to the muscles, vessels, viscera and glands. The adjustment of the organism to the given surroundings is the most important function

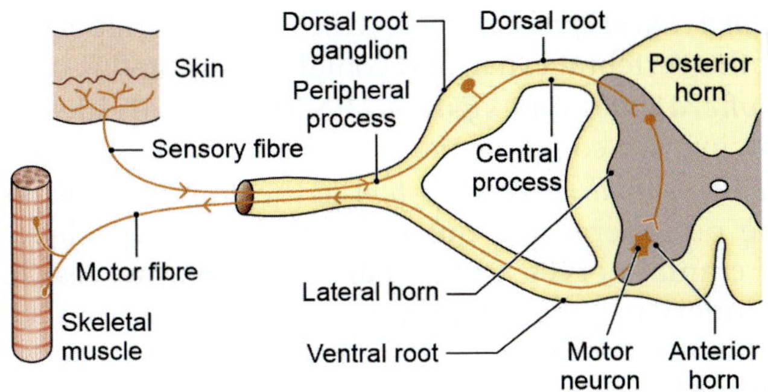

Fig. 7.1: Afferent and efferent pathways through the spinal cord

of the nervous system, without which it will not be possible for the organism to survive.

> *Competency achievement:* The student should be able to:
> AN 7.1 Describe general plan of nervous system with components of central, peripheral and autonomic nervous systems

PARTS OF NERVOUS SYSTEM

The nervous system is broadly divided into central and peripheral parts which are continuous with each other. Further subdivisions of each part are given below.

A. ***Central nervous system (CNS) includes:***

1. *Brain or encephalon*, which occupies cranial cavity, and contains the higher governing centres (Fig. 7.2).

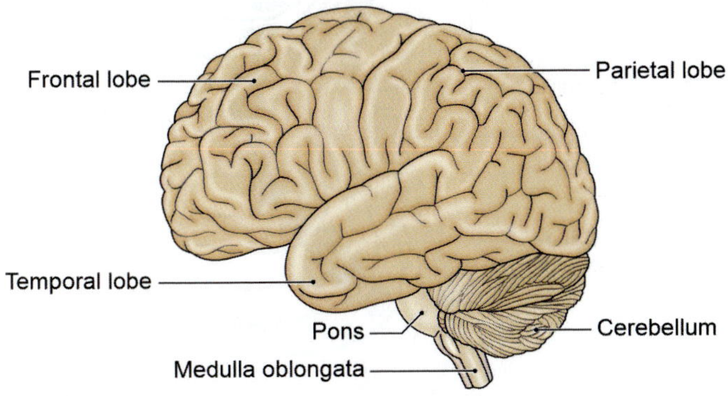

Fig. 7.2: Superolateral surface of cerebral hemisphere, pons, medulla oblongata and cerebellum

2. *Spinal cord or spinal medulla*, which occupies upper two-thirds of the vertebral canal, and contains many reflex centres.

B. ***Peripheral nervous system (PNS)*** is subdivided into the following two components.

1. *Cerebrospinal nervous system* is the somatic component of the peripheral nervous system, which includes 12 pairs of cranial nerves and 31 pairs of spinal nerves (Fig. 7.3). It innervates the somatic structures of the head and neck, limbs and body wall, and mediates somatic sensory and motor functions.

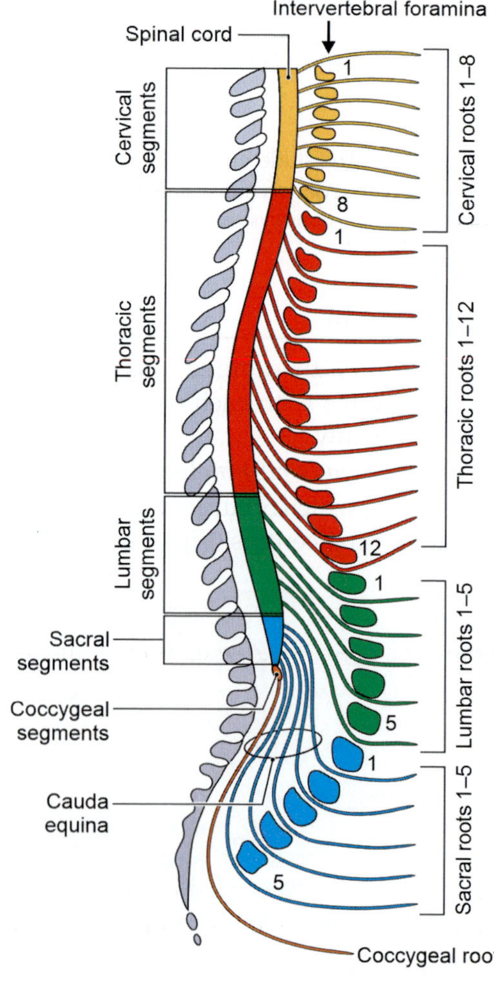

Fig. 7.3: Segments of spinal cord with 31 pairs of spinal nerves

Table 7.1: Comparison of cerebrospinal and peripheral autonomic nervous systems	
Cerebrospinal nervous system	*Peripheral autonomic nervous system*
The somatic efferent pathway is made up of one neuron which passes directly to the effector organ (skeletal muscles) Neuron ↓ axon Skeletal muscle	The autonomic efferent pathway is made up of two neurons (preganglionic and postganglionic) with an intervening ganglion for the relay of the preganglionic fibre. The effector organ (viscera) is supplied by the postganglionic fibre

2. *Peripheral autonomic nervous system* is the visceral component of the peripheral nervous system, which includes the visceral or splanchnic nerves that are connected to the CNS through the somatic nerves. It innervates the viscera, glands, blood vessels and nonstriated muscles, and mediates the visceral functions.

The cerebrospinal and autonomic nervous systems differ from each other in their efferent pathways. Table 7.1 shows comparison of the two systems.

Competency achievement: The student should be able to:
AN 7.2 List components of nervous tissue and their functions
AN 7.3 Describe parts of a neuron and classify them based on number of neurites, size and function

CELL TYPES OF NERVOUS SYSTEM

The nervous tissue is composed of two distinct types of cells:

a. The excitable cells are the nerve cells or neurons; and
b. The non-excitable cells constitute neuroglia and ependyma in the CNS, and Schwann cells in the PNS.

1. Neuron

Each nerve cell or neuron has:

a. A cell body or *perikaryon* or somata having a central nucleus and Nissl granules in its cytoplasm (Fig. 7.4). The neurons of only females contain Barr body. This Barr body is a planoconvex heterochromatin mass present close to the nuclear membrane.

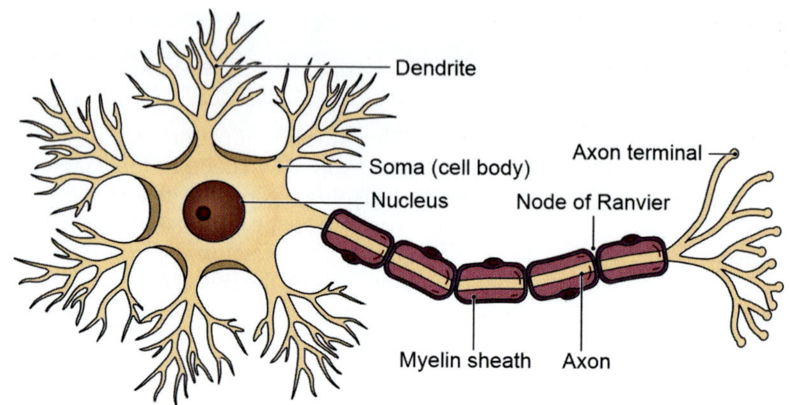

Fig. 7.4: Components of a neuron with a peripheral nerve

b. Cell processes called neurites, which are of two types.

   Many short afferent processes, which are freely branching and varicose, are called *dendrites*.

A single long efferent process called axon, arising from axon hillock. It may give off occasional branches (collaterals) and is of uniform diameter.

The terminal branches of the axon are called axon terminals or telodendria.

The cell bodies (somata) of the neurons form grey matter and nuclei in the CNS, and ganglia in the PNS. The cell processes (axons) form tracts in the CNS, and nerves in the PNS.

Table 7.2 shows the differences between axon and dendrite.

Table 7.2: Comparison of axon and dendrite

Axon	*Dendrite*
1. Only one axon is present in a neuron.	Usually multiple in a neuron.
2. Thin long process of uniform thickness and smooth surface.	These are short multiple processes. Their thickness diminishes as these divide repeatedly. The branches are studded with spiny projections.
3. The branches of axon are fewer and at right angles to the axon.	The dendrites branch profusely and are given off at acute angles.
4. Axon contains neurofibrils and no Nissl granules.	Dendrites contain both neurofibrils and Nissl granules.
5. Forms the efferent component of the impulse.	Forms the afferent component of the impulse.

Types of neurons: Neurons can be classified in several ways.

I. According to the number of their processes (neurites) they may be:
   a. *Unipolar*, e.g. mesencephalic nucleus
   b. *Pseudounipolar*, e.g. sensory ganglia or spinal ganglia (Fig. 7.5)
   c. *Bipolar*, e.g. spiral and vestibular ganglia and bipolar neurons of retina.
   d. *Multipolar*, neurons in cerebrum and cerebellum.

II. According to the length of axon, the neurons are classified as pyramidal cells, Purkinje cell
   a. *Golgi type I* neurons, with a long axon, pyramidal cells, Purkinje cells; and
   b. *Golgi type II* neurons (microneurons), with a short axon, e.g. granule cell of cerebellum.

III. According to function: Sensory, motor and internuncial.

Motor are multipolar: Upper motor neuron—within brain; lower motor neuron—in anterior grey column of spinal cord.

Dynamic polarity: The neurons show dynamic polarity in their processes. The impulse flows toward the soma in the dendrites, and

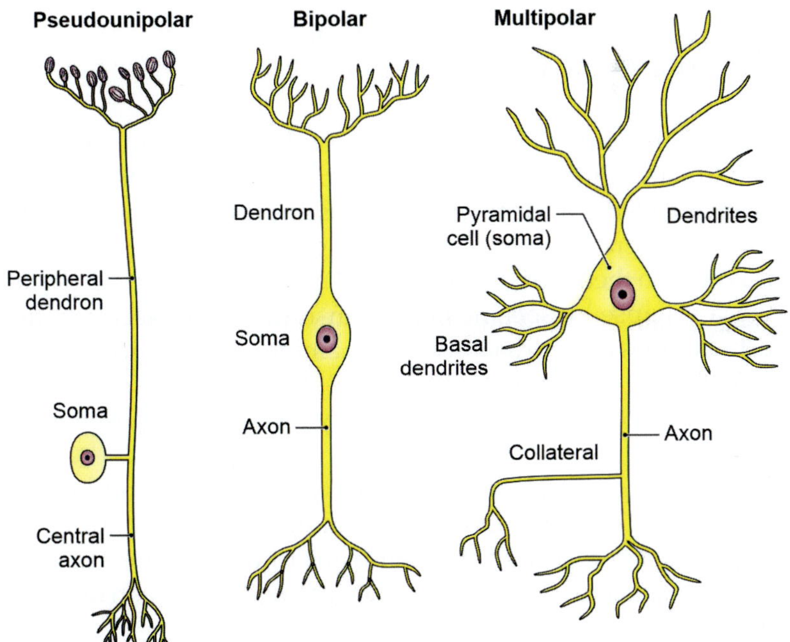

Fig. 7.5: Types of neurons

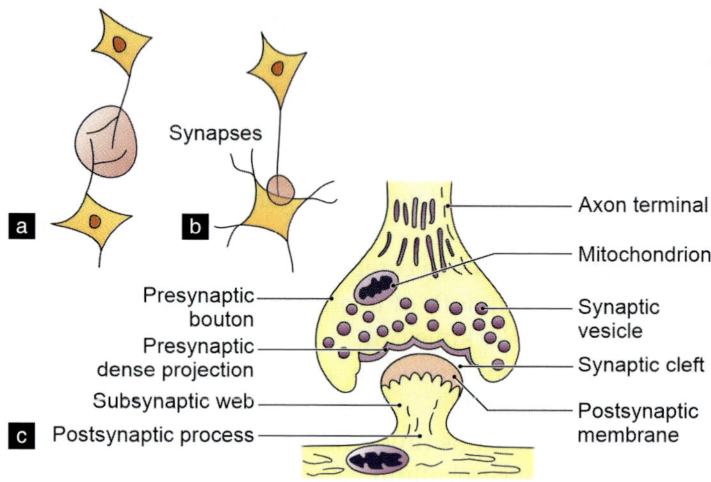

Fig. 7.6: Types of synapses: (a) Axodendrite, (b) axosomatic, and (c) structure of a synapse

away from the soma in the axon. However, in certain microneurons, where the axon is absent, the impulse can flow in either direction through their dendrites.

Competency achievement: The student should be able to:
AN 7.7 Describe various types of synapse

Synapse: The neurons form long chains along which the impulses are conducted in different directions. Each junction between the neurons is called a synapse (Fig. 7.6). It is important to know that the contact between the neurons is by contiguity and not by continuity. This is neuron theory of Waldeyer (1891). The impulse is transmitted across a synapse by specific neurotransmitters, like acetylcholine, catecholamines (noradrenalin and dopamine), serotonin, histamine, glycine, GABA and certain polypeptides. The neurotransmitter enter into synaptic cleft and are picked up by receptors on postsynaptic membrane.

The most common types of the synapse are axodendritic, axo-somatic, (Fig. 7.6a and b). In synaptic glomeruli, groups of axons make contact with the dendrites of one or more neurons for complex interactions. Figure 7.6c shows the ultrastructure of a synapse.

Functionally, a synapse may either be inhibitory or excitatory.

2. Neuroglia

The non-excitable supporting cells of the nervous system form a major component of the nervous tissue. These cells include the following:

1. *Neuroglial cells,* found in the parenchyma of brain and spinal cord.
2. *Ependymal cells* lining the internal cavities or ventricles.
3. *Capsular* or *satellite cells,* surrounding neurons of the sensory and autonomic ganglia.
4. *Schwann cells,* forming sheaths for axons of peripheral nerves.
5. Several types of *supporting cells,* ensheathing the motor and sensory nerve terminals, and supporting the sensory epithelia.

The neuroglial cells, found in the parenchyma of brain and spinal cord, are broadly classified as:

A. *Macroglia,* of ectodermal (neural) origin, comprising astrocytes, oligodendrocytes, and glioblasts.
B. *Microglia,* of mesodermal origin.

All glial cells are much smaller but far more numerous than the nerve cells.

a. ***Astrocytes:*** As the name suggests, these cells are star-shaped because of their numerous processes radiating in all directions. Astrocytes are of two types.

   Protoplasmic astrocytes, with thick and symmetrical processes are found in the grey matter.

   Fibrous astrocytes, with thin and asymmetrical processes, are found in the white matter.

   The processes of astrocytes often end in plate-like expansions on the blood vessels, ependyma, and pial surface of the CNS (Fig. 7.7).

b. ***Oligodendrocytes:*** As the name suggests these cells have fewer cell processes. According to their distribution, the oligodendrocytes may be intrafascicular or perineuronal.

   The *intrafascicular cells* are found in the myelinated tracts.

   The *perineuronal cells* are seen on the surface of the somata of neurons.

c. ***Glioblast:*** These are stem cells which can differentiate into macroglial cells. They are particularly numerous beneath the ependyma.

d. ***Microglia:*** These are the smallest of the glial cells which have a flattened cell body with a few short, fine processes.

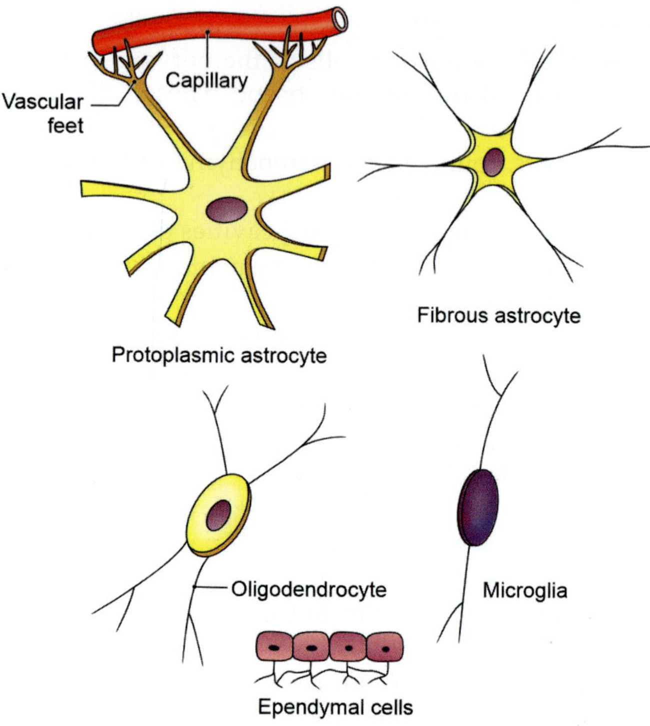

Fig. 7.7: Types of neuroglia

They are often related to capillaries, and are said to be phagocytic in nature.

Microglial cells are possibly derived from the circulating monocytes which migrate into the CNS during the late foetal and early postnatal life.

Functions of Glial and Ependymal Cells

1. They provide mechanical support to neurons.
2. Because of their non-conducting nature, the glial cells act as insulators between the neurons and prevent neuronal impulses from spreading in unwanted directions.
3. They can remove the foreign material and cell debris by phagocytosis.
4. They can repair the damaged areas of nervous tissue. By proliferation (gliosis) they form glial scar tissue, and fill the gaps left by degenerated neurons.

5. Glial cells can take up and store neurotransmitters released by the neighbouring synapses. These can either be metabolized or released again from the glial cells.
6. They help in neuronal functions by maintaining a suitable metabolic and ionic environment for the neurons.
7. Oligodendrocytes myelinate tracts.
8. Ependymal cells are concerned with exchanges of materials between brain and CSF.

BLOOD–BRAIN BARRIER

Certain dyes, when injected intravenously, fail to stain the parenchyma of brain and spinal cord, although they pass easily into the non-nervous tissues. However, the same dyes, when injected into the ventricles, enter the brain substances easily. This indicates that a barrier exists at the capillary level between the blood and nerve cells. The possible structures constituting the blood–brain barrier are as follows.

a. Capillary endothelium without fenestrations.
b. Basement membrane of the endothelium.
c. The end feet of astrocytes covering the capillary walls.

The barrier permits a selective passage of blood contents to the nervous tissue, and thus the toxic and harmful substances are ordinarily prevented from reaching the brain.

REFLEX ARC

A reflex arc is the basic functional unit of the nervous system which can perform an integrated neural activity. A monosynaptic reflex arc is the simplest and is made up of:

a. A receptor, e.g. skin;
b. A sensory or afferent neuron;
c. A motor or efferent neuron; and
d. An effector, e.g. muscle.

An involuntary motor response of the body is called a reflex action. The stretch reflexes (tendon jerks) are the examples of monosynaptic reflexes (Fig. 7.8).

The complex forms of reflex arc are polysynaptic due to addition of one or more internuncial neurons (interneurons) in between the afferent and efferent neurons (Fig. 7.9). Withdrawal reflex response to a painful stimulation is polysynaptic reflex.

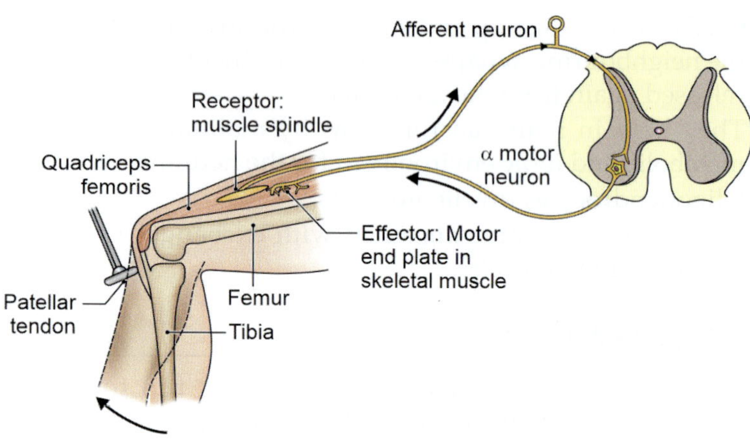

Fig. 7.8: Monosynaptic reflex arc

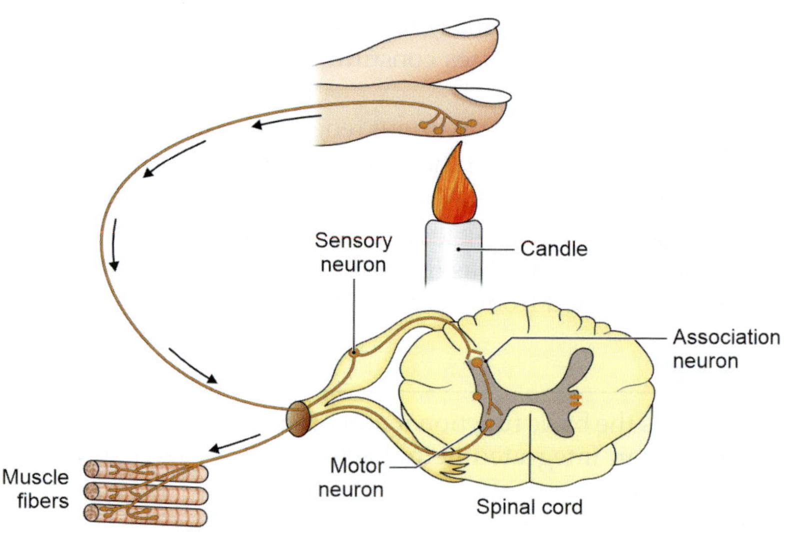

Fig. 7.9: Polysynaptic reflex arc

PERIPHERAL NERVES

The nerves are solid white cords composed of bundles (fasciculi) of nerve fibres.

Each motor nerve fibre is an axon with its coverings.

The nerve fibres are supported and bound together by connective tissue sheaths at different levels of organization of the nerve. The whole nerve trunk is ensheathed by *epineurium*, each fasciculus by

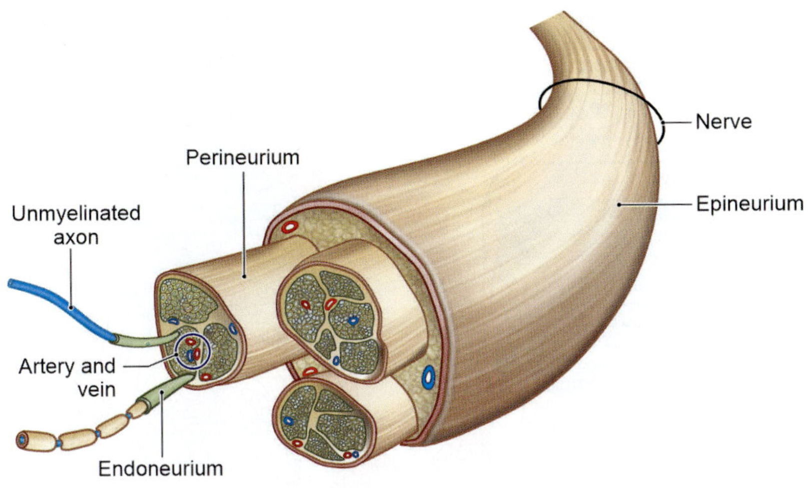

Fig. 7.10: Fibrous support of the nerve fibres

perineurium, and each nerve fibre by a delicate *endoneurium*. The toughness of a nerve is due to its fibrous sheaths, otherwise the nerve tissue itself is very delicate and friable (Fig. 7.10).

Competency achievement: The student should be able to:
AN 4.1 Describe dermatomes in body
AN 7.4 Describe structure of a typical spinal nerve

SPINAL NERVES

There are 31 pairs of spinal nerves, including 8 cervical, 12 thoracic, 5 lumbar, 5 sacral and 1 coccygeal.

Area of skin supplied by a single segment of spinal cord giving origin to one pair of spinal nerves is called a *dermatome*.

The distribution of dermatomes to the skin is shown in Fig. 7.11. Each spinal nerve is connected with the spinal cord by two roots, a *ventral root* which is motor, and a dorsal root which is sensory (Fig. 7.12).

The *dorsal root* is characterized by the presence of a *spinal ganglion* at its distal end. In the majority of nerves the ganglion lies in the intervertebral foramen.

The ventral and dorsal nerve roots unite together within the intervertebral foramen to form the *spinal nerve*.

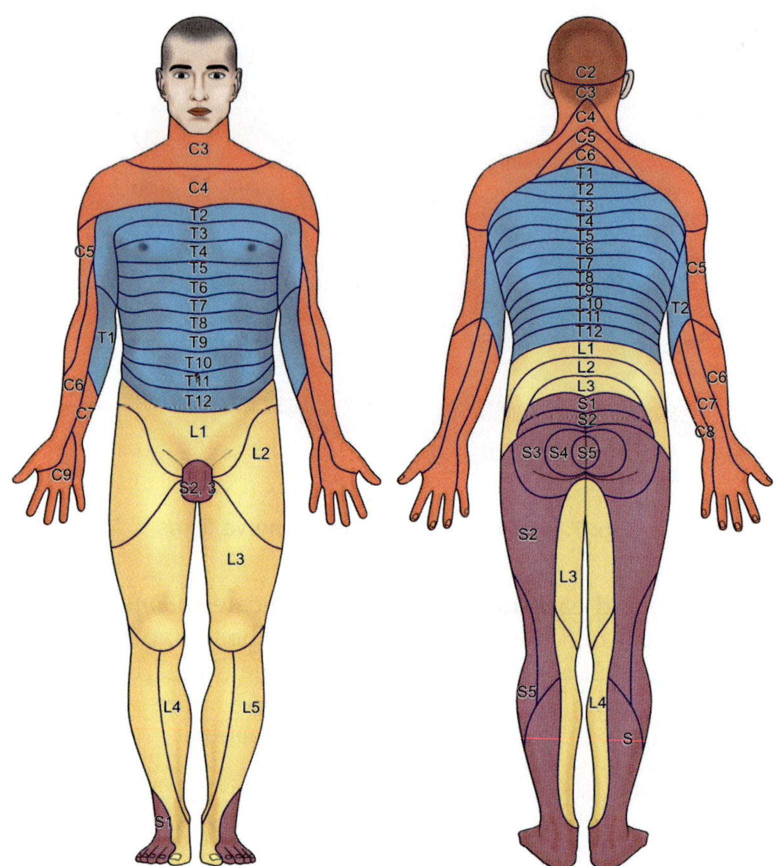

Fig. 7.11: Dermatomes: (a) Anterior aspect, and (b) posterior aspect

The nerve emerges through the intervertebral foramen, gives off recurrent meningeal branches, and then divides immediately into a *dorsal* and a *ventral ramus*.

The *dorsal ramus* passes backwards and supplies the intrinsic muscles of the back, and the skin covering them.

The *ventral ramus* is connected with the sympathetic ganglion, and is distributed to the limb or the anterolateral body wall.

In case of a typical (thoracic) spinal nerve, the ventral ramus does not mix with neighbouring rami, and gives off several muscular branches, a lateral cutaneous branch, and an anterior cutaneous branch. However, the ventral rami of other spinal nerves are plaited to form the nerve plexuses for the limbs, like the brachial plexus, lumbar plexus, etc.

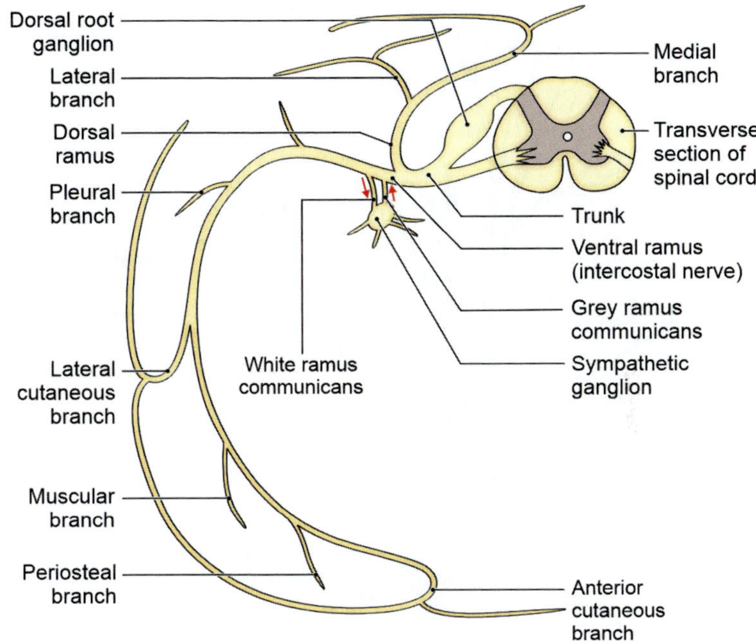

Fig. 7.12: Course of typical thoracic nerve

Nerve Plexuses for Limbs

All nerve plexuses are formed only by the ventral rami, and never by the dorsal rami.

These supply the limbs.

Against each plexus the spinal cord is enlarged, e.g. 'cervical enlargement' for the brachial plexus, and 'lumbar enlargement' for the lumbosacral plexus. Plexus formation resembles a tree (Fig. 7.13).

Various nerve plexuses are:

Cervical: Formed by C1, C2, C3 and C4 ventral primary rami.

Brachial: Formed by C5, C6, C7, C8 and T1 ventral primary rami.

Lumbar: Formed by L1, L2, L3 and part of L4 ventral primary rami.

Sacral plexus: Formed by part of L4, L5, S1, S2 and S3 ventral primary rami.

Each nerve root of the plexus (ventral ramus) divides into a ventral and a dorsal division.

The ventral division supplies the flexor compartment, and the dorsal division, the extensor compartment, of the limb.

The flexor compartment has a richer nerve supply than the extensor compartment. The flexor skin is more sensitive than

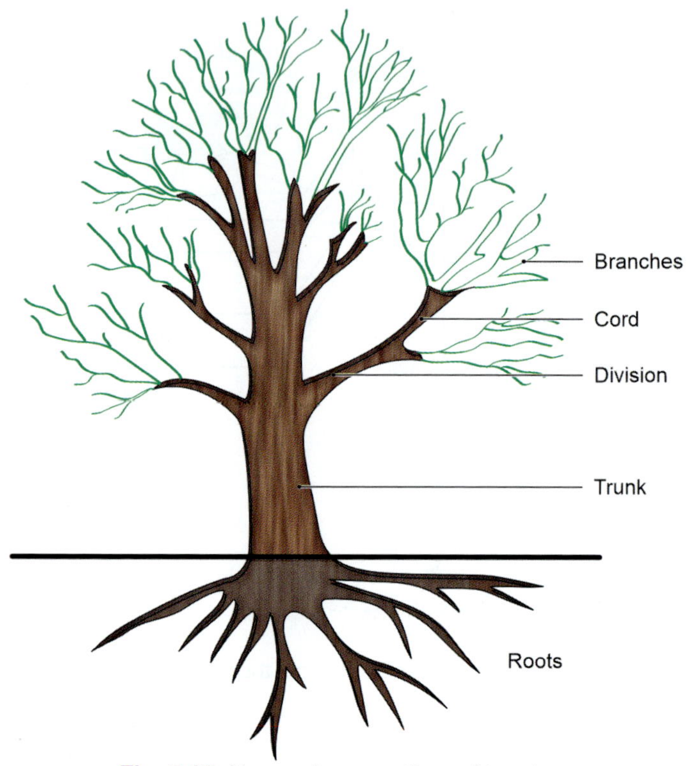

Fig. 7.13: Nerve plexuses likened to a tree

the extensor skin, and the flexor muscles (antigravity, bulkier muscles) are more efficient and are under a more precise control than the coarse extensor muscles.

The plexus formation (Fig. 7.14) is a physiological or functional adaptation, and is perhaps the result of the following special features in the limbs.

1. Overlapping of dermatomes
2. Overlapping of myotomes
3. Composite nature of muscles
4. Possible migration of muscles from the trunk to the limbs
5. Linkage of the opposite groups of muscles in the spinal cord for reciprocal innervation.

Blood and Nerve Supply of Peripheral Nerves

The peripheral nerves are supplied by vessels, called vasa nervorum, which form longitudinal anastomoses on the surface of the nerves.

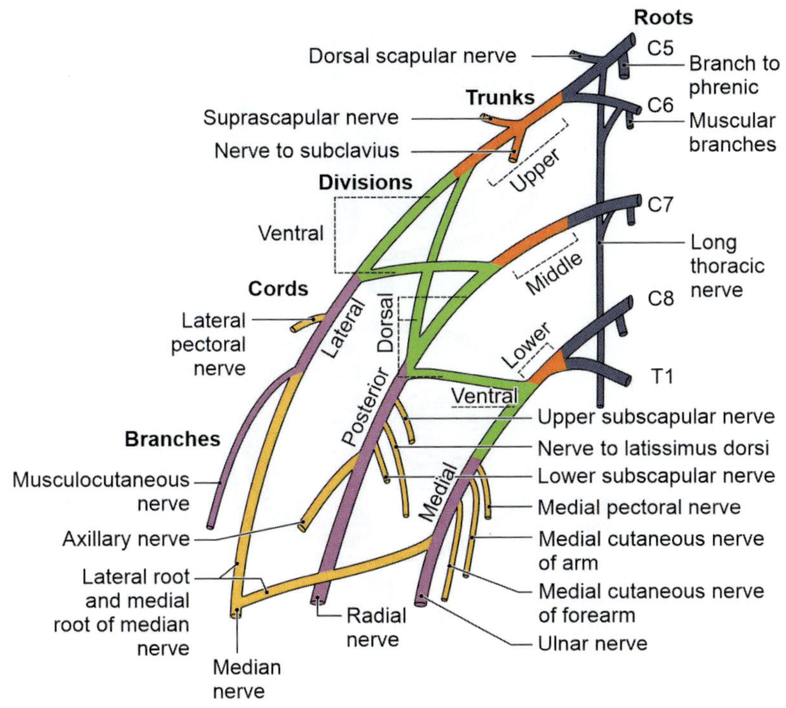

Fig. 7.14: Brachial plexus

The nerves distributed to the sheaths of the nerve trunks are called nervi nervorum.

NERVE FIBRES

Each motor nerve fibre is an axon with its coverings.

Larger axons are covered by a myelin sheath and are termed *myelinated* or *medullated fibres* (Fig. 7.15a).

The fatty nature of myelin is responsible for the glistening whiteness of the peripheral nerve trunks and white matter of the CNS.

Thinner axons, of less than one micron diameter, have thin layers of myelin sheath and are therefore termed *nonmyelinated* or *nonmedullated* (Fig. 7.15b).

However, all the fibres whether myelinated or nonmyelinated have a *neurolemmal* sheath, which is uniformly absent in the tracts. In peripheral nerves, both the myelin and neurolemmal sheaths are derived from Schwann cells.

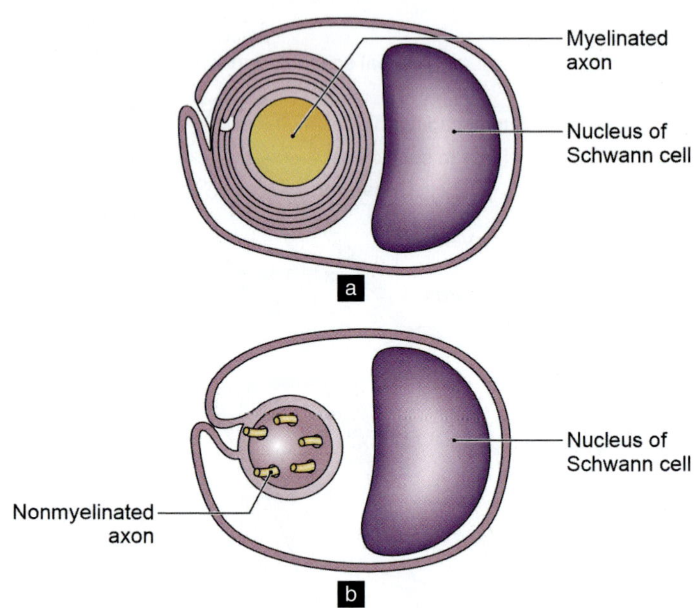

Fig. 7.15: (a) Myelinated, and (b) nonmyelinated axon

Myelinated Fibres

Myelinated fibres form the bulk of the somatic nerves. Structurally, they are made up of following parts from within outwards:

1. *Axis cylinder* forms the central core of the fibre. It consists of axoplasm covered by axolemma (Fig. 7.16).
2. *Myelin sheath*, derived from Schwann cells, surrounds the axis cylinder. It is made up of alternate concentric layers of lipids and proteins formed by spiralization of the mesaxon; the lipids include cholesterol, glycolipids and phospholipids.

   Myelin sheath is interrupted at regular intervals called the *nodes of Ranvier* where the adjacent Schwann cells meet.

   Collateral branches of the axon arise at the nodes of Ranvier.

   Thicker axons possess a thicker coat of myelin and longer internodes.

   Each *internode* is myelinated by one Schwann cell. Oblique clefts in the myelin, called *incisures of Schmidt Lantermann*, provide conduction channels for metabolites into the depth of the myelin and to the subjacent axon.

   Myelin sheath acts as an insulator for the nerve fibres.
3. *Neurolemmal sheath* (sheath of Schwann) surrounds the myelin sheath.

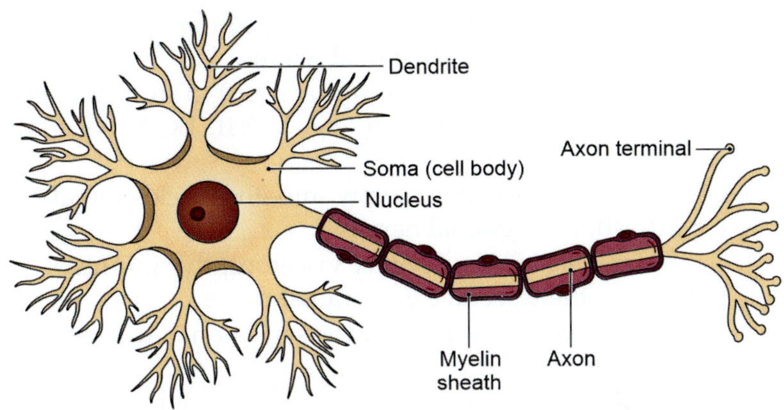

Fig. 7.16: Neuron and the formation of a peripheral motor nerve

It represents the plasma membrane (basal lamina) of the Schwann cell.

Beneath the membrane there lies a thin layer of cytoplasm with the nucleus of the Schwann cell.

The sheaths of two cells interdigitate at the nodes of Ranvier. Neurolemmal sheath is necessary for regeneration of a damaged nerve.

Tracts do not regenerate because of absence of neurolemmal sheath.

4. *Endoneurium* is a delicate connective tissue sheath which surrounds the neurolemmal sheath.

Nonmyelinated Fibres

Nonmyelinated fibres comprise the smaller axons of the CNS, in addition to peripheral postganglionic autonomic fibres, several types of fine sensory fibres (C fibres of skin, muscle and viscera), olfactory nerves, etc. Structurally, a 'nonmyelinated fibre' consists of a group of small axons (0.12–2 microns diameter) that have invaginated separately a single Schwann cell (in series) without any spiralling of the mesaxon (Fig. 7.15). The endoneurium, instead of ensheathing individual axons, surrounds all the neurolemmal sheath by virtue of which the nonmyelinated fibres, like the myelinated fibres, can regenerate after damage.

Classification of Peripheral Nerve Fibres

A. *According to their function*, the cranial nerves have the following nuclear columns:

1. *General somatic efferent* to supply striated muscles of somatic origin, e.g. III, IV, VI, XII cranial nerves.
2. *Special visceral efferent* (*branchial efferent*) to supply striated muscles of branchial origin, e.g. V, VII, IX, X, XI cranial nerves.
3. *General visceral efferent* to supply smooth muscles and glands, e.g. III, VII, IX, X cranial nerves.
4. *General visceral afferent* to carry visceroceptive impulses (like pain) from the viscera, e.g. X cranial nerve.
5. *Special visceral afferent* to carry the sensation of taste, e.g. VII, IX, X cranial nerves.
6. *General somatic afferent* to carry exteroceptive impulses from the skin of face and proprioceptive impulses from the muscles, tendons and joints (Fig. 7.17a and b), e.g. V cranial nerve.

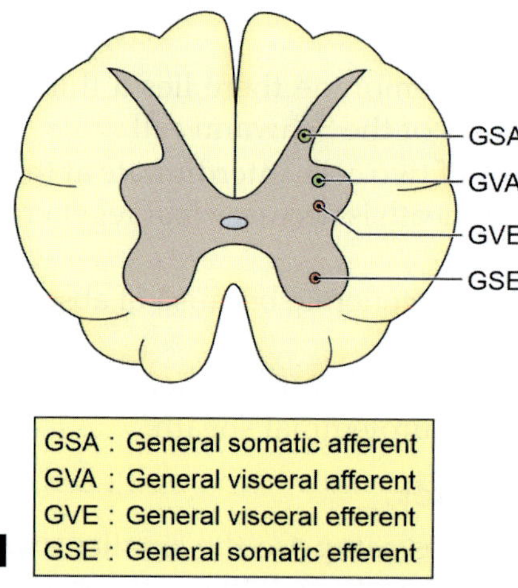

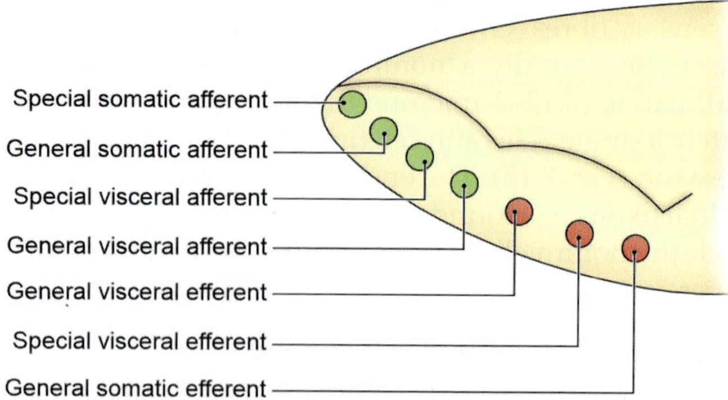

Fig. 7.17: Nuclear columns of (a) spinal cord, and (b) medulla oblongata

7. *Special somatic afferent* to carry the sensations of hearing and equilibrium, e.g. VIII cranial nerve.

B. ***According to their size and speed of conduction***, the nerve fibres are divided into three categories, namely A, B and C. These have been compared in Table 7.3.

Table 7.4 shows the summary of cranial nerves.

Table 7.3: Comparison of types of nerve fibres

Group A fibre	*Group B fibre*	*Group C fibre*
1. Thickest and fastest	Medium size	Thinnest and slowest
2. Myelinated	Myelinated	Non-myelinated
3. Diameter: 1.5–22 microns	Diameter: 1.5–3.4 microns	Diameter: 0.1–0.2 microns
4. Speed: 4–120 metres/sec e.g. skeletomotor fibre, fusimotor fibre afferent to skin, muscles and tendons	Speed: 3–15 metres/sec, e.g. preganglionic autonomic efferents	Speed: 0.5–4 metres/sec, e.g. postganglionic autonomic efferents, afferent fibre to skin, muscle and viscera
5. Fast conduction	Slow conduction	Very slow conduction

Table 7.4: Summary of the cranial nerves

Nerve	*Function*	*Details*
I. Olfactory	Smell	20 rootless, pass through root of nose to reach temporal lobe of brain
II. Optic	Vision	From the retina via optic chiasma and lateral geniculate body to the occipital lobe of brain
III. Oculomotor	Motor + para sympathetic	Supplies 4½ extraocular muscles. Also two sets of muscles which help in accommodation
IV. Trochlear	Motor	One muscle of eyeball (superior oblique)
V. Trigeminal	Sensory + motor	Most of the skin of face, nasal mucous membrane, conjunctiva; motor to muscles of mastication
VI. Abducent	Motor	Motor to one muscle of eye (lateral rectus)

(Contd.)

Table 7.4: Summary of the cranial nerves (*Contd.*)		
Nerve	*Function*	*Details*
VII. Facial	Motor + special sense + parasympathetic	Motor to muscles of the face those around eyes and mouth; taste from anterior 2/3rd of tongue; secretomotor to submandibular, lacrimal, nasal glands, etc.
VIII. Vestibulocochlear	Hearing and balance	Vestibular part for balancing the body and maintenance of posture; cochlear part for hearing, appreciated in temporal lobe
IX. Glossopharyngeal	Special sense + motor + parasympathetic	Taste from posterior 1/3rd of tongue, motor to one muscle of pharynx and secretory to parotid gland
X. Vagus + Cranial root of XI. Accessory	Motor + special sense + parasympathetic	Taste from posterior most part of tongue, motor to muscles of soft palate, pharynx, larynx, stomach and intestines and secretory to glands of respiratory and most part of digestive system
Spinal root	Motor	Motor to two important muscles of neck, i.e. sternocleidomastoid and trapezius
XII. Hypoglossal	Motor	To seven out of eight muscles of tongue

AUTONOMIC NERVOUS SYSTEM

Autonomic nervous system controls involuntary activities of the body, like sweating, salivation, peristalsis, etc. It differs fundamentally from the somatic nervous system in having:

a. Preganglionic fibres arising from the CNS
b. Ganglia for relay of the preganglionic fibres
c. Postganglionic fibres arising from the ganglia which supply the effectors (smooth muscles, cardiac muscles and glands).

In contrast, the somatic nerves after arising from the CNS reach their destination without any interruption (Fig. 7.1).

Autonomic nervous system is divided into two more or less complementary parts, the sympathetic and parasympathetic systems.

The sympathetic activities are widespread and diffuse, and combat the acute emergencies.

The parasympathetic activities are usually discrete and isolated, and provide a comfortable environment.

Both systems function in absolute coordination and adjust the body involuntarily to the given surroundings.

SYMPATHETIC NERVOUS SYSTEM

1. It is also known as '*thoracolumbar*' outflow because it arises from Tl to L2 segments of the spinal cord (Fig. 7.18).
2. The medullated preganglionic fibres (*white rami communicantes*) arise-from the lateral column of the spinal cord, emerge through the ventral rami where the white rami are connected to the ganglia of the sympathetic chain (Fig. 7.18). Sympathetic fibres hitch-hike along the spinal nerve.
3. Preganglionic fibres relay either in the *lateral ganglia* (sympathetic chain) or in the *collateral ganglia*, e.g. the coeliac ganglion. The nonmedullated postganglionic fibres (*grey rami communicantes*) run for some distance before reaching the organ of supply. The adrenal medulla is a unique exception in the body; it is supplied by the preganglionic fibres (Fig. 7.18).

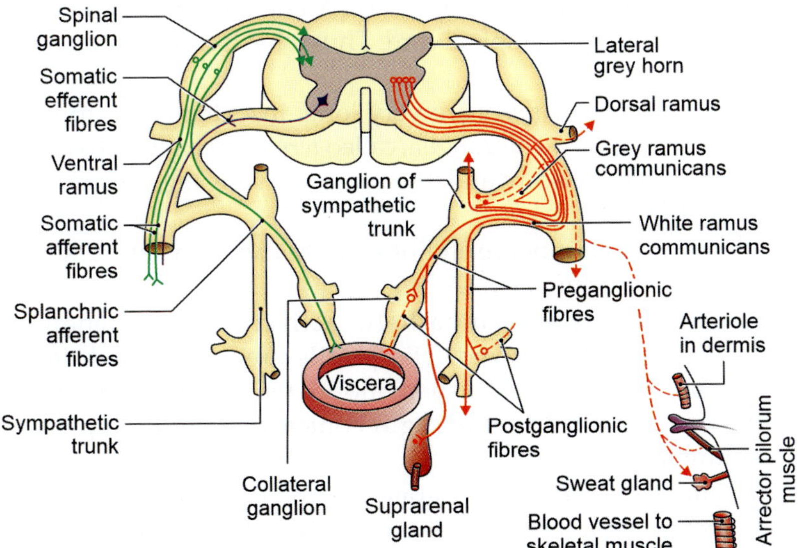

Fig. 7.18: Course of sympathetic fibres

4. Sympathetic nerve endings are *adrenergic* in nature, meaning thereby that noradrenalin is produced for neurotransmission. The only exception to this general rule are the cholinergic sympathetic nerves supplying the sweat glands and skeletal muscle vessels for vasodilatation.
5. *Functionally*, sympathetic nerves are vasomotor (vasoconstrictor), sudomotor (secretomotor to sweat glands), and pilomotor (contract the arrector pili and cause erection of hair) in the skin of limbs and body wall (Fig. 7.18). In addition, sympathetic activity causes dilation of pupil, pale face, dry mouth, tachycardia, rise in blood pressure, inhibition of hollow viscera, and closure of the perineal sphincters.

   The blood supply to the skeletal muscles, heart and brain is markedly increased.

Thus, sympathetic reactions tend to be 'mass reactions', widely diffused in their effect and that they are directed towards mobilization of the resources of the body for expenditure of energy in dealing with the emergencies or emotional crises (fright, fight, flight).

PARASYMPATHETIC NERVOUS SYSTEM

1. It is also known as *craniosacral outflow* because it arises from the brain (mixed with III, VII, IX and X cranial nerves) and sacral 2–4 segments of the spinal cord. Thus it has a cranial and a sacral part.
2. The *preganglionic fibres* are very long, reaching right up to the viscera of supply. The ganglia, called *terminal ganglia*, are situated mostly on the viscera and, therefore, the *postganglionic fibres* are very short.
3. Parasympathetic nerve endings are *cholinergic* in nature, similar to the somatic nerves.
4. *Functionally*, parasympathetic activity is seen when the subject is fully relaxed. His pupils are constricted, lenses accommodated, face flushed, mouth moist, pulse slow, blood pressure low, bladder and gut contracting, and the perineal sphincters relaxed.

In general the effects of parasympathetic activity are usually discrete and isolated, and directed towards conservation and restoration of the resources of energy in the body.

ANS can be studied from *Appendices 2 of volumes 1 and 2, and Appendix of volume 3 of BD Chaurasia's Human Anatomy, 9th edition.*

Table 7.5 shows the comparison between the two divisions of autonomic nervous system.

Table 7.5: Comparison of sympathetic and parasympathetic nervous systems

Sympathetic nervous system	*Parasympathetic nervous system*
All neurons forming this system originate from T_1 to L_2 segment of spinal cord. So it is called "thoraco-lumbar outflow"	All neurons forming this system originate from brain (III, VII, IX, X cranial nerves) and S2–S4 segment of spinal cord. So it is called "cranio sacral outflow"
Preganglionic fibres are short, relay either in lateral ganglia or collateral ganglia (Fig. 7.19) or adrenal medulla Post-ganglionic fibres are long	Preganglionic fibres are very long reaching up to terminal ganglia mostly on viscera Postganglionic fibres are short (Fig. 7.20)
Nerve endings are adrenergic in nature except in sweat gland and skeletal muscle fibres	Nerve endings are cholinergic in nature
Functionally, sympathetic nerves are vasomotor, sudomotor and pilomotor to skin. It is seen when subject is in fear, fight and flight position. It dilates skeletal muscle blood vessels	Functionally, it is seen when subject is fully relaxed. Parasympathetic system has no effect on skin
Effect is widely diffused and directed towards mobilization of resources and expenditure of energy during emergency and emotional crisis	Effect is discrete, isolated, directed towards conservation and restoration of the resources of energy in the body
It supplies visceral blood vessels, and skin.	It only supplies viscera (Fig. 7.20)
Viscera usually have low amount of sensory output, whereas skin is an area of high amount of sensory output. So pain arising from low sensory output area is projected as coming from high sensory output area. This is the basis of *referred pain*	

Neurotransmitters

Following neurotransmitters are released at various autonomic nerve endings:

- ***Preganglionic parasympathetic:*** Acetylcholine
- ***Preganglionic sympathetic:*** Acetylcholine
- ***Postganglionic parasympathetic:*** Acetylcholine
- ***Postganglionic sympathetic:*** Norepinephrine except those supplying arrector pili muscles and sweat glands which release acetylcholine.

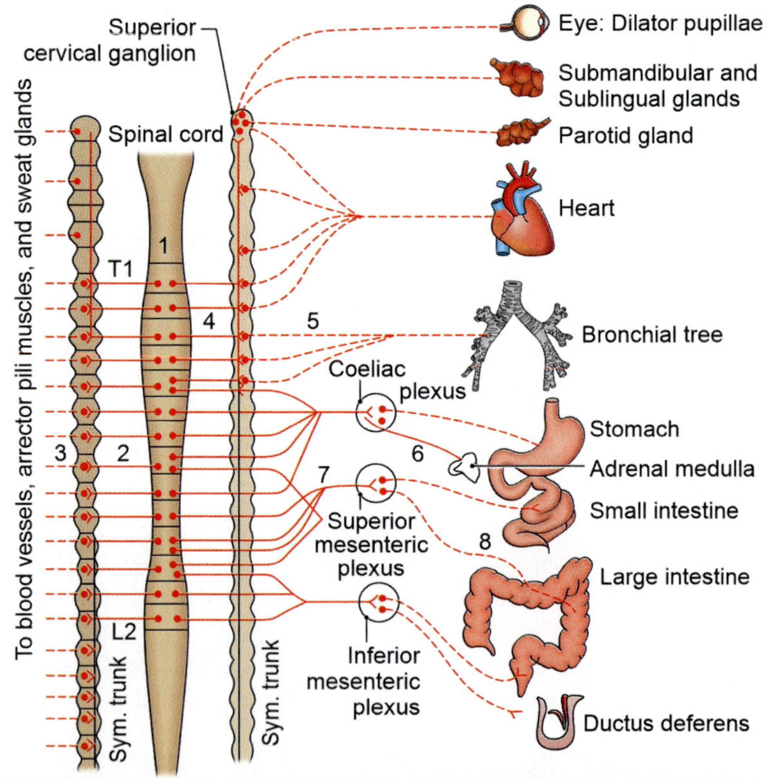

1. Spinal cord, T1 to L2 segments of spinal cord; 2. White ramus communicans to sympathetic ganglia; 3. Grey ramus communicans to structures in skin; 4. Preganglionic fibres for thoracic viscera; 5. Postganglionic fibres for thoracic viscera; 6. Preganglionic fibres for adrenal medulla 7. Preganglionic fibres for abdominal and pelvic viscera; 8. Long post-ganglionic fibres for abdominal and pelvic viscera

Fig. 7.19: Distribution of sympathetic nervous system

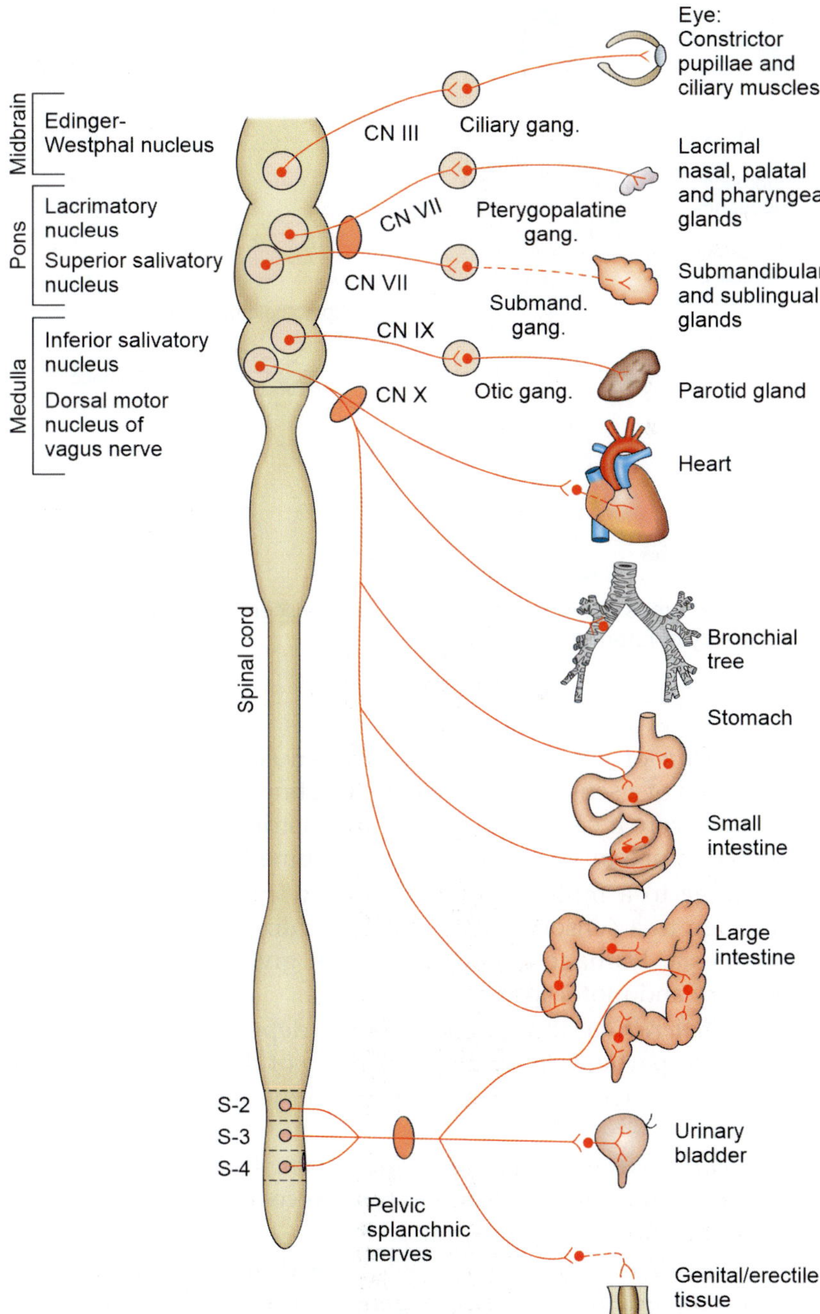

Fig. 7.20: Distribution of parasympathetic nervous system

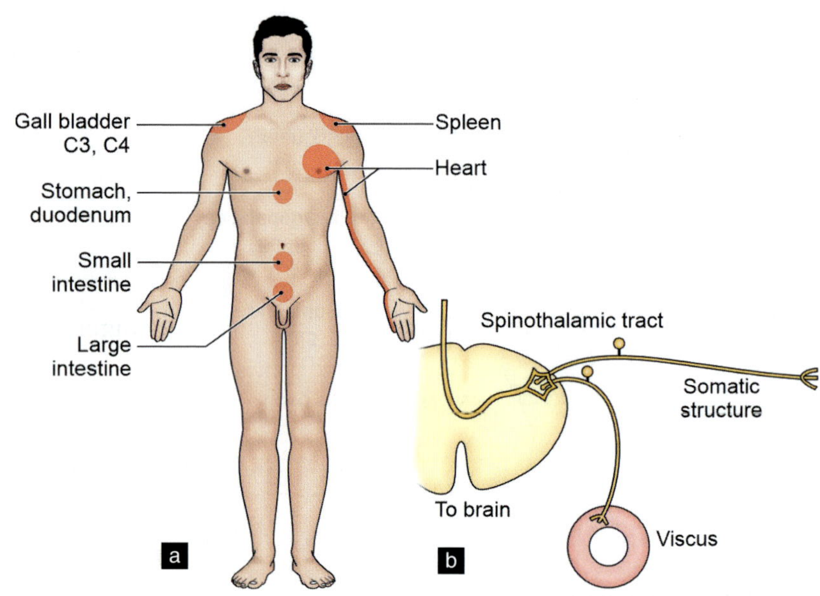

Fig. 7.21: (a) Areas of skin where referred pain of viscera is felt, and (b) convergence theory of referred pain

Clinical Anatomy of Nervous System

- ***Irritation*** of a motor nerve causes muscular spasm. Mild irritation of a sensory nerve causes tingling and numbness, but when severe it causes pain along the distribution of the nerve. Irritation of a mixed nerve causes combined effects.
- ***Damage*** to a motor nerve causes muscular paralysis, and damage to a sensory nerve causes localized anaesthesia and analgesia. Damage to a mixed nerve gives rise to both the sensory and motor losses.

  Regeneration of a damaged nerve depends on the degree of injury, particularly on the continuity of the nerve. Different degrees of nerve injury are expressed by the following three terms.

  a. *Neuropraxia* is a minimal lesion causing transient functional block without any degeneration. Recovery is spontaneous and complete, e.g. sleeping foot.
  b. *Axonotmesis* is a lesion where, although continuity is preserved, true Wallerian degeneration occurs. Regeneration takes place in due course.

7

c. *Neurotmesis* is the complete division of a nerve. For regeneration to occur the cut ends must be sutured (Fig. 7.22).

- Severe pain along the distribution of a nerve is called neuralgia. Inflammation of a nerve is marked by neuralgia with sensory and motor deficits, and is called neuritis.
- ***Denervation*** of a part produces *trophic changes*. The skin becomes dry (no sweating), smooth (loss of hair) and glazed; trophic ulcers may develop which do not heal easily. In patients with leprosy, repeated painless injuries to the tips of the fingers and toes makes them worn out and blunted.

  A joint after denervation becomes a *neuropathic* (*Charcot's*) *joint*, which shows painless swelling, excessive mobility and bony destruction. The common medical diseases associated with trophic changes are leprosy, tabes dorsalis, and syringomyelia. The bedsores in paralysed patients are examples of the trophic ulcers. In general the ulcers and wounds in the denervated skin do not heal easily (Fig. 7.23).
- ***Neuropathies*** is a group of diseases of peripheral nerves. It is of two types:
  - *Polyneuropathy:* Several neurons are affected and usually long neurons like those supplying the feet and legs are affected first. This occurs mostly due to nutritional deficiencies (folic

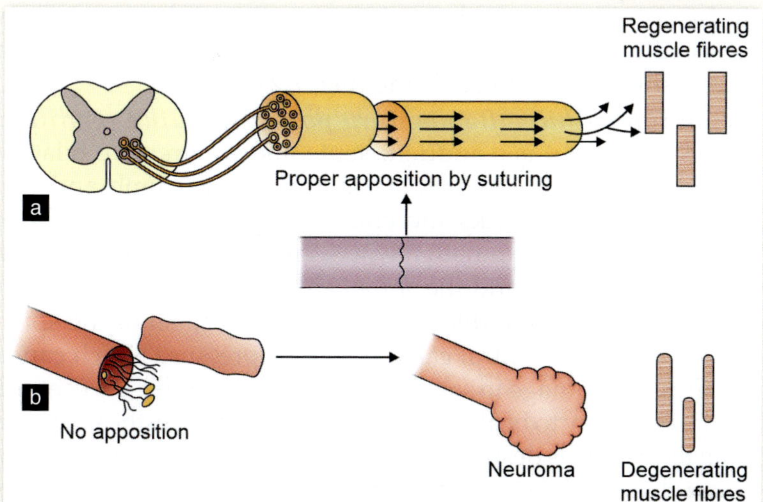

Fig. 7.22: (a) Effect of proper apposition of cut ends, and (b) no apposition of cut ends of nerves leading to degenerating muscle fibres

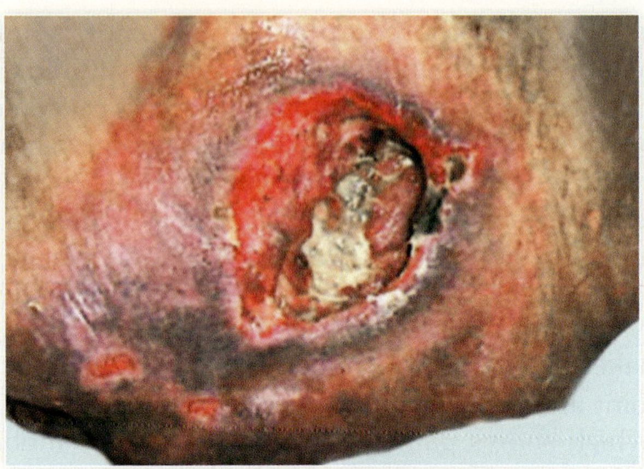

Fig. 7.23: Bedsore

acid and vitamin B), metabolic disorders (diabetes mellitus), chronic diseases (renal and hepatic failure and carcinoma), infections (influenza, measles and typhoid fever) and toxic reactions (arsenic, lead, mercury and carbon tetrachloride).

– *Mononeuropathy:* Usually one neuron is affected and most common cause is ischaemia due to pressure. The resultant dysfunction depends on site and degree of injury.

- ***Bell's palsy*** is the compression of a facial nerve in or just outside stylomastoid foramen due to inflammation and oedema of the nerve. This causes paralysis of facial muscles and loss of facial expression on the affected side (Fig. 7.24).
- ***Acute idiopathic inflammatory polyneuropathy (Guillain-Barré syndrome)*** is a sudden, acute and progressive bilateral ascending paralysis which starts at the lower limb and then spreads to arms, trunks and cranial nerves. It is characterized by widespread inflammation with some demyelination of spinal and cranial nerves and the spinal ganglia.
- ***Syringomyelia*** is the dilation of the central canal of the spinal cord. Dilation of central canal develops pressure which causes progressive damage to sensory and motor neurons. Early effects are insensibility to heat and pain (dissociated anaesthesia) and in long term there is destruction of motor and sensory tracts leading to paralysis and loss of sensations and reflexes. This occurs most commonly in the cervical region and is associated with congenital abnormality of the distal end of the fourth ventricle.

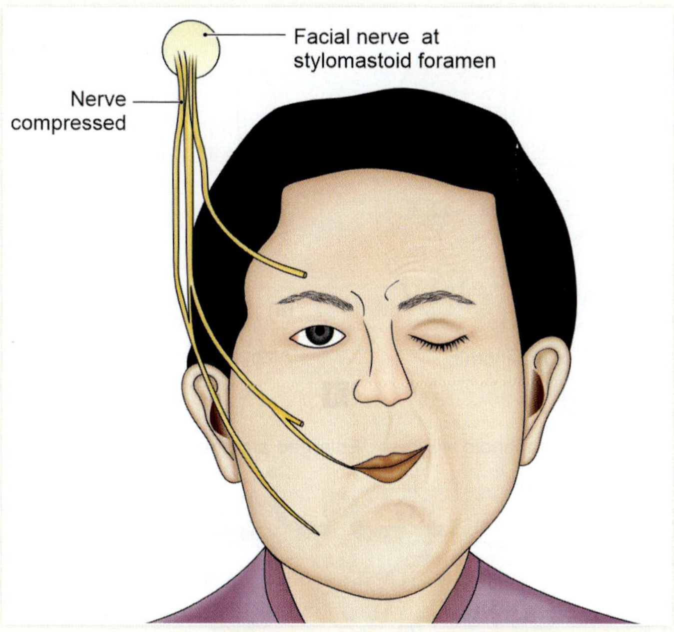

Fig. 7.24: Bell's palsy on right half of the face, no wrinkling of forehead, eye remains open, nasolabial fold obliterated, lowered angle of mouth

- ***Ageing:*** Usually after 60–70 years or so there are changes in the brain. These are:
  a. Prominence of sulci due to cortical shrinkage.
  b. The gyri get narrow and sulci get broad.
  c. The subarachnoid space becomes wider.
  d. There is enlargement of the ventricles.
- ***Dementia:*** In this condition, there is slow and progressive loss of memory, intellect and personality. The consciousness of the subject is normal. Dementia usually occurs due to Alzheimer's disease.
- ***Alzheimer's disease:*** The changes of normal ageing are pronounced in the parietal lobe, temporal lobe, and in the hippocampus (Fig. 7.25a and b).
- ***Infections of brain:*** (a) Bacterial, (b) Viral, (c) Miscellaneous types.
  a. **Bacterial** (through blood) may cause meningitis or brain abscess. Otitis media may cause meningitis or temporal lobe

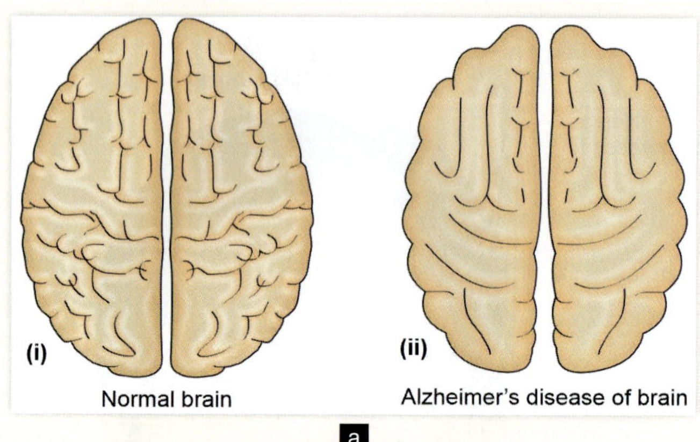

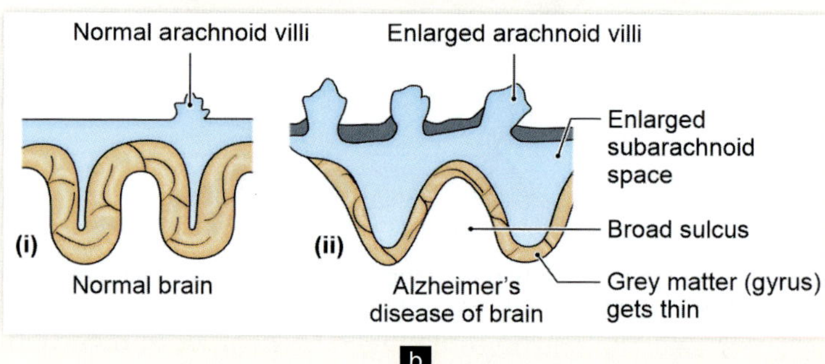

Fig. 7.25: (a) (i)Normal brain and (ii) Alzheimer's disease of brain, (b) (i) Normal arachnoid villi and (ii) Arachnoid villi in Alzheimer's disease

abscess. Tuberculosis: TB meningitis is due to blood-borne infection.

b. **Viral infections:** Most viruses enter the body through blood. Viruses may cause meningitis or encephalitis.

Herpes simplex virus and encephalitis: This virus usually causes vesicles at angles of the mouth and alae of the nose, following cold or any other disease. In some cases it may cause encephalitis.

Chickenpox: The varicella zoster virus (V2V) initially causes *chickenpox*. This virus persists in latent form in dorsal root ganglia of spinal nerves.

Herpes zoster is seen in elderly and younger patients with immune deficiency. It presents as a vesicular rash affecting one or more dermatomes. This condition is very painful

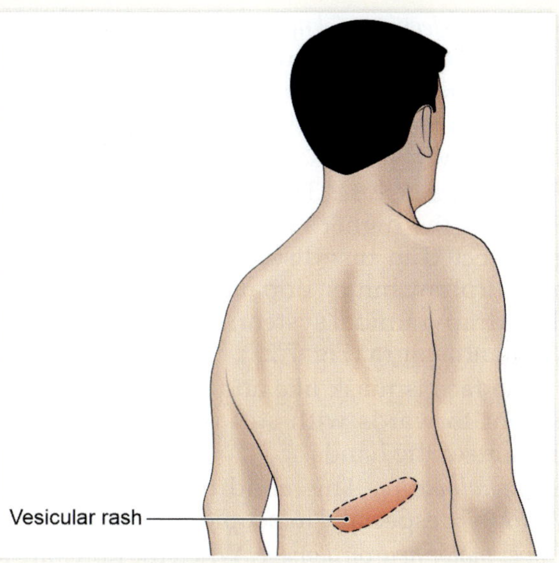

Fig. 7.26: Rash in herpes zoster

(Fig. 7.26). Thoracic dermatomes are mostly affected. It may affect ophthalmic branch of trigeminal nerve as well. Vesicles appear on cornea and it may lead to blindness. If geniculate ganglion of VII nerve is affected, it may cause Ramsay Hunt syndrome of VII nerve palsy. In this syndrome ipsilateral side taste is lost, with buccal ulceration and rash in external auditory meatus. It may be mistaken for Bell's palsy.

Poliomyelitis: The virus has attraction for anterior (motor) horn cells, especially of the spinal cord which get damaged. The nerves arising from these neurons get affected resulting in paresis or paralysis. There may be partial or complete recovery. Under Polio Eradication Programme, India has been declared "polio free" in March 2014—a great achievement.

c. **Miscellaneous types**, i.e. infestations and infections.
   1. *Fungal infections:* Primary infections of fungus of brain in healthy adults are rare. The fungus infections usually occur in AIDS (acquired immunodeficiency syndrome).
   2. *Protozoal infections:*
      - *Malaria:* Acute malaria by *P. falciparum* may cause cerebral malaria. It is very serious condition and may cause death unless treated well in time.

7

- *African sleeping sickness:* The tsetse fly transmits *T. brucei* infection in man resulting in meningoencephalitis.
- *Cysticercosis:* The larvae of tapeworm (*Taenia solium*) may form a cyst in the brain. This cyst may cause epilepsy.

3. *Parkinson's disease:* The extrapyramidal system which connects the higher centers and the anterior horn cells get affected in this disease. There is usually deficiency of neurotransmitter dopamine in the affected nuclei of the extrapyramidal system, including depigmentation of substantia nigra (Fig. 7.27).

   The face is mask like and expressionless, the posture is bent forwards with stiff pill-rolling movements and tremors of the hands.
4. *Encephalopathy:* This condition occurs due to lack of vitamin B, especially in people who are chronic alcoholics.
5. *Upper motor neuron damage:* When the fibres are interrupted from their cortical origin till these synapse with anterior

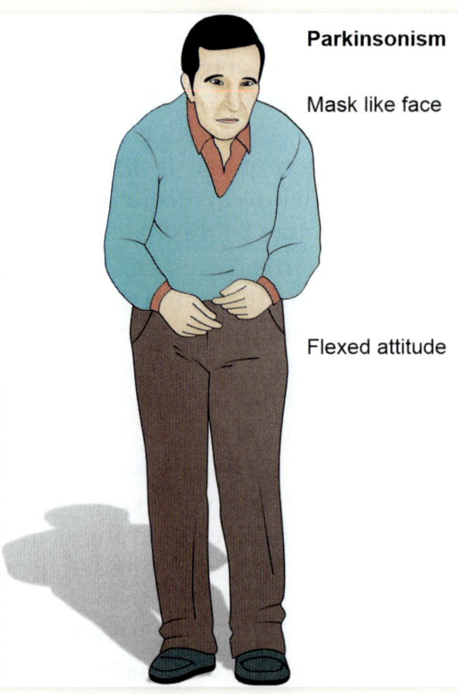

Fig. 7.27: Gait in parkinsonism

horn cells of the spinal cord, it is called upper motor neuron damage. The tendon jerks are exaggerated and the plantar reflex is of the extensor type.

6. *Lower motor neuron damage:* When the anterior horn cells (motor neurons) are affected, usually by poliomyelitis virus, there is paresis or paralysis of the muscles supplied by the nerves arising from the affected neurons. The affected muscles atrophy, and reflexes are absent.
7. *Leprosy:* There is chronic inflammation of the nerve sheaths. It is mostly associated with fibrosis and degeneration of the nerve fibres and autoamputation (Fig. 7.28).
8. *Epilepsy:* Epilepsy occurs in 1% population. There is focus of hyperexcitable neurons, which get induced by various types of stimuli, causing seizures. 25% cases of epilepsy are associated with some known disease, while 75% do not show any genetic influence.

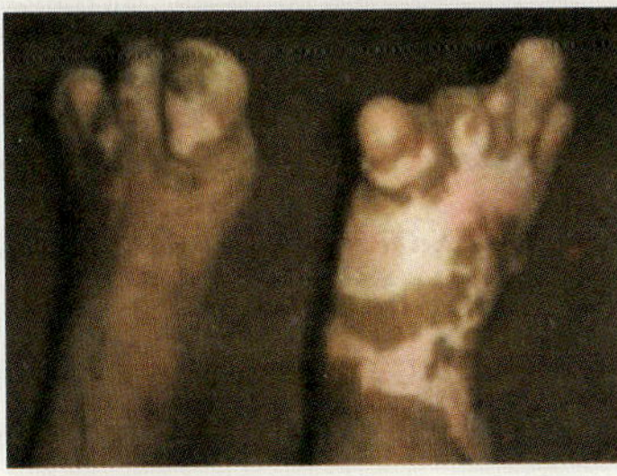

Fig. 7.28: Changes in leprosy

Points to Remember

- Neuron is the unit of nervous tissue.
- Neuron has only one axon while the dendrites are variable.
- At synapse there is only contiguity of cell membranes. There is no continuity of cytoplasm at the synapse.
- Astrocytes form part of "blood–brain barrier."
- Cervical (spinal) nerves are 8 while cervical vertebrae are 7 only.
- Coccygeal nerve is one while coccygeal vertebrae are 4.
- Limbs are mostly supplied by ventral primary rami of the spinal nerves.
- Endoneurium surrounds each nerve fibre, perineurium is around the nerve fascicle, epineurium is around the entire nerve.
- Nerve plexuses are only formed by ventral primary rami of the spinal nerves.

- Plexuses are cervical, brachial, lumbosacral and coccygeal.
- Sympathetic nervous system is thoracolumbar outflow.
- Parasymphathetic nervous system is craniosacral outflow.
- Sympathetic nervous system supplies the whole body from head to toes, while parasympathetic nerves only supply the viscera.
- Sympathetic is sudomotor, vasomotor and pilomotor to skin.
- Sympathetic is unsympathetic to the digestive system.
- Sympathetic nerves are mostly responsible for the referred pain.

Multiple Choice Questions

1. Number of spinal nerves in cervical region is:
a. 7 nerves b. 8 nerves c. 6 nerves d. 9 nerves

2. Axon has all features *except*:
a. Only one axon is present in a neuron
b. Branches of axon are fewer and at right angles to the axon
c. Axon forms effector component of the impulse
d. Axon contains Nissl granules

3. Bipolar neurons are present in:
a. Spiral ganglia
b. Vestibular ganglia
c. Olfactory cells
d. Neurons in posterior horn of spinal cord

4. Neuroglial cells are derived from neuroectoderm *except*:
a. Astrocytes b. Microglia
c. Oligodendrocytes d. Glioblasts

5. Blood–brain barrier is formed by following structures *except*:
a. Capillary endothelium without fenestrations
b. Basement membrane of the endothelium
c. End feet of astrocytes covering the capillary wall
d. Capillary endothelium with fenestrations

6. Reflex arc is made up of all parts *except*:
a. Receptors, e.g. skin b. Afferent neuron
c. Efferent neuron d. Gland

7. Supporting tissue around nerve fibres are following *except*:
a. Endoneurium b. Perineurium
c. Epineurium d. Epimysium

7

8. Nerve plexuses are only formed by:

a. Dorsal rami b. Ventral rami
c. Dorsal roots d. Ventral roots

9. Myelinated nerve fibres are formed by all components *except*:

a. Axis cylinder b. Myelin sheath
c. Neurilemmal sheath d. Epineurium

10. Cranial nerve nuclei belonging to general somatic efferent column are all *except*:

a. III nerve b. VI nerve c. XII nerve d. IX nerve

11. Nuclei of general visceral efferent column are all *except*:

a. Edinger Westphal b. Lacrimatory
c. Salivatory d. Nucleus ambiguus

12. Thoracolumbar outflow arises from lateral horns of one of the following segments of spinal cord:

a. T1 – L2 segments b. T1 – L1 segments
c. T1 – L1 segments d. T1 – S1 segments

13. Parasympathetic outflow does not arise from which of the following nerves:

a. III nerve b. VII nerve
c. XII nerve d. S2 – S4 nerves

14. Referred pain of myocardial ischemia is mostly felt at:

a. Precordium aspect of left upper limb
b. Lateral aspect of left upper limb
c. Right shoulder region
d. Left shoulder region

Answers

1. b **2.** d **3.** d **4.** b **5.** d **6.** d **7.** d **8.** b
9. d **10.** d **11.** d **12.** a **13.** c **14.** a

Chapter 8

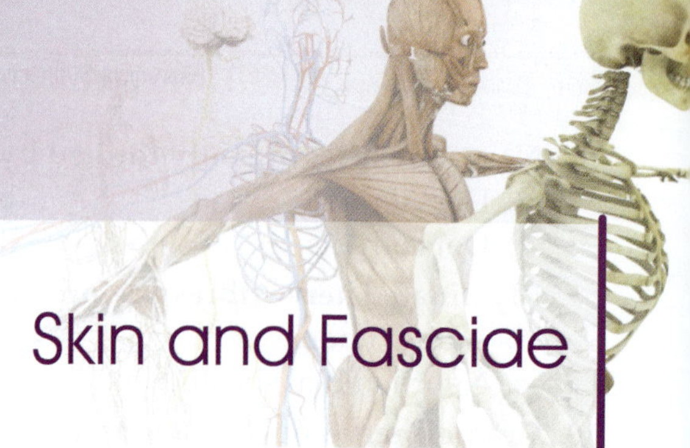

Skin and Fasciae

"Winners don't do different things. They do things differently." **—William James**

SKIN

Synonyms

1. Cutis (L); 2. Derma (G); 3. Integument. Compare with the terms cutaneous, dermatology and dermatomes.

Definition

Skin is the general covering of the entire external surface of the body, including the external auditory meatus and the outer surface of tympanic membrane.

It is continuous with the mucous membrane at the orifices of the body.

Because of a large number of its functions, the skin is regarded as an important organ of the body (Fig. 8.1).

SURFACE AREA

In an adult the surface area of the skin is 1.5–2 (average 1.7) sq. metres. In order to assess the area involved in burns, one can follow the rule of nine: Head and neck 9%; each upper limb 9%; the front of the trunk 18%; the back of the trunk (including buttocks) 18%; each lower limb 18%; and perineum 1% (Fig. 8.2a). The percentage of area in a child is shown in Fig. 8.2b.

The surface area of an individual can be calculated by Du Bois formula. Thus, $A = W \times H \times 71.84$, where A = surface area in sq. cm, W = weight in kg, and H = height in cm.

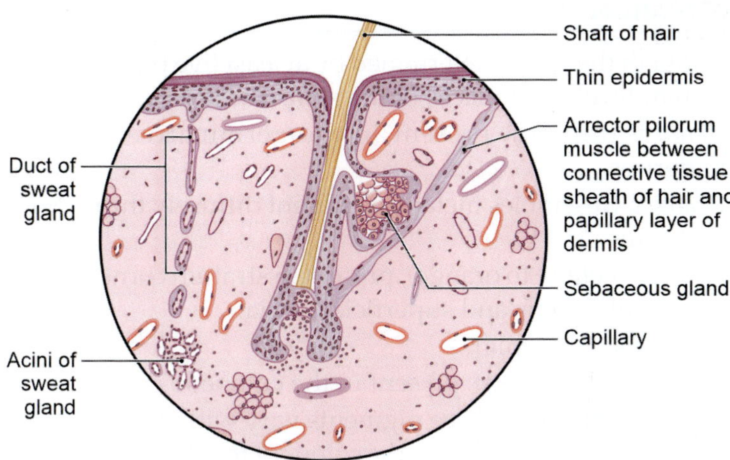

Fig. 8.1: Histological structure of thin skin

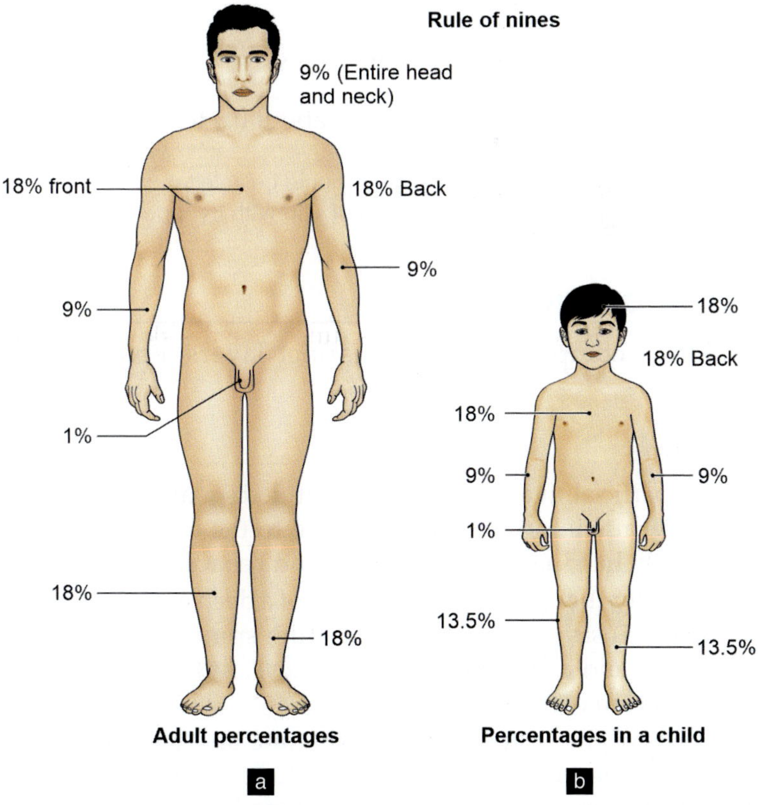

Rule of nines

9% (Entire head and neck)

18% front

18% Back

9%

9%

1%

18%

18%

18%

18% Back

18%

9%

9%

1%

13.5%

13.5%

Adult percentages

Percentages in a child

a

b

Fig. 8.2: Percentages of area in burn: (a) Adult, and (b) child

PIGMENTATION OF SKIN

The colour of the skin is determined by at least five pigments present at different levels and places of the skin. These are:

1. *Melanin* (brown), present in the germinative zone of the epidermis.
2. *Melanoid* (resembles melanin), present diffusely throughout the epidermis.
3. *Carotene* (yellow to orange), present in stratum corneum and the fat cells of dermis and superficial fascia.
4. *Haemoglobin* (purple).
5. *Oxyhaemoglobin* (red), present in the cutaneous vessels.

The amounts of first three pigments vary with the race, age, and part of the body. In white races, the colour of the skin depends chiefly on the vascularity of the dermis and thickness (translucency) of the keratin. The colour is red where keratin is thin (lips), and it is white where keratin is thick (palms and soles).

Thickness

The thickness of the skin varies from about 0.5 to 3 mm.

> *Competency achievement:* The student should be able to:
> AN 4.2 Describe structure and function of skin with its appendages

STRUCTURE OF SKIN

The skin is composed of two distinct layers, epidermis and dermis.

A. Epidermis

It is the superficial, avascular layer of stratified squamous epithelium. It is ectodermal in origin and gives rise to the appendages of the skin, namely hair, nails, sweat glands and sebaceous glands.

Structurally, the epidermis is made up of a deep **germinative zone**, comprising (i) stratum basale, (ii) stratum spinosum, (iii) stratum granulosum and a superficial *cornified zone*, (iv) stratum lucidum, and (v) stratum corneum.

The cells of the deepest layer proliferate and pass towards the surface to replace the cornified cells lost due to wear and tear. As the cells migrate superficially, they become more and more flattened, and lose their nuclei to form the flattened dead cells of the stratum corneum.

In the germinative zone, there are (i) 'dopa' positive melanocytes (melanoblasts, dendritic cells, or clear cells) of neural crest origin, which synthesize melanin. (ii) Langerhans cells which are phagocytic in nature. (iii) Merkel's cells which are sensory receptor cells in stratum basale.

B. Dermis or Corium

Dermis or corium is the deep, vascular layer of the skin, derived from mesoderm.

It is made up of connective tissue (with variable elastic fibres) mixed with blood vessels, lymphatics and nerves. The connective tissue is arranged into a superficial *papillary layer* and a deep *reticular layer*.

The papillary layer forms conical, blunt projections (dermal papillae) which fit into reciprocal depressions on the undersurface of the epidermis. The reticular layer is composed chiefly of the white fibrous tissue arranged mostly in parallel bundles.

The direction of the bundles, constituting flexure or *cleavage lines* (Langer's lines), is longitudinal in the limbs and horizontal in the trunk and neck (Fig. 8.3).

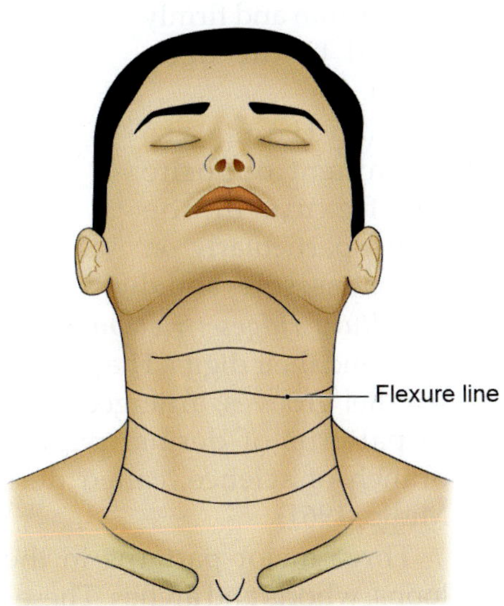

Fig. 8.3: Flexure/Langer's lines

In old age the elastic fibres atrophy and the skin becomes wrinkled. Overstretching of the skin may lead to rupture of the fibres, followed by scar formation. These scars appear as white streaks on the skin (e.g. linea gravidarum).

At the *flexure lines* of the joints, the skin is firmly adherent to the underlying deep fascia. Dermis is the real skin, because, when dried it makes green hide, and when tanned it makes leather. Its deep surface is continuous with the superficial fascia.

SURFACE IRREGULARITIES OF THE SKIN

The skin is marked by three types of surface irregularities, the tension lines, flexure lines and papillary ridges (Montagna and Lobitz, 1964).

1. ***Tension lines:*** Form a network of linear furrows which divide the surface into polygonal or lozenge-shaped areas. These lines to some extent correspond to variations in the pattern of fibres in the dermis. These are seen clearly on dorsum of hand.
2. ***Flexure lines (skin creases or skin joints):*** Are certain permanent lines along which the skin folds during habitual movements (chiefly flexion) of the joints.

   The skin along these lines is thin and firmly bound to the deep fascia.

   The lines are prominent opposite the flexure of the joints, particularly on the palms, soles and digits (Fig. 8.4).

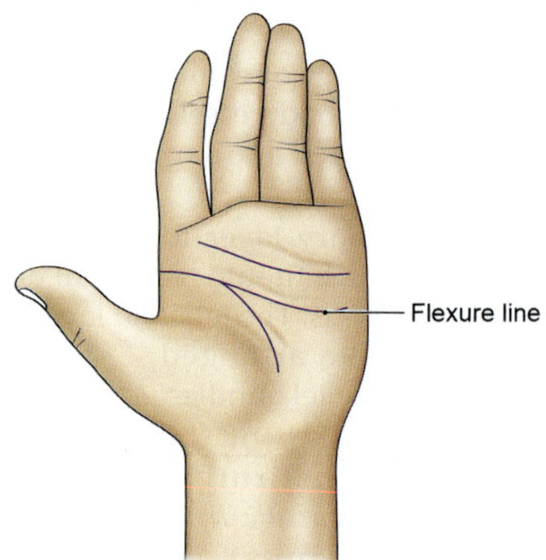

Fig. 8.4: Flexure lines in palm and digits

3. ***Papillary ridges (friction ridges):*** Are confined to palms and soles and their digits. They form narrow ridges separated by fine parallel grooves, arranged in curved arrays. They correspond to patterns of dermal papillae. Their study constitutes a branch of science, called dermatoglyphics (Cummins and Midlo, 1961).

   Three major patterns in the human fingerprints include loops, whorls and arches. These patterns and many other minor features are determined genetically by multifactorial inheritance (Fig. 8.5). These do not change throughout life, except to enlarge. This serves as a basis for identification through fingerprints or footprints.

Skin of palm and sole is thick, rest of the body has thin skin. Table 8.1 compares the two types of skin.

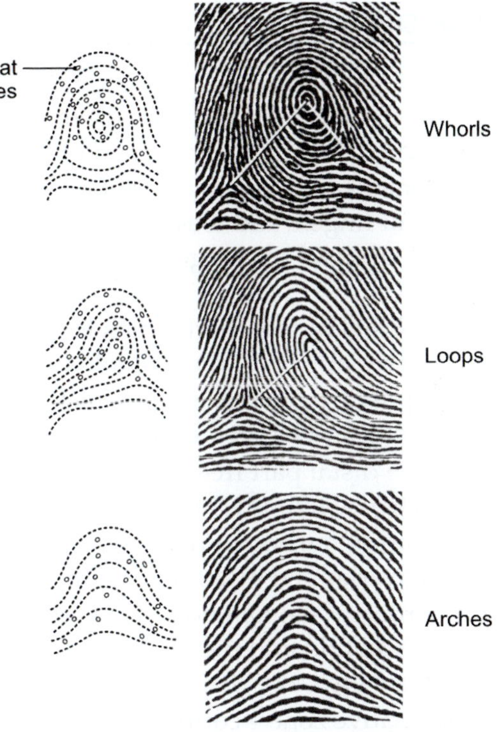

Fig. 8.5: Types of papillary ridges

Table 8.1: Comparison of thick and thin skin		
Features	*Thick skin*	*Thin skin*
Epidermal layers	Comprises 5 layers stratum basale stratum spinosum stratum granulosum stratum lucidum stratum corneum	Comprises 4 layers stratum basale stratum spinosum stratum granulosum stratum corneum
Epidermal ridges	Present	Absent
Sebaceous gland hair follicle and arrector pili muscle	Absent	Present
Sweat gland	Many	Few
Sensory receptors	Many	Few
Location	Palm and sole and palmar aspects of digits	All parts of body except palm, sole and palmar aspects of digits

APPENDAGES OF SKIN

1. Nails

Synonyms. (a) Onych or onycho (G); and (b) ungues (L). Compare with the terms paronychia, koilonychia and onychomycosis.

Nails are hardened keratin plates (cornified zone) on the dorsal surface of the tips of fingers and toes, acting as a rigid support for the digital pads of terminal phalanges. Each nail has the following parts.

a. *Root* is the proximal hidden part which is burried into the nail groove and is overlapped by the nail fold of the skin (Fig. 8.6).
b. *Body* is the exposed part of the nail which is adherent to the underlying skin; a and b together form *nail plate.*
c. *Free border* is the distal part free from the skin. It is attached to the under surface by hyponychium.

The proximal part of the body presents a white opaque crescent called *lunule*. It is overlapped by a fold of skin, the eponychium.

Each lateral border of the nail body is overlapped by a fold of a skin, termed the *nail* fold and the groove between nail body and nail fold is called *nail groove.*

The skin (germinative zone + corium) beneath the root and body of the nail is called *nail bed*. The germinative zone of the nail bed beneath the root and lunule is thick and proliferative (germinal matrix), and is responsible for the growth of the nail.

The rest of the nail bed is thin (sterile matrix) over which the growing nail glides.

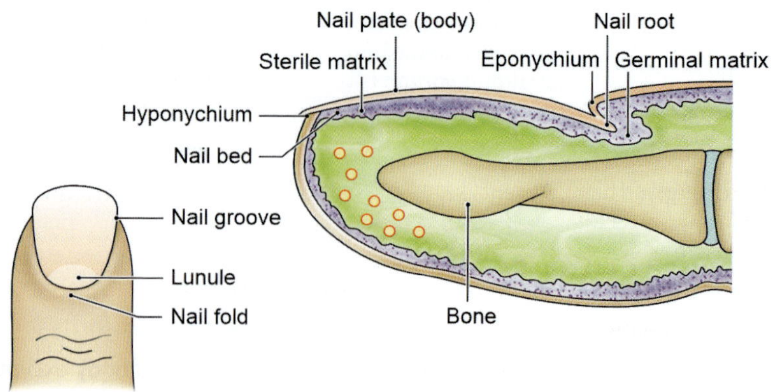

Fig. 8.6: Parts of a nail

Under the translucent body (except lunule) of the nail, the corium is very vascular. This accounts for their pink colour.

Nail of middle finger grows the fastest.

2. Hair

Hair are keratinous filaments derived from invaginations of the germinative layer of epidermis into the dermis.

These are peculiar to mammals (like feathers to the birds), and help in conservation of their body heat.

However, in man the heat loss is prevented by the cutaneous sensation of touch.

Hair are distributed all over the body, except for the palms, soles, dorsal surface of distal phalanges, umbilicus, glans penis, inner surface of prepuce, the labia minora, and inner surface of labia majora. The length, thickness and colour of the hair vary in different part of the body and in different individuals.

Structure of Hair

Each hair has an implanted part called the **root**, a **bulb** and a projecting part, called the **shaft**.

Layers of Shaft

Innermost is:

i. The medulla, comprising of cells with eleidin granules and air spaces.
ii. The cortex is the middle part made of elongated cells with melanin pigment.
iii. Cuticle is a single layer of flat keratinised cells.

The root is surrounded by a **hair follicle** (a sheath of epidermis and dermis), and is expanded at its proximal end to form the **hair bulb**. Each hair bulb is invaginated at its end by hair papilla (vascular connective tissue) which forms the neurovascular hilum of the hair and its sheath.

Hair follicle surrounds the hair. Wall of the follicle comprises: (i) Inner root sheath, (ii) outer root sheath and (iii) connective tissue sheath (Fig. 8.7).

i. Inner root sheath surrounds the beginning of the shaft. Its cells degenerate above the sebaceous gland.
ii. Outer root sheath is continuous with epidermal cells and it shows all the layers of epidermis.
iii. Connective tissue sheath is derived from the dermis.

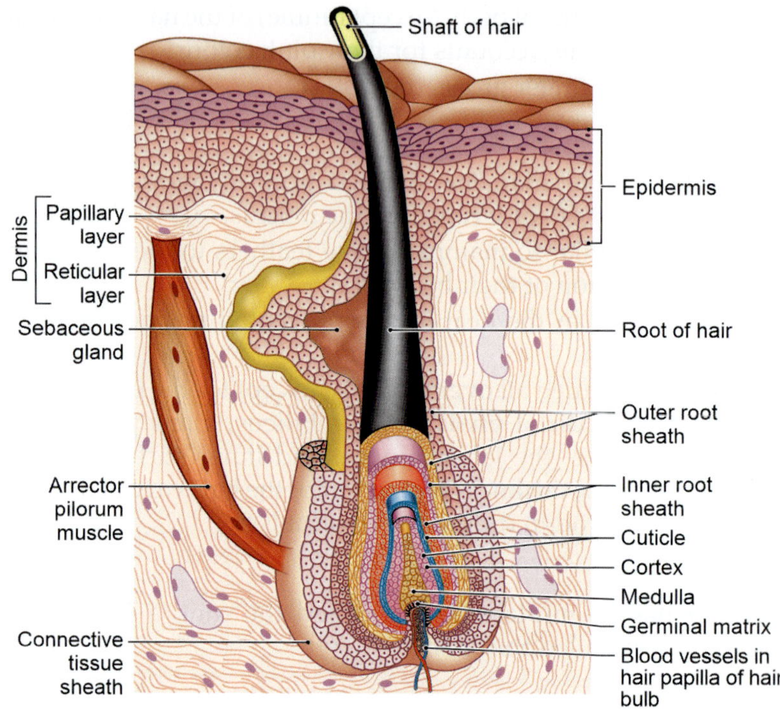

Fig. 8.7: Hair follice with arrector pilorum muscle

Hair grows at the hair bulb, by proliferation of its cells capping the papilla.

The hair follicles, enclosing hair roots lie obliquely to the surface of the skin, which is responsible for the characteristic hair streams in different parts of the body.

The arrectores pilorum muscles (smooth muscles supplied by sympathetic nerve) connect the undersurface of the follicles to the superficial part of the dermis. Arrector pili muscles are absent in a few regions like hair of face, axilla, eyelashes, eyebrows, hair of anterior nares and of external auditory meatus.

Development of Hair

The foetal skin is covered by fine hair called *lanugo* (primary hair). These are mostly shed by birth, and are replaced during infancy by another set of fine hair called *vellus* (secondary hair).

The secondary hair are retained in most parts of the body, but are replaced by the thick and dark *terminal hair* of the scalp and eyebrows, and other hairy areas of the adult skin.

Growth of Hair

The hair grow at the rate of about 1.5–2.2 mm per week; their growth is controlled by hormones.

The life span of the hair varies from 4 months (eyelashes, axillary hair) to 4 years (scalp hair).

Colour of Hair

Colour of hair depends upon the amount and type of melanin pigment.

3. Sweat Glands

Sudoriferous or sweat glands are distributed all over the skin, except for the lips, glans penis, and nail bed. These glands are of two types, *eccrine* and *apocrine* (Table 8.2) (Zelickson, 1971).

Eccrine Glands

The eccrine glands are much more abundant and distributed in almost every part of the skin.

Each gland is a single tube, the deep part of which is coiled into a ball. The coiled part, called the *body* of the gland, lies in the deeper part of corium or in the subcutaneous tissue. The straight part, called the *duct*, traverses the dermis and epidermis and opens on the surface of the skin.

Location: The glands are large in the axilla and groin, most numerous in the palms and soles, and least numerous in the neck and back.

The eccrine glands are *merocrine* in nature, i.e. produce the thin watery secretion without any disintegration of the epithelial cells.

Control: They are supplied and controlled by *cholinergic sympathetic nerves*.

Table 8.2: Comparison between types of sweat glands

Features	*Eccrine sweat gland*	*Apocrine sweat gland*
Activity	Throughout life	Active at puberty and remain active throughout life
Opening on surface	Through the sweat pore	Around hair shaft
Function	Maintain temperature	Provides peculiar odour
Nervous control	Postganglionic sympathetic neurons, which are cholinergic	Postganglionic sympathetic neurons which are adrenergic
Secretion	Watery with salts	Viscid with lipids and proteins

Functions: The glands help in regulation of the body temperature by evaporation of sweat, and also help in excreting the body salts. In dogs, sweat glands are confined to foot pads. Therefore, dogs do not sweat, they pant.

Apocrine Glands

Apocrine glands are confined to axilla, eyelids (Moll's glands), nipple and areola of the breast, perianal region, and the external genitalia.

Structure: They are larger than eccrine glands and produce a thicker secretion having a characteristic odour. They develop in close association with hair and their ducts typically open into the distal ends of the hair follicles.

Ceruminous glands of the external auditory meatus are modified apocrine sweat glands.

Nervous control: The apocrine glands also are merocrine in nature, but are regulated by a dual autonomic control. Some workers are not inclined to call them as sweat glands at all because they do not respond sufficiently to temperature changes.

Functions: In animals they produce chemical signals or pheromones, which are important in courtship and social behaviour.

On an average one litre of sweat is secreted per day; another 400 ml of water is lost through the lungs, and 100 ml through the faeces.

This makes a total of about 1500 ml, a rough estimate of the invisible loss of water per day.

However, in hot climates the secretion of sweat may amount to 3–10 litres per day, with a maximum of 1–2 litres per hour.

So long as the sweat glands are intact, the skin can regenerate. If the sweat glands are lost, skin grafting becomes necessary.

4. Sebaceous Glands

Location: Sebaceous glands, producing an oily secretion, are widely distributed all over the dermis of the skin (Figs 8.1 and 8.7), except for the palms and soles. They are especially abundant in the scalp and face, and are also very numerous around the apertures of the ear, nose, mouth and anus.

Structure: Sebaceous glands are small and sacculated in appearance, made up of a cluster of about 2–5 piriform alveoli.

Most of their ducts open into the hair follicles. But the ducts of sebaceous glands of lips, glans penis, inner surface of prepuce, labia minora, nipple and areola of the breast, and tarsal glands of the eyelids, open on the surface of the skin.

Sebaceous glands are *holocrine* in nature, i.e. they produce their secretion by complete fatty degeneration of the central cells of the alveolus, which are then replaced by the proliferating peripheral cells.

Nervous control: The secretion is under *hormonal control*, especially the androgens.

The oily secretion of sebaceous glands is called *sebum*.

Functions: It lubricates skin and protects it from moisture, desiccation, and the harmful sun rays. Sebum also lubricates hair and prevents them from becoming brittle.

In addition, sebum also has some bactericidal action.

Sebum makes the skin waterproof. Water evaporates from the skin, but the fats and oils are absorbed by it.

Functions of Skin

1. ***Protection:*** Skin protects the body from mechanical injuries.
   i. *Physical barrier*. Due to stratum corneum, skin acts as a barrier against bacterial infections, heat and cold, wet and drought, acid and alkali.
   ii. *Immune properties*. Langerhans cells phagocytose antigen and take it to T lymphocytes.
   iii. *Reflex action*. Sensory nerve endings start reflex action against painful stimuli and prevent it from damage.
   iv. The actinic rays of the sun are absorbed by melanocytes.
2. ***Sensory.*** Skin is sensory to touch, pain and temperature.
3. ***Regulation of body temperature.*** Heat is lost through evaporation of sweat. It is conserved by the fat and hair.
4. ***Absorption.*** Oily substances are freely absorbed by the skin.
5. ***Secretion.*** Skin secretes sweat and sebum.
6. ***Excretion.*** The excess of water, salts and waste products are excreted through the sweat.
7. ***Regulation of pH.*** A good amount of acid is excreted through the sweat.
8. ***Synthesis.*** In the skin, vitamin D is synthesized from ergosterol by the action of ultraviolet rays of the sun.
9. ***Storage.*** Skin stores chlorides.
10. ***Reparative.*** The cuts and wounds of the skin are quickly healed.

11. ***Water balance.*** Skin does not permit water to pass in and out of skin. Thus it maintains the water balance of the body.

Blood Supply

The dermis is vascular while epidermis is avascular. Epidermal cells especially those of stratum basale are supplied nourishment by diffusion.

Nerve Supply

There are motor and sensory nerves. The motor nerve fibres are autonomic nerve fibres which are sudomotor (increase the sweat) and vasomotor. The sensory nerves endings in the skin are of the following types:

i. Free nerve endings in the epidermis for perception of pain.
ii. Merkel's disc end on Merkel's cells situated in stratum basale, acting as mechanoreceptors.
iii. Meissner's corpuscles are present in dermal papillae, acting as mechanoreceptors.
iv. Pacinian corpuscles are sensitive to deep pressure.
v. Ruffini's endings are sensitive to heat.
vi. Krause's bulbs in dermis detects cold. The plexuses of free nerve endings around hair follicles detect pain and movement.

Clinical Anatomy of Skin

- In anaemia the nails are pale and white.
- In iron deficiency anaemia the nails become thin, brittle and spoon-shaped (koilonychia, Fig. 8.8).

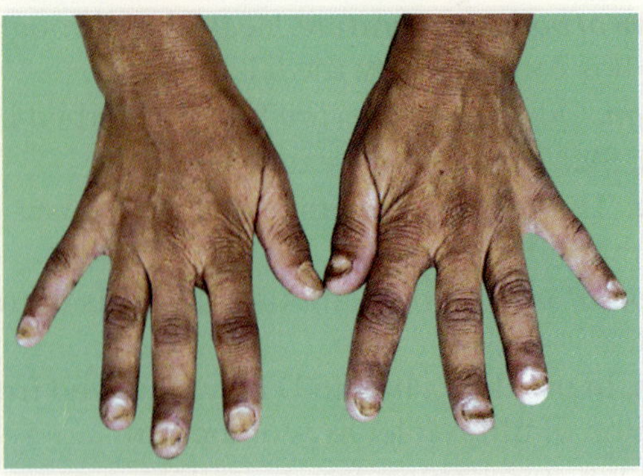

Fig. 8.8: Koilonychia of the nails

Competency achievement: The student should be able to:
AN 4.5 Explain principles of skin incisions

Skin incisions for surgery are given along flexure lines. Thus the incisions look like "a flexure line only." Healing is better and gives cosmetic value.

- Hypertrophy of the nail bed (*clubbing*) occurs in chronic suppurative disease (lung abscess, bronchiectasis, osteomyelitis) and in severe type of cyanosis (Fallot's tetralogy, chronic congestive cardiac failure) (Fig. 8.9).
- Disturbances of nail growth due to acute illness or trauma give rise to transverse grooves in the nail substance, which move distally with the nail growth. Since the average rate of growth is about 0.1 mm per day or 3 mm per month, the date of the past illness can be estimated.
- It takes about 90–120 days for the whole nail (body) to grow. Therefore, in fungal diseases of the nails the course of treatment should last for not less than this period. The growth is faster in summer than in winter, in the fingers than in toes, and in the longer fingers than in the shorter ones.
- Hairs exhibit alterations in certain diseases. In malnutrition hairs become thin, dry and sparse; in hypothyroidism they become coarse and dry.
- Excessive growth of hair (*hirsutism*) occurs in adrenogenital syndrome. Loss of hair is known as alopecia.
- Skin is dry in 'Dhatura' poisoning, heat stroke, and diabetic coma; it is unusually moist in hypoglycaemic coma, and peripheral failure.

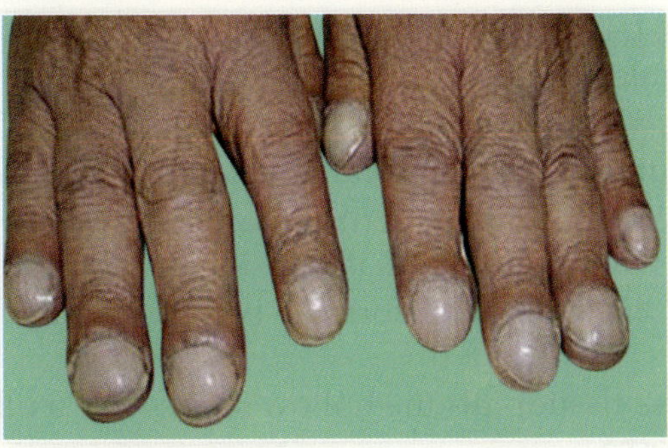

Fig. 8.9: Clubbing of the nails

- In *ichthyosis* (characterized by abnormally dry skin), the sebaceous glands are few and small, and the secretion of sebum is markedly reduced. Excessive oiliness of skin, due to overactivity of sebaceous glands, is called seborrhoea. It may occur from puberty onwards, but diminishes with advancing age.
- *Acne vulgaris* is a common complication of seborrhoea. Seborrhoeic skin is susceptible to infections (*seborrhoeic dermatitis* or *furunculosis*) and to chemical irritants (chemical folliculitis and dermatitis).

FASCIAE

Fasciae are of two types: Superficial fascia and deep fascia.

> *Competency achievement:* The student should be able to:
> AN 4.3 Describe superficial fascia along with fat distribution in body

SUPERFICIAL FASCIA

Definition

Superficial fascia is a general coating of the body beneath the skin, made up of loose areolar tissue with varying amounts of fat.

Distribution of Fat in this Fascia

1. *Fat is abundant* in the gluteal region (buttocks), lumbar region (flanks), front of the thighs, anterior abdominal wall below the umbilicus, mammary gland (Fig. 8.10), postdeltoid region, and the cervicothoracic region.
2. In *females*, fat is more abundant and is more evenly distributed than in males.
3. Fat is *absent* from the eyelids, external ear, penis, and scrotum.
4. The subcutaneous layer of fat is called the *panniculus adiposus*.

In females fat is in the superficial fascia of the lower abdomen, upper thigh, whereas in males it is inside the abdominal cavity.

In general, in women fat forms a thicker and more even layer than in men.

Fat (adipose tissue) fills the hollow spaces like axilla, orbits and ischiorectal fossa.

Fat present around the kidneys in abdomen, supports these organs.

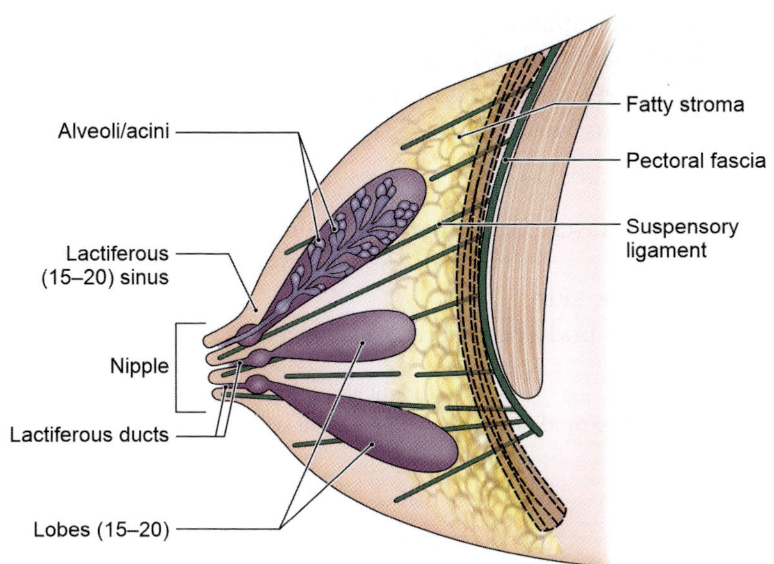

Fig. 8.10: Fat in mammary gland

Types of Fats

There are two types of fat, i.e. yellow and brown fat.

Most of the body fat is yellow, only in hibernating animals it is brown. The cells of brown fat are smaller with several small droplets, and multiple mitochondria.

Fat cells are specialised cells, and the size of fat cells increases during accumulation of fat, rather than the number of cells.

Any attempt to reduce excessive fat (obesity) must be slow and steady and not drastic, as the latter may cause harm to the body.

Important Features

1. Superficial fascia is *most distinct* in the lower part of the anterior abdominal wall, perineum, and the limbs.
2. It is *very thin* on the dorsal aspect of the hands and feet, sides of the neck, face, and around the anus.
3. It is *very dense* in the scalp, palms, and soles.
4. Superficial fascia shows *stratification* (into two layers) in the lower part of anterior abdominal wall, perineum, and uppermost part of the thighs.
5. It contains:
    a. Subcutaneous muscles in the face (muscles of facial expression), neck (platysma) and scrotum (dartos).

b. Mammary gland
c. Deeply situated sweat glands
d. Localized groups of lymph nodes
e. Cutaneous nerves and vessels.

Functions

1. Superficial fascia facilitates movements of the skin.
2. It serves as a soft medium for the passage of the vessels and nerves to the skin.
3. It conserves body heat because fat is a bad conductor of heat.

> *Competency achievement:* The student should be able to:
> AN 4.4 Describe modifications of deep fascia with its functions

DEEP FASCIA

Definition

Deep fascia is a tough inelastic fibrous sheet which invests the body beneath the superficial fascia. It is devoid of fat.

Distribution

1. Deep fascia is *best defined* in the limbs where it forms tough and tight sleeves, and in the neck where it forms a collar.
2. It is absent on the trunk and face. On the trunk its absence permits expansion of organs. On the face its absence allows movements of facial expression and of mastication.

Important Features

1. *Extensions* (*prolongations*) of the deep fascia form:
   a. The intermuscular septa which divide the limb into compartments (Fig. 8.11).
   b. The fibroareolar sheaths for the muscles, vessels and nerves.
2. *Thickenings* of the deep fascia form:
   a. Retinacula (retention bands) around certain joints like wrist (Fig. 8.12) and ankle.
   b. The palmar and plantar aponeuroses (Fig. 8.13), for protection of nerves and blood vessels.
3. *Interruptions* in the deep fascia on the subcutaneous bones.

   Deep fascia never crosses a subcutaneous bone. Instead it blends with its periosteum and is bound down to the bone.

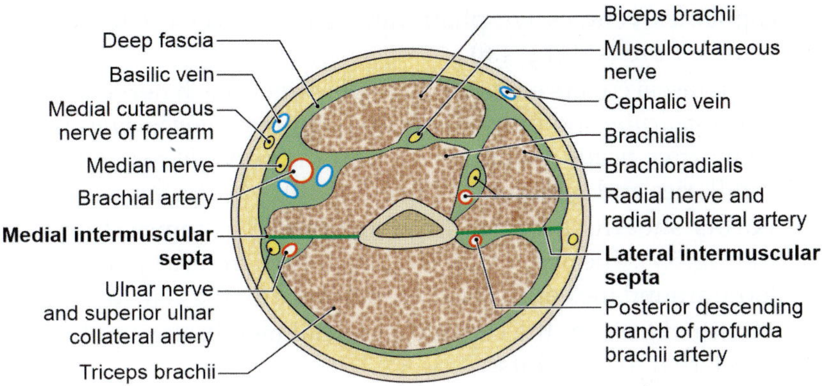

Fig. 8.11: Fascial compartments

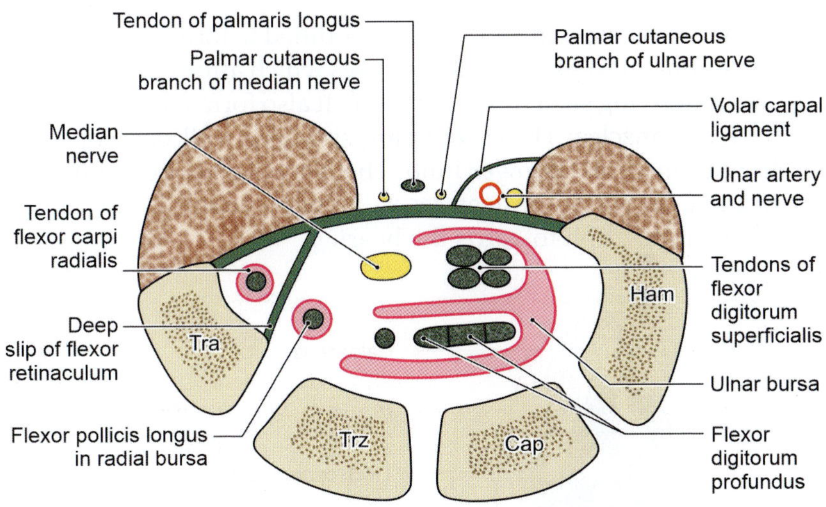

Fig. 8.12: Flexor retinaculum of wrist

MODIFICATIONS OF DEEP FASCIA

1. Forms the intermuscular septa separating functionally different group of muscles into separate compartments (Fig. 8.11).
2. Covers each muscle as *epimysium* which sends in the septa to enclose each muscle fasciculus known as *perimysium*. From the perimysium septa pass to enclose each muscle fibre. These fine septa are the *endomysium*. Through all these connective tissue septa, e.g. epimysium, perimysium and endomysium, arterioles,

capillaries, venules, lymphatics and nerves traverse to reach each muscle fibre (*see* Fig. 4.6).

3. Deep fascia covers each nerve as *epineurium*, each nerve fascicle as *perineurium* and individual nerve fibre as *endoneurium*. These connective tissue coverings support the nerve fibres and carry capillaries and lymphatics (*see* Fig. 7.10).
4. Forms sheaths around large arteries, e.g. femoral sheath (*see* Fig. 5.7). The deep fascia is dense around the artery and rather loose around the vein to give an allowance for the vein to distend.
5. Modified to form the capsule, synovial membrane and bursae in relation to the joints.
6. Forms tendon sheaths wherever tendons cross over a joint like radial/ulnar bursa. This mechanism prevents wear and tear of the tendon (Fig. 8.12).
7. In the region of palm and sole it is modified to form aponeuroses, e.g. palmar and plantar aponeuroses which afford protection to the underlying structures (Fig. 8.13). It also forms septa between various muscles. These septa are specially well developed in the calf muscles of lower limb. The contraction of calf muscles in the tight sleeve of deep fascia helps in pushing the venous blood and lymph towards the heart.

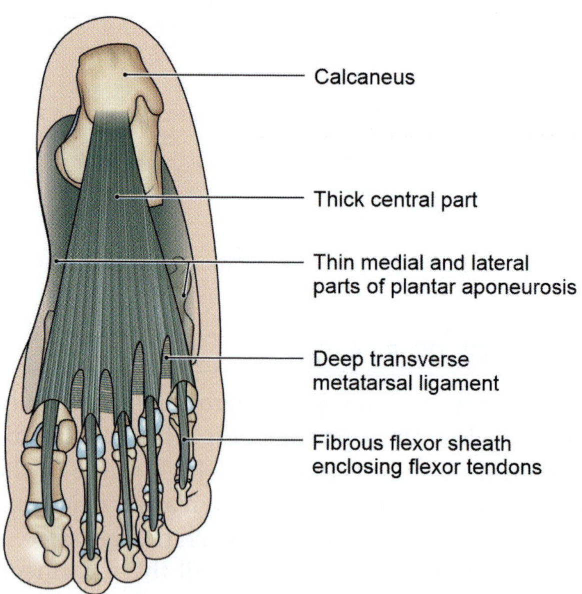

Fig. 8.13: Plantar aponeurosis

Thus the deep fascia helps in venous and lymphatic return from the lower limb (see Fig. 5.12).

8. In the forearm and leg, the deep fascia is modified to form the *interosseous membrane*, which keeps:
   a. The two bones at optimum distance.
   b. Increases surface area for attachment of muscles (*see* Fig. 3.12b).
   c. Transmits weight from one bone to other.

Functions

1. Deep fascia keeps the underlying structures in position and preserves the characteristic surface contour of the limbs and neck.
2. It provides extra surface for muscular attachments.
3. It helps in venous and lymphatic return.
4. It assists muscles in their action by the degree of tension and pressure it exerts upon their surfaces.
5. The retinacula act as pulleys and serve to prevent the loss of power. In such situations the friction is minimized by the synovial sheaths of the tendons (Fig. 8.12).

Clinical Anatomy of Skin

Skin is the outer garment of the body and is subjected to following maladies.

- ***Dermatitis or eczema:*** There is redness, swelling, itching and exudation in acute cases. It usually becomes chronic. Dermatitis may be allergic due to soaps and cosmetics.
- ***Albinism:*** There is no melanin pigment. It is usually an inherited condition.
- ***Herpes zoster virus:*** This virus causes vesicular lesion around the nasal and oral orifices and along a dermatome (*see* Fig. 7.26). It is also responsible for causing chickenpox.
- ***Pressure sores:*** The skin slowly dies over the pressure sites, e.g. pressure sores in the lower back when patient lies on the back for prolonged periods due to illness (*see* Fig. 7.23).
- ***Burns:*** It is a condition which occurs due to too much heat or cold, acids, alkalies and electricity, etc. If only epidermis is affected, the burn is called *superficial*. If both dermis and epidermis are affected, the burn is called *deep*. Burn results in dehydration, shock and contractures.

- ***Benign pigmented naevus or mole:*** Melanin pigment cells are found in small numbers in the basal layer of skin. These neuroectodermal cells may proliferate at the dermoepidermal junction, in the dermis, to form naevi of different sizes and forms.
- ***Colour:*** Skin is pale in anaemia, yellow in jaundice and blue in cyanosis.
- ***Boil (furuncle):*** Boil is an infection and suppuration of the hair follicle and the sebaceous gland.
- ***Skin incisions:*** These should be made parallel to the lines of cleavage. This will result in small scars (Fig. 8.3).
- ***Sebaceous cyst*** is common in the scalp. It is due to obstruction of the duct of a sebaceous gland, caused either by trauma or infection (Fig. 8.14). If the duct of sebaceous gland of cheek is blocked, it leads to closed comedones or acne (Fig. 8.15). If the condition gets severe, the condition is acne vulgaris (Fig. 8.16).
- ***Scabies*** is a mite infection. It is commonly seen in genital region (Fig. 8.17) and in interdigital cleft (Fig. 8.18).
- ***Keloid*** is overgrowth of connective tissue at site of injury or burn (Fig. 8.19).
- ***Fungal infection of nail*** is common (Fig. 8.20). It may occur in between the toes also.
- ***Vitiligo*** is an autoimmune disease leading to white patches on skin (Fig. 8.21).
- ***Baldness*** is related to hormones. Alopecia areata (Fig. 8.22) is an autoimmune disease.
- Deep fascia of the leg helps in **venous return** from the legs. The muscular contractions press on the deep veins and form an effective mechanism of venous return. This contraction becomes more effective within the tight sleeve of deep fascia.
- ***Planes:*** The deep fascia forms planes and the fluid or pus tracks along these fascial planes. The tubercular abscess of the cervical vertebrae passes along the prevertebral fascia into the posterior triangle of neck or into the axilla.
- ***Retinacula*** keep the tendons and nerves in position. Sometimes the delicate nerve may get compressed as it traverses under the retinacula. Median nerve may get compressed deep to the flexor retinaculum, leading to the *carpal tunnel syndrome* (Fig. 8.12).
- Similarly tibial nerve may get compressed under the flexor retinaculum of leg leading to *tarsal tunnel syndrome*.

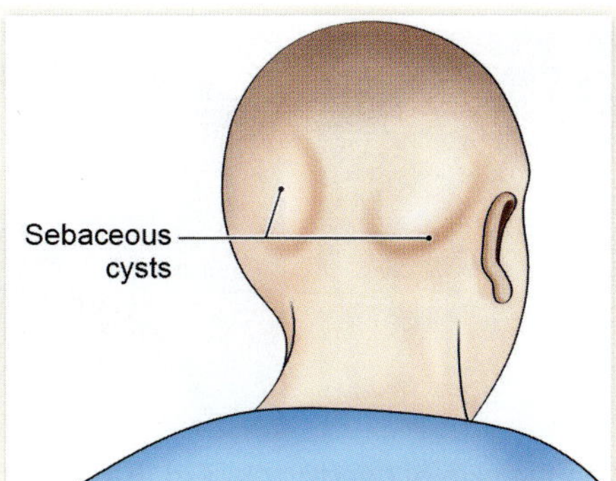

Fig. 8.14: Sebaceous cysts on the scalp

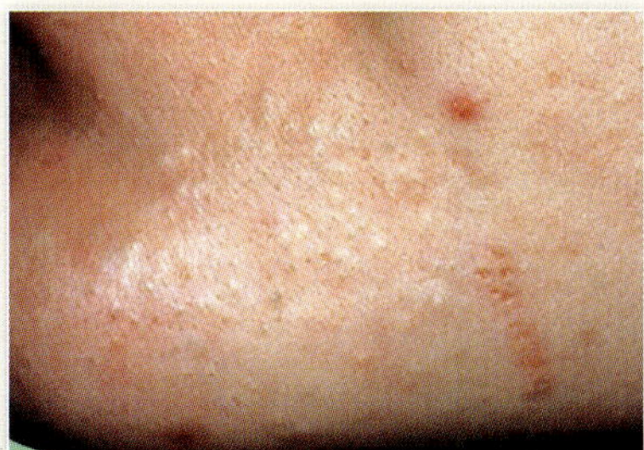

Fig. 8.15: Comedones or acne on the chin

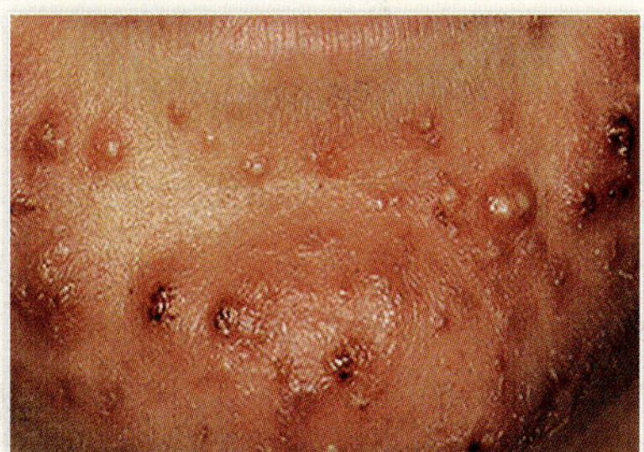

Fig. 8.16: Acne vulgaris

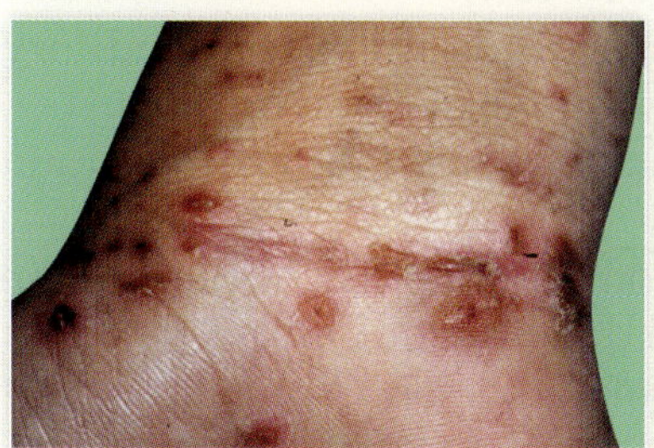

Fig. 8.17: Scabies—wrist region

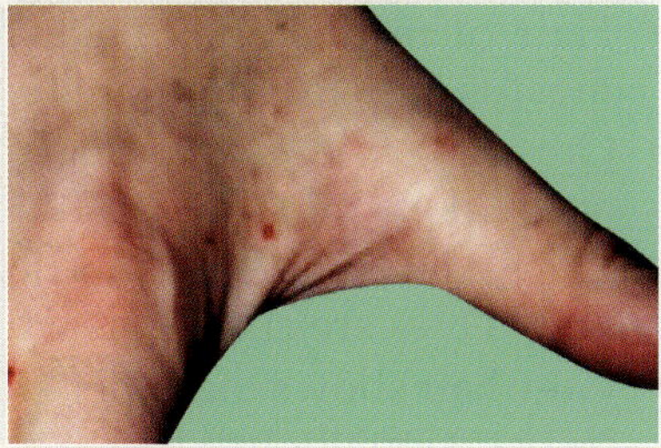

Fig. 8.18: Scabies—interdigital cleft

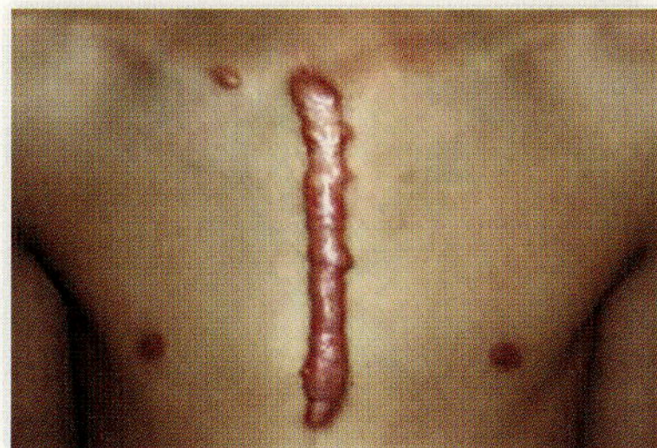

Fig. 8.19: Keloid after surgery

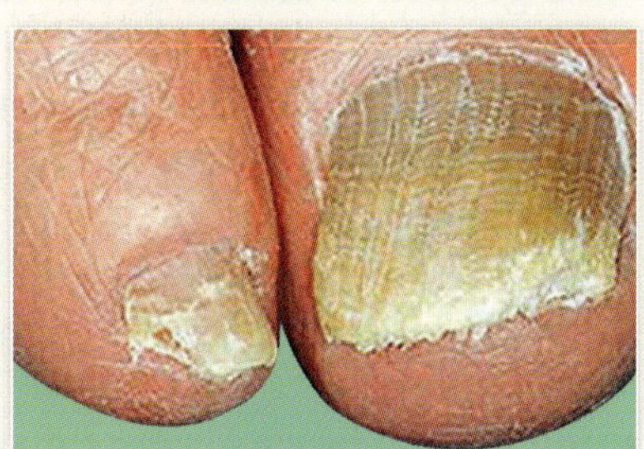

Fig. 8.20: Fungal infection of toe nails

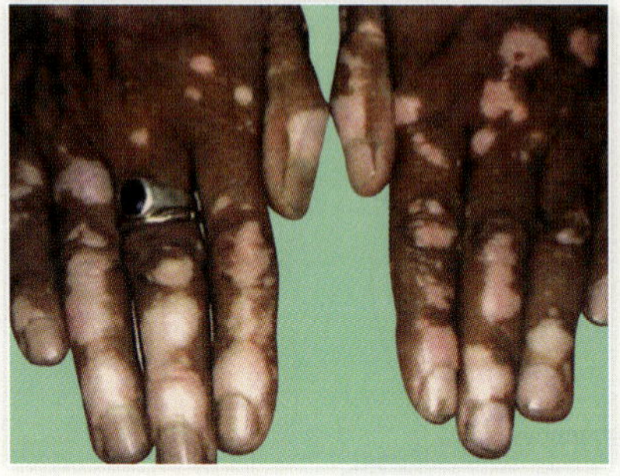

Fig. 8.21: Vitiligo on the skin of hands

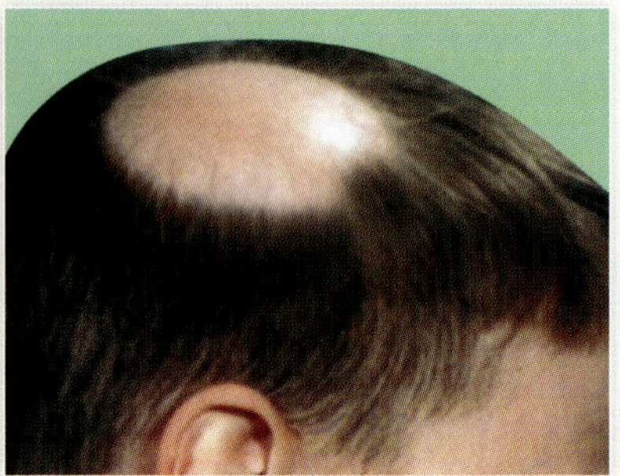

Fig. 8.22: Alopecia-areata

Courtesy (Figs 8.15 to 8.22): Dr Anuradha and Dr Praveen Aggarwal of Aggarwal Medical Centre, Delhi.

Points to Remember

- "Rule of 9" is taken for counting percentages of burn.
- Dermis is processed/tanned to make leather.
- Epidermis contains mainly free nerve endings.
- Skin is the largest organ of the body in terms of surface area and sensory nerve endings.
- Nails take nearly 4 months to grow fully.
- Hair of face, axilla, eyelashes, eyebrows, external auditory meatus and anterior nares lack arrector pilorum muscles.
- Grey hair with lack of melanin and more of air after a certain age make a person graceful.
- Grey hair are lighter and float on the scalp like "clouds in the sky." Dyes are chemicals which do harm the body.
- Grey hair shows the experience of the person. Cosmetics should be occasionally used.
- Finger prints are unique to each and every person.
- Acne occurs due to blockage of the duct of sebaceous gland.
- Hair contain sulphur and emits peculiar smell on burning.
- Long hair are present on the scalp while short hair are situated on the eyelids.
- Sweat glands are maximum in palm/sole. These are supplied by sympathetic fibres. Sympathetic stimulation makes the palm wet.
- Superficial fascia is very thin on dorsum of hands, feet, face and neck, while it is very dense in scalp, palms and soles.

- Mammary gland is situated in the superficial fascia and is largest modified gland.
- Deep fascia helps in venous and lymphatic return.
- It is modified to form numerous structures around the joints.
- Deep fascia in temporal region is the toughest. It is absent on face and anterior abdominal wall.

Multiple Choice Questions

1. Appendages of skin are all *except*:
   a. Hair
   b. Nail
   c. Sebaceous glands
   d. Arrectore pilorum muscles

2. Full nail grows in:
   a. 30–60 days b. 60–90 days
   c. 90–120 days d. 120–160 days

3. Arrector pilorum is a:
   a. Skeletal muscle
   b. Smooth muscle
   c. Cardiac muscle
   d. Mixture of skeletal and smooth muscles

4. Following are the effects of sympathetic stimulation on the skin *except*:
   a. Vasomotor
   b. Sudomotor
   c. Pilomotor
   d. Increased pigmentation

5. Hair are not present in following areas *except*:
   a. Palm
   b. Sole
   c. Dorsal surface of distal phalanges
   d. Dorsal surface of middle phalanges

6. Hair are of following types *except*:
   a. Primary hair or lanugo
   b. Secondary hair or vellus
   c. Terminal dark hair
   d. Terminal hair with multiple divisions

7. Following *except* one are subcutaneous muscles:
   a. Dartos
   b. Muscles of facial expression
   c. Palmaris brevis
   d. Palmaris longus

8. Carotid sheath is thin:
   a. Around artery
   b. Around vein
   c. Around nerve
   d. Around all structures

9. Functions of interosseous membrane are all *except*:
   a. Keeps the bones at optimum distance
   b. Increases surface area for attachment of the muscles
   c. Direction of fibres is from ulna to radius
   d. Has foramina for passage of structures

10. Deep fascia in the leg helps in:
   a. Making compartments in the leg
   b. Forms an effective mechanisms of venous return
   c. Forms sheath around blood vessels
   d. Forms aponeurosis

Answers

1. d **2.** c **3.** b **4.** d **5.** d **6.** d **7.** d **8.** b
9. c **10.** d

Chapter 9

Connective Tissue, Ligaments and Raphe

"Give a man a fish and you feed him for one day. Teach a man to fish and you feed him for a lifetime."
—Lao Tzu

CONNECTIVE TISSUE

INTRODUCTION

Connective tissue is a widely distributed general type of tissue which supports, binds and protects the special (well differentiated) tissues of the body.

It has both the cellular and extracellular components.

The cellular component of connective tissue plays the role of active defence, whereas the extracellular component (fibres and ground substance) serves a number of mechanical functions of support and protection against the mechanical stresses and strains.

The ordinary type of connective tissue is distributed all over the body, but the special type of connective tissue forms certain well-differentiated tissues, like the bone and cartilage.

The greater part of connective tissue develops from embryonic mesoderm.

A number of cell types is also found in the connective tissue the blood and lymph.

The cells of the connective tissue are widely separated by the abundance of extracellular matrix.

CONSTITUENT ELEMENTS

Connective tissue is made up of cells and extracellular matrix.

A. Cells

Cells are fibroblast, fat cell, plasma cell, macrophage, mast cell, and pigment cell.

B. Extracellular Matrix

The matrix has a fibrous and a non-fibrous element. The fibrous element has three types of fibres—collagen, elastin and reticulin. The non-fibrous element is formed by the ground substance.

TYPES OF CONNECTIVE TISSUE

Different types of connective tissue are found in different parts of the body according to the local functional requirements. These types are based on predominance of the cell type, concentration and arrangement of the fibre type, and character of ground substance. The connective tissues are classified as follows.

I. Loose Connective Tissue

Its types are: Areolar tissue, adipose tissue, myxomatous tissue and reticular tissue.

II. Dense Irregular Connective Tissue

1. Ordinary—tendon
2. Specialised—cartilage and bone.

The details of cells, matrix and types of connective tissue are described in the Histology, 6th edition *by K Garg, Gayatri Rath* and *Mithlesh Chandra*.

Functions of Connective Tissue

1. As a packing material, connective tissue provides a *supporting matrix* for many highly organized structures.
2. It forms *restraining mechanism* of the body in the form of retinacula, check ligaments (Fig. 9.1) and fibrous pulley (Fig. 9.2).
3. The ensheathing layer of *deep fascia* preserves the characteristic contour of the limbs and aids circulation in the veins and lymphatics (*see* Fig. 5.12).
4. It provides surface coating of the body in the form of *superficial fascia* which stores fat and conserves body heat.
5. It provides *additional surface* for the attachment of muscles in the form of deep fascia, intermuscular septa and interosseous membranes (*see* Figs 3.12b and 8.11).
6. It forms *fascial planes* which provide convenient pathways for vessels (blood vessels and lymphatics) and nerves.

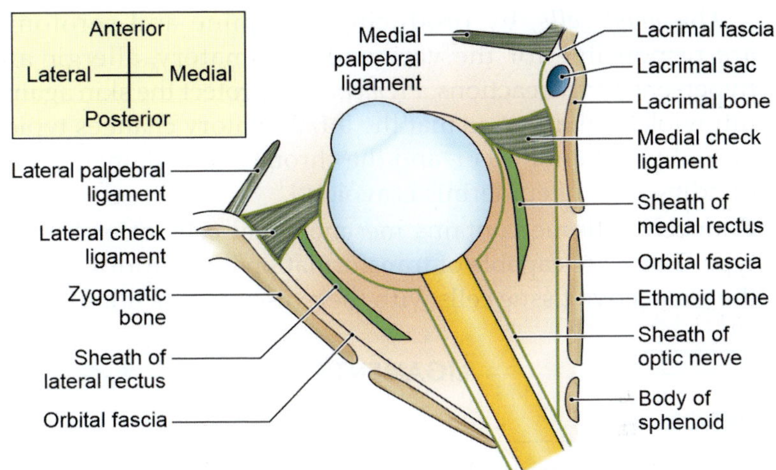

Fig. 9.1: Check ligaments of the orbit

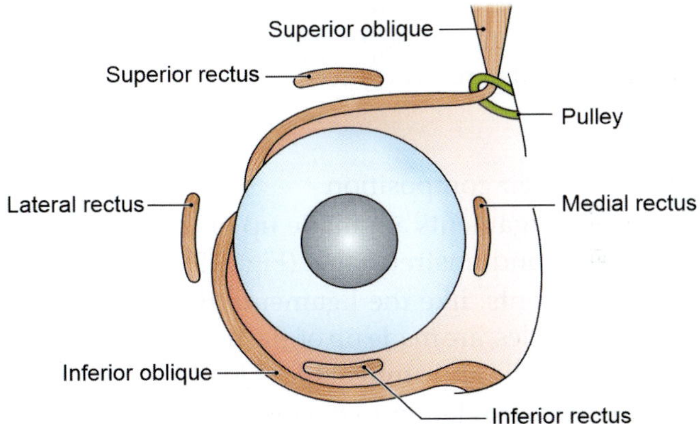

Fig. 9.2: Fibrous pulley to change the direction of muscle

7. In places where it is loose in texture (loose connective tissue) it *facilitates movements* between the adjacent structures, and by forming bursal sacs it minimizes friction and pressure effects (*see* Fig. 8.12).
8. Connective tissue helps in the *repair of injuries* whereby the fibroblasts lay down collagen fibres to form the scar tissue.
9. The *macrophages* of connective tissue serve a defensive function against the bacterial invasion by their phagocytic activity. They also act as scavengers in removing the cell debris and foreign material.

   The *plasma cells* are capable of producing antibodies against specific antigens (foreign proteins).

The *mast cells*, by producing histamine and serotonin, are responsible for the various inflammatory, allergic and hypersensitivity reactions. *Pigment cells* protect the skin against ultraviolet radiation, so that the inflammatory changes typical of sunburn do not occur, and the chromosomal damage in the dividing cells of epidermis is avoided.

10. Connective tissue contains mesenchymal cells of embryonic type. These are capable of transformation into various types of the connective tissue cells with their discrete functions.

LIGAMENTS

DEFINITION

Ligaments are fibrous bands which connect the adjacent bones, forming integral parts of the joints. They are tough and unyielding, but at the same time are flexible and pliant, so that the normal movements can occur without any resistance, but the abnormal movements are prevented.

Types of Ligaments

A. According to their composition
   1. Most of the ligaments are made up of collagen fibres. These are inelastic and unstretchable (Fig. 9.3).
   2. A few ligaments, like the ligamenta flava and ligaments of auditory ossicles, are made up of elastic fibres (predominantly). These are elastic and stretchable (Fig. 9.4).

B. According to their relation to the joint
   1. Intrinsic ligaments surround the joint, and may be intracapsular.

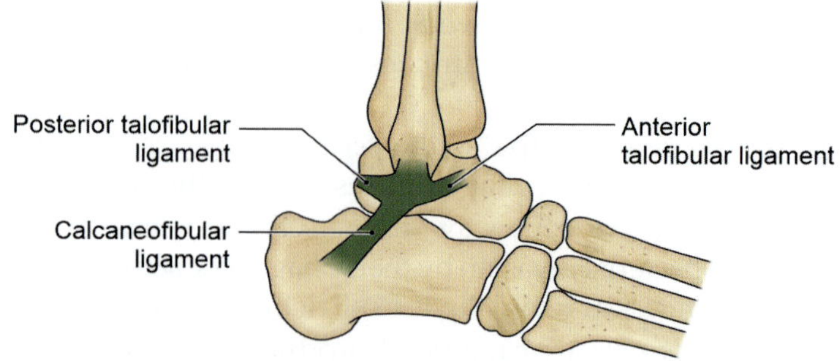

Fig. 9.3: Lateral ligament of ankle joint (collagenous)

2. Extrinsic ligaments are independent of the joint; and lie little away from it (Fig. 9.5).

Morphology

Ligaments in some areas are considered as degenerated tendons of the related muscles.

1. Tibial collateral ligament is degenerated tendon of adductor magnus muscle.

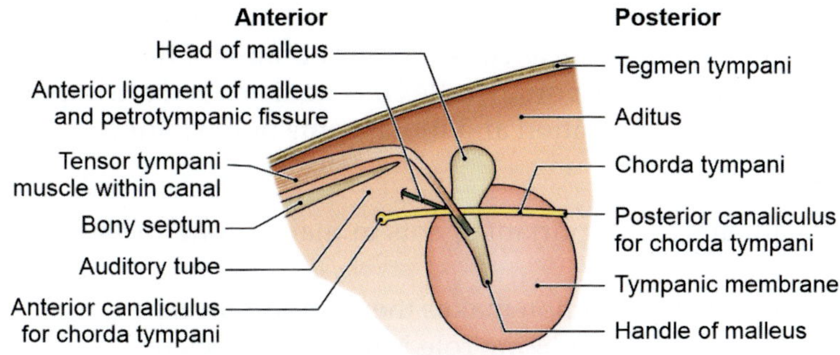

Fig. 9.4: Anterior ligament of malleus (elastin)

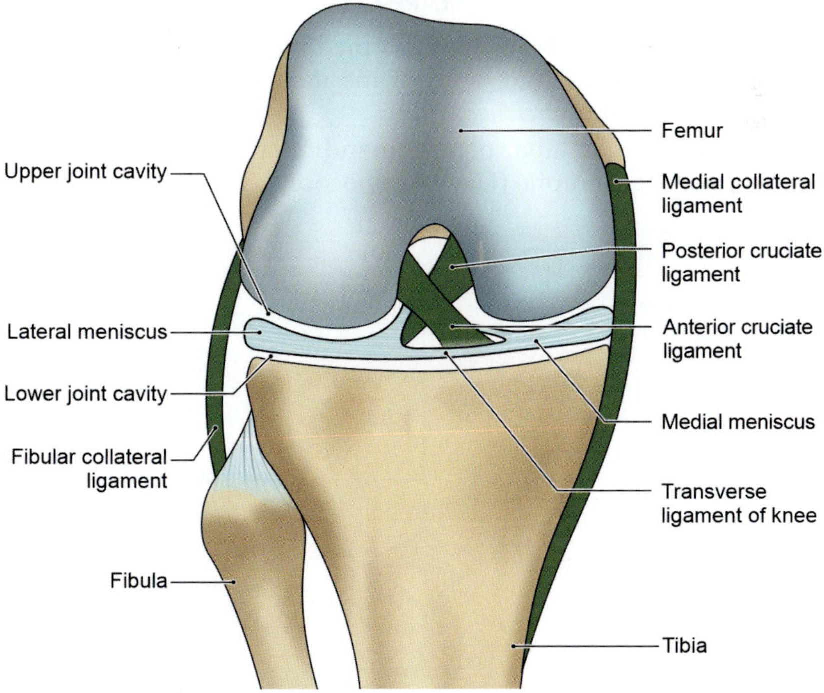

Fig. 9.5: Some of the extrinsic and intrinsic ligaments of knee joint

2. Sacrotuberous ligament is degenerated tendon of long head of biceps femoris.
3. Sacrospinous ligament is degenerated part of coccygeus muscle.
4. Long plantar ligament is part of peroneus longus.

Their tendinous nature is evident in some animal ancestors.

Blood and Nerve Supply

The blood vessels and nerves of the joint ramify on its ligaments and supply them.

Most ligaments serve as sense organs because of their rich nerve supply. They act as important reflex mechanisms and are important in monitoring the position and movements of the joint.

Functions

1. Ligaments are important agents in maintaining the stability at the joint.
2. Their sensory function makes them important reflex organs, so that their joint stabilizing role is far more efficient.

RAPHE

A raphe is a linear fibrous band formed by interdigitation of the tendinous or aponeurotic ends of the muscles. It differs from a ligament in that it is *stretchable*.

Examples: Linea alba, pterygomandibular raphe, mylohyoid raphe, pharyngeal raphe (Fig. 9.6), anococcygeal raphe, etc.

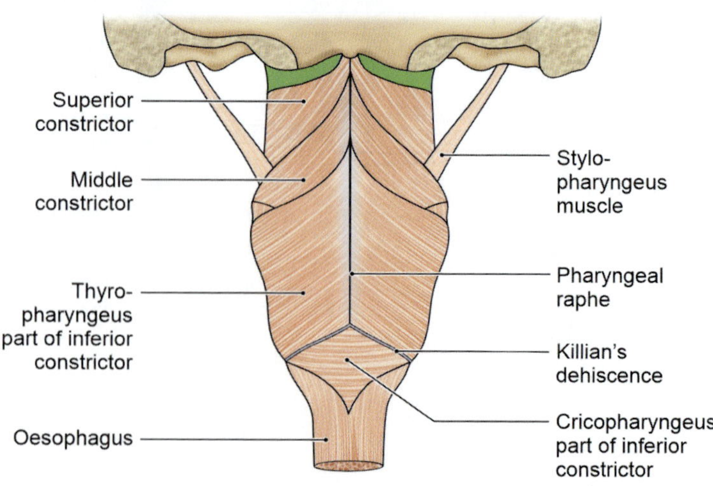

Fig. 9.6: Pharyngeal raphe

Clinical Anatomy of Connective Tissue

- ***Collagen diseases*** include rheumatic fever, rheumatoid arthritis, disseminated lupus erythematosus, scleroderma, dermatomyositis, polyarteritis nodosa, and serum sickness. These are the diseases of connective tissue characterized by its fibrinoid necrosis.
- ***Scleroderma*** is a slowly progressive rheumatic disease accompanied by vascular lesions, especially in the skin, lungs and kidneys. It is characterized by deposition of fibrous tissue in the skin. This leads to thickness and firmness of the affected areas. It is an autoimmune disease of connective tissue.
- ***Dupuytren's contracture:*** Occurs due to contraction of fibrous tissue of palmar aponeurosis. The disease results in flexion deformities of fingers, especially ring finger and little finger (Fig. 9.7).
- ***Inflammations*** (*fibrositis*) and injuries (*pulls* and *sprains*) of the connective tissue are very painful because of its rich nerve supply or the associated muscle spasm. Relief (healing) of pain in these disorders is markedly delayed due to poor blood supply of the connective tissue.
- ***Marfan's syndrome*** is a hereditary disease causing mesodermal and ectodermal dysplasia. It is characterized by excessive height, arachnodactyly, high arched palate, dislocated eye lenses, and congenital heart disease.
- Tendons at the back of wrist are enveloped by synovial sheath. At times the sheath may form a swelling at back of wrist. This is called the "ganglion" (Fig. 9.8).

  Ganglion is a cystic swelling resulting from mucoid degeneration of synovial sheaths around the tendons.

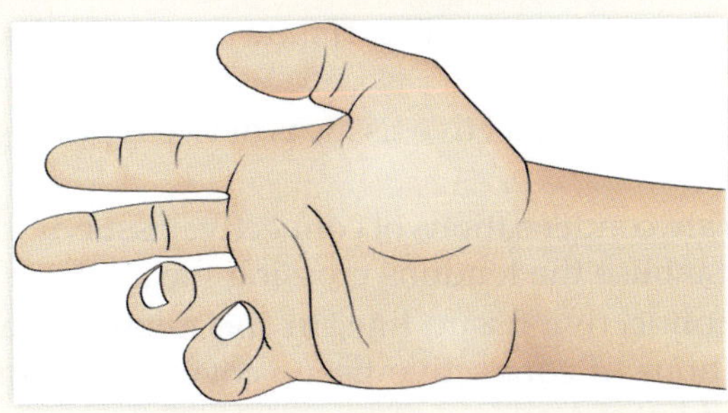

Fig. 9.7: Dupuytren's contracture

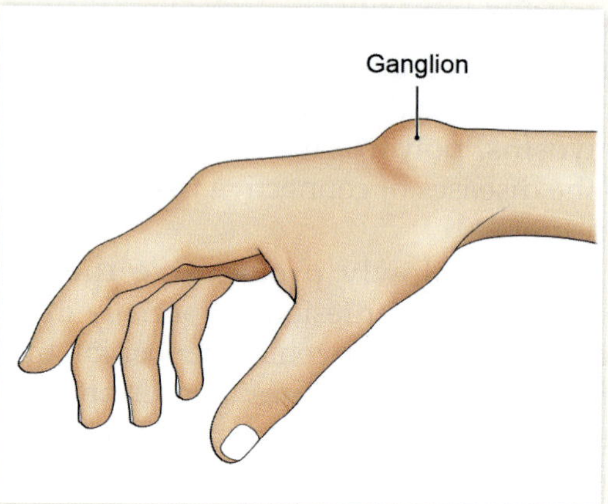

Fig. 9.8: Ganglion on the dorsum of wrist

- Undue stretching and tearing of the fibres of a ligament due to an injury is known as 'sprain'. It causes severe pain and effusion into the ligament and joint. The bones are normal as seen in the X-ray film.
- The joint stability is lost in the neuropathic joints, as occurs in tabes dorsalis, syringomyelia, leprosy, etc.

Points to Remember

- Various cells of connective tissue are fibroblast, adipose cell, macrophages, plasma cells, white blood cells, etc.
- Various types of fibres are collagen fibres, elastic fibres and reticular fibres.
- Types of connective tissue are loose connective tissue and dense connective tissue. Dense connective tissue may be ordinary dense connective tissue or specialised dense connective tissue.
- Specialised dense connective tissue is of two types, e.g. cartilage and bone.
- Retinacula are condensations of connective tissue at wrist, ankle, etc. These stablise the tendons crossing the joint.
- Raphe is connective tissue line, in the median plane due to interdigitations of connective tissue coverings of the muscles of right and left sides.

Multiple Choice Questions

1. **Which of the following cells of general connective tissue act as defensive cells in the body?**
   a. Fibroblasts
   b. Fat cells
   c. Macrophages
   d. Mesenchymal stem cells
2. **Which of the following cells produce antibodies?**
   a. Plasma cells
   b. Adipocytes
   c. Macrophages
   d. Mast cells
3. **Which cells are responsible for various allergic responses?**
   a. Macrophages
   b. Mast cells
   c. Pigment cells
   d. Mesenchymal cells
4. **Which one of the following is not the fibrous element of the connective tissue?**
   a. Collagen fibres
   b. Elastic fibres
   c. Reticular fibres
   d. Hyaline cartilage
5. **Which of the following ligaments is chiefly elastic in nature?**
   a. Ligamentum flava
   b. Ligamentum patellae
   c. Capsular ligament
   d. Deltoid ligament

Answers

1. c **2.** a **3.** b **4.** d **5.** a

Chapter 10

Respiratory System

Which is the longest word in English? "SMILES", because there is a "MILE" gap between S and S. So let's keep smiling.

Respiratory system consists of organs which provide the pathway for supply of oxygen to the body and expulsion of carbon dioxide from the body to the surrounding atmosphere. Oxygen is required for the chemical reactions releasing energy used for the proper functioning of the cells.

Respiration involves exchange of gases and is a twofold process:

1. *External respiration* is the exchange of gases between the blood and the alveoli of the lungs.
2. *Internal respiration* is the interchange of gases in the tissues.

ORGANS OF RESPIRATION

Organs of respiration include organs which help in the mechanism of respiration. These are as follows:

- Nose: External nares, nasal cavity and posterior nares
- Paranasal sinuses
- Nasopharynx
- Larynx
- Trachea and bronchi (Fig. 10.1)
- Lungs in the pleural cavity
- Respiratory muscles: The diaphragm and intercostal muscles.

Nose

It is comprised of a pair of external nares, through which air is inhaled in and exhaled out. Nose is the prominence on the face in

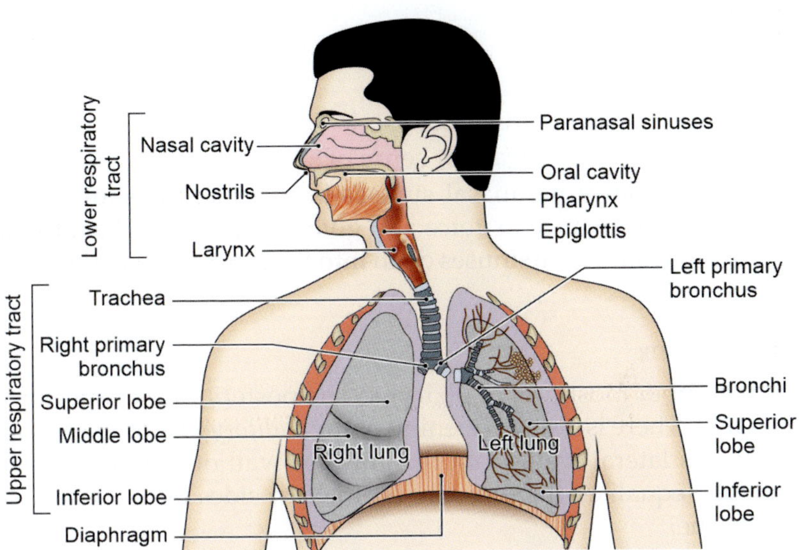

Fig. 10.1: Components of the respiratory system

between and below the eyes. It is made of small flat *nasal bones* and *nasal cartilages*. The lower lateral part is made up of fibrous tissue and is called the *'ala'* of the nose.

The nasal cavity is divided into two halves by a nasal septum formed by *ethmoid, vomer* and *septal cartilage*. Roof is formed by *nasal, frontal, ethmoid* and *sphenoid bones*. Floor is formed by *hard palate and soft palate*. In the lateral wall of each cavity, there are three *conchae* or projections of bone, which divide the cavity into *meatuses*. The frontal, ethmoid, sphenoid and maxillary bones have air sinuses. Their openings are present in the meatuses. In sinusitis, there is excessive drainage of fluid from the nasal cavity.

The *nasolacrimal duct* draining the lacrimal fluid (tears) also drains into the nasal cavity, while in crying the tears also drain out from the nasal cavity.

The nasal cavity posteriorly shows two *posterior nasal apertures*. The air passes through them to reach the nasopharynx.

- Nose is lined by highly vascular ciliated columnar epithelium (mucous membrane) which contains mucus secreting goblet cells.

Paranasal air sinuses are air containing spaces between the two tables of sphenoid, ethmoid, frontal and maxilla bones of the skull.

Functions of nose:

- Filtration of air
- Humidification of air
- Heating/cooling of inspired air
- Olfaction: It is the organ for sense of smell.

The function of paranasal sinuses is to make the skull bones lighter, give resonance to voice and give humidity and heat to the dry and cold air. These sinuses open into the lateral wall of the nasal cavity.

Nasopharynx

It is the upper most part of pharynx. The posterior nasal apertures open in it. There is also an opening of the *auditory tube* or *Eustachian tube*, in its lateral wall, from the anterior wall of the middle ear. This tube equalises the pressure on the two sides of the tympanic membrane.

On the posterior wall of nasopharynx *pharyngeal tonsils* (adenoids) are present. These consist of lymphoid tissue. They are prominent in children up to 14–16 years of age and thereafter they gradually atrophy.

Air passes from nasopharynx into the larynx. Air and fluids/food cross each other in the oropharynx (Fig. 10.2a and b). If one shouts or laughs aloud while eating/drinking, the food/fluid may enter the larynx. This produces a protective bout of cough as food/fluid is forbidden inside the larynx/trachea. Pharynx also functions in speech, giving the voice its individual characteristic note.

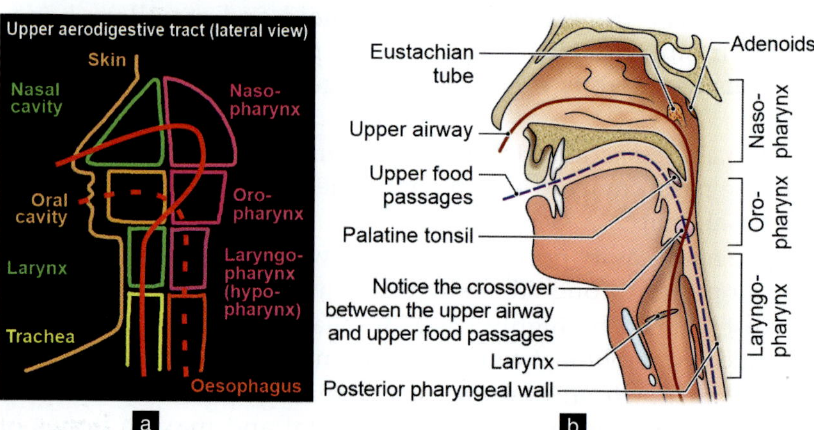

Fig. 10.2a and b: Parts of pharynx

Larynx

It is also called 'voice-box' and extends from 3rd cervical to 6th cervical vertebrae. It is made up of cartilages and membranes.

Cartilages of the larynx are:

- Thyroid (1)
- Cricoid (1)
- Epiglottis (1)
- Arytenoids (2).

Membrane of the larynx is folded to form *two vocal cords*. There are muscles which move these cords. Vibrations of these vocal cords produce voice.

Thyroid cartilage is very prominent in males and is called 'Adam's apple'.

Inlet of larynx acts as a sphincter preventing fluid/food from entering the larynx, trachea and lungs. Larynx at the level of 6th cervical vertebra continues as trachea.

Trachea and Bronchi

Trachea is a musculocartilaginous tube extending from 6th cervical vertebra to 6th thoracic vertebra where it divides into *two primary bronchi* one each for the right and left lungs. The right bronchus is wider, shorter and is in line with trachea. Right bronchus is 2.5 cm while left bronchus is 5 cm in length. Trachea contains hyaline cartilage incomplete rings (U-shaped) to keep the tube patent as air is constantly passing in and out of lungs.

On each side of the trachea in the neck lie the *carotid sheath* containing palpable common carotid artery with internal jugular vein and vagus nerve.

Lungs

Lungs are two voluminous cone-shaped organs occupying most of the thoracic cavity leaving a small space for the heart. Each lung is enclosed in a serous pleural cavity. The *pleural cavity* contains serous fluid which helps in expansion and contraction of the lung.

> *Competency achievement:* The student should be able to:
> AN 24.1 Mention the blood supply, lymphatic drainage and nerve supply of pleura, extent of pleura and describe the pleural recesses and their applied anatomy

Pleura: It is a closed serous sac which encloses the lung. It has two layers. The *parietal pleura* which lines the inner surface of the chest wall and thoracic surface of the diaphragm. It is reflected at the *hilum* to become the *visceral pleura*. The visceral pleura lines the outer surface of lung and its fissures (Fig. 10.3a and b).

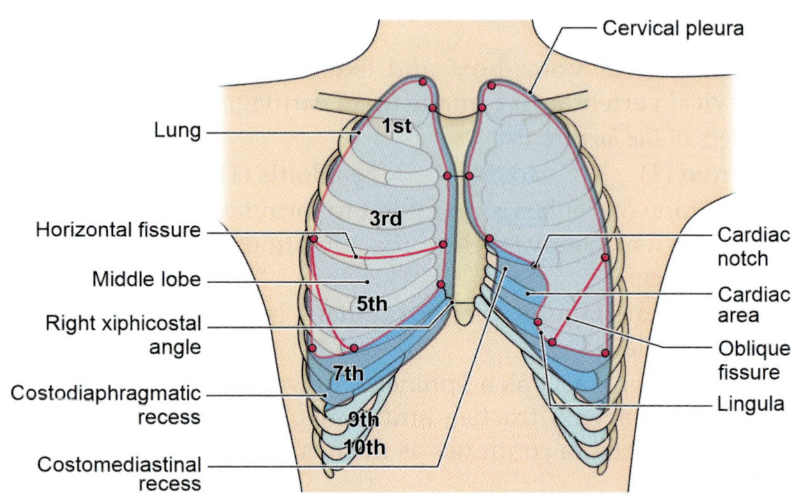

Fig. 10.3a: Surface marking of the parietal pleura and visceral pleura/lung—anterior aspect

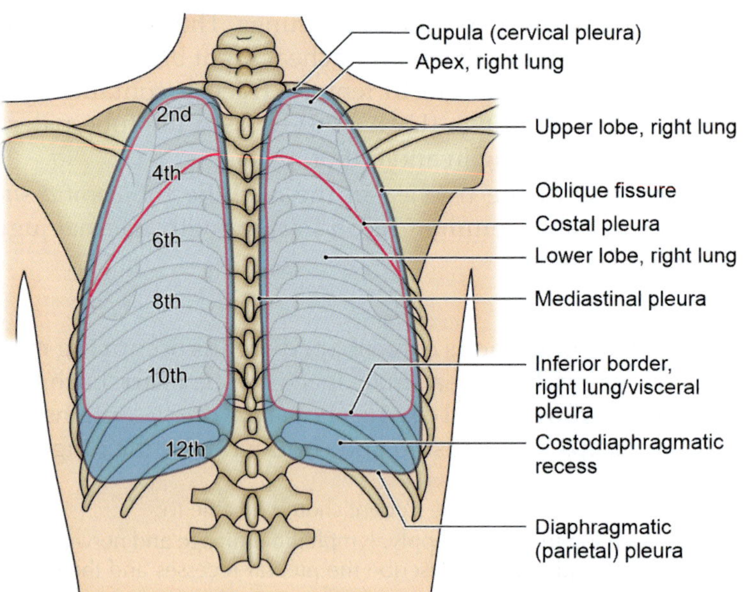

Fig. 10.3b: Surface marking of the parietal pleura and visceral pleura/lung—posterior aspect

The pleural cavity: It is a potential space between the two pleurae. They are separated by a thin film of serous fluid, sufficient to prevent friction between them during breathing.

Competency achievement: The student should be able to:
AN 24.2 Identify side, external features and relations of structures which form root of lung & bronchial tree and their clinical correlate
AN 24.3 Describe a bronchopulmonary segment

Parts of Lung

- ***Apex:*** It is rounded and rises into the root of neck about 2.5 cm above the level of the medial third of clavicle. It is related with blood vessels and nerves of the neck.
- ***Base*** is concave and closely related with the upper surface of diaphragm.
- ***Costal surface:*** It is convex and related with the costal cartilages, ribs and intercostal muscles. This surface has impressions of the ribs.
- ***Medial/mediastinal surface:*** It is concave and has the hilum. The structures which leave and enter form the root of each lung. These are:
  - Bronchus/bronchi
  - Pulmonary artery
  - Pulmonary veins
  - Bronchial artery and bronchial vein
  - Lymphatic vessels
  - Nerves
- The lung has a *thin anterior border* and a *thick posterior border*
- Table 10.1 shows the differences between right and left lungs.

Lungs are made up of two portions, a conducting portion and a respiratory portion.

Conducting portion: The primary bronchus enters the lung at the *hilum*. In the *right lung* it divides into *three secondary bronchi* for

Table 10.1: Difference between small and large intestines	
Right lung	*Left lung*
1. It has 2 fissures and 3 lobes	1. It has one fissure and 2 lobes
2. Anterior border is straight	2. Anterior border is interrupted by the cardiac notch
3. Larger and heavier, weighs about 700 g	3. Smaller and lighter, weighs about 600 g
4. Shorter and broader	4. Longer and narrower

each of the *three lobes of the right* lung, i.e. upper, middle and lower separated by the oblique and horizontal fissures (Fig. 10.4). The three secondary bronchi divide into 10 segmental bronchi.

Left lung contains two lobes, i.e. upper and lower lobes, separated by oblique fissure. So, there are only *two secondary bronchi*. But, the segmental bronchi are 10 in this lung also, five for upper lobe and five for lower lobe (Fig. 10.5).

Each segmental bronchus divides repeatedly till its diameter becomes 1.0 mm. At this level, it is called the *terminal bronchiole*, with no cartilage plates or glands in it.

Respiratory portion: Terminal bronchiole divides further and forms *respiratory bronchiole*, *alveolar sac*, and finally the *alveoli*. Here, the wall becomes thinner. Alveoli are lined by two types of cells. *Type I* cells are the sites for exchange of gases. *Type II* cells secrete *phospholipid surfactant*. This keeps the alveoli patent. In this portion, the exchange of gases occurs. So, it is called the respiratory portion.

Hilum of lung contains bronchus/bronchi, one pulmonary artery, two pulmonary veins, nerve plexuses, lymph vessels and lymph nodes (Fig. 10.6).

Bronchi conduct air to and from lungs. Pulmonary artery carries deoxygenated blood from the right ventricle for purification into the lungs. The oxygenated blood is returned via four pulmonary veins (two from each lung) to left atrium.

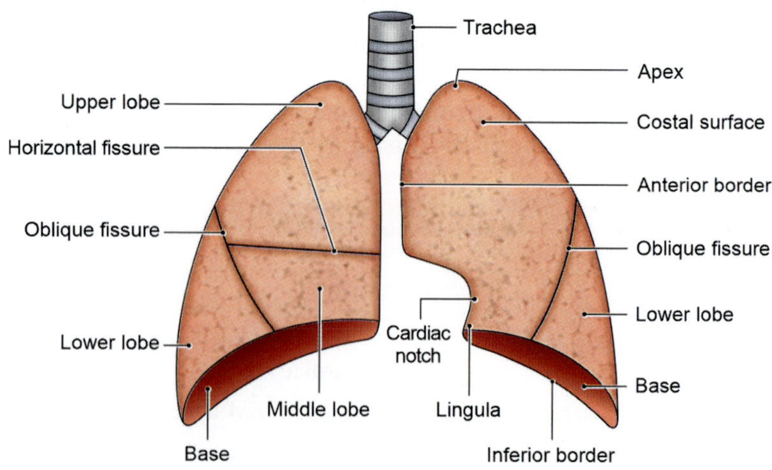

Fig. 10.4: Lungs

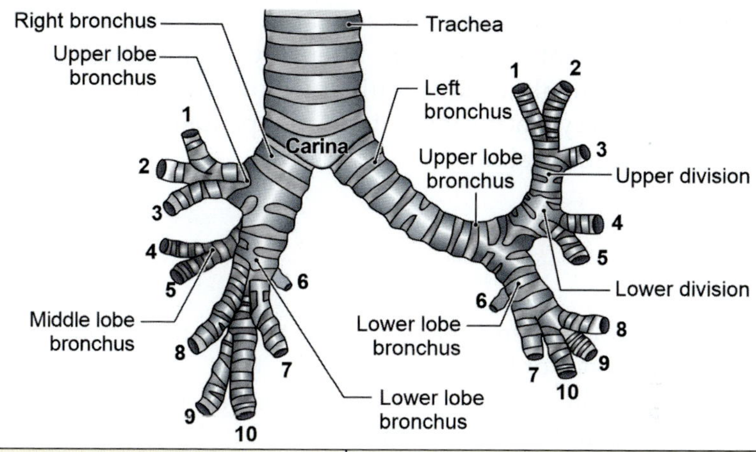

Right lung		Left lung	
Lobes	**Segments**	**Lobes**	**Segments**
A. Upper	1. Apical	A. Upper	1. Apical
	2. Posterior	• Upper division	2. Posterior
	3. Anterior		3. Anterior
B. Middle	4. Lateral	• Lower division	4. Superior lingular
	5. Medial		5. Inferior lingular
C. Lower	6. Superior	B. Lower	6. Superior
	7. Medial basal		7. Medial basal
	8. Anterior basal		8. Anterior basal
	9. Lateral basal		9. Lateral basal
	10. Posterior basal		10. Posterior basal

Fig. 10.5: Bronchopulmonary segments of the lungs

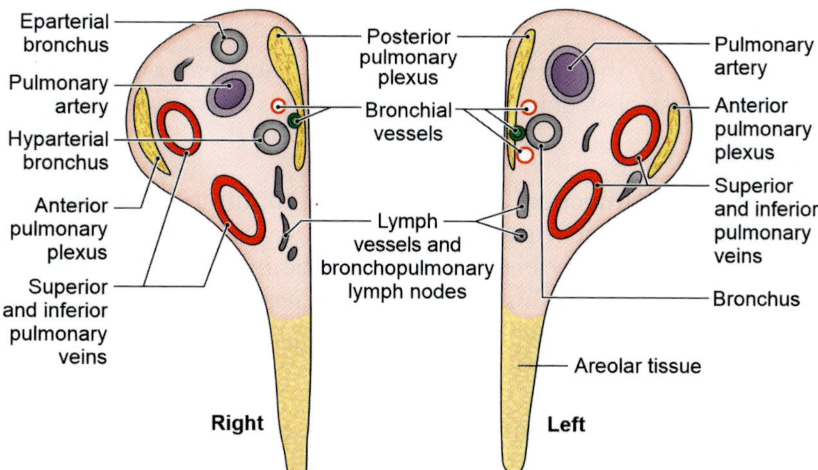

Fig. 10.6: Structures passing through the hila of right and left lungs

Definition of bronchopulmonary segments: These are well-defined anatomical segments, aerated by a tertiary/segmental bronchus. These are pyramidal in shape with apex towards hilum and base towards periphery. Each segment has independent artery, but the vein is inter-segmental.

Clinical Anatomy of Respiratory System

Nose

- The nasal bone often gets *fractured* as the two nasal bones form the prominence of the nose.
- The nasal septum may be *deviated* to one or other side, causing asymmetry in the size of nasal cavity.
- Picking of the lower part of nasal septum may cause bleeding from the nose, called the epistaxis.
- *Nasal cavity* is prone to *common cold*. It is caused by the rhinovirus and is a mild, but irritating disease.
- *The paranasal sinuses* are draining into the nasal cavity. The infection from the nasal cavity reaches the sinuses to cause *sinusitis*. Maxillary sinusitis does not heal fully as it is not able to drain completely. Postural drainage is advised in addition to other treatment.
- Infection of palatine tonsils is called *'tonsillitis'*. Infection of nasopharyngeal tonsil is called *'adenoids'*. The adenoids obstruct normal passage of air, so the child breathes through the mouth.

Diphtheria

It is caused by the bacteria *C. diphtheriae*. The membrane formed in the disease obstructs the air passage and is a serious condition.

Bronchitis

The bacterial infection associated with common cold extends down into the trachea and the bronchi, causing 'bronchitis'. It may be acute or may become chronic. The infection may extend further down into the lungs causing *bronchopneumonia*. Bronchitis is common in smokers.

Pneumonia

Develops due to colonisation of the lungs by microorganisms. It may develop due to impaired coughing, damage to ciliary epithelium of respiratory tract, pulmonary oedema and decreased resistance to infection.

Lobar pneumonia results from infection of one or more lobes of lung by *Streptococcus pneumoniae*. It is treated by antibacterial drugs.

Bronchopneumonia results from spread of infection from bronchi to terminal bronchioles and alveoli.

Asthma

Asthma starts as an allergic process with superadded inflammatory reaction. Person finds expiration rather difficult, due to bronchospasm (contraction of bronchial muscle) and excessive secretion of mucus in the bronchial tree.

Tuberculosis

This is extremely common in our country due to poor hygiene, malnutrition and living in overcrowded colonies. Tuberculosis (TB) is caused by *Mycobacterium tuberculosis*. Cough of more than 3–4 weeks of duration should be investigated for TB. The patient also develops weight loss, malaise, haemoptysis (expectoration of blood stained sputum).

It needs treatment for 6–8 months under medical supervision. TB may spread from lungs to intestine also.

Cancer of the Lung

Cancer of the bronchi is common in active or passive smokers. In smokers, the cancer of lung is far more common than non-smokers. The cancer cells may spread to lung tissue, liver, brain and bones. It is usually fatal.

Points to Remember

1. Respiratory system is for exchange of carbon dioxide of the body with oxygen.
2. Soft palate prevents bolus of food from entering into the nasal cavity.
3. Right lung has 3 lobes while left lung has 2 lobes only.
4. There are 10 segmental bronchi in both right and left lungs.

Multiple Choice Questions

1. **Which of these body systems is involved in the removal of carbon dioxide?**
   a. Respiratory system
   b. Digestive system
   c. Urinary system
   d. Nervous system
2. **Normal tidal volume in adult is about:**
   a. 300 ml
   b. 500 ml
   c. 1200 ml
   d. 3600 ml
3. **Muscles used in quiet respiration are all *except*:**
   a. Internal intercostal muscle
   b. External intercostal muscle
   c. Diaphragm
   d. Sternocleidomastoid
4. **The actual gas exchange with blood occurs in the:**
   a. Bronchi
   b. Respiratory bronchioles
   c. Terminal bronchioles
   d. Alveolar ducts and alveoli

Answers

1. a **2.** b **3.** d **4.** d

Chapter 11

Digestive System

Coffee never knew it will taste nice and sweet, before it met sugar and milk. We are good as individuals but become better when we blend with the right people.

The digestive system is concerned with the ingestion and breakdown of food including its absorption.

Digestive system is responsible for maintaining a continuous supply of required elements for the cellular metabolism in every tissue, organ and system of body.

The main components of the digestive system are the *digestive tract/alimentary* canal. The tract begins at mouth where food is taken in and ends at the anus from where the unwanted material is eliminated (Fig. 11.1).

Associated with the tracts are a number of glands which help in the digestive process. These are the salivary glands, liver, gall-bladder, bladder, pancreas and intestinal glands.

The activities of the digestive system can be grouped as:

1. ***Ingestion:*** Taking in of food in the digestive tract.
2. ***Digestion:*** During this process food is broken down into smaller pieces by mastication and various enzymes secreted by glands of digestive system. Enzymes of salivary glands, gastric juice, intestinal juice, pancreatic juice, and bile aid the digestive process.
3. ***Absorption:*** The digested food products are absorbed from the walls of intestine to be deposited in liver.
4. ***Elimination:*** Substances which cannot be digested or absorbed are expelled out from anal canal as faecal matter.

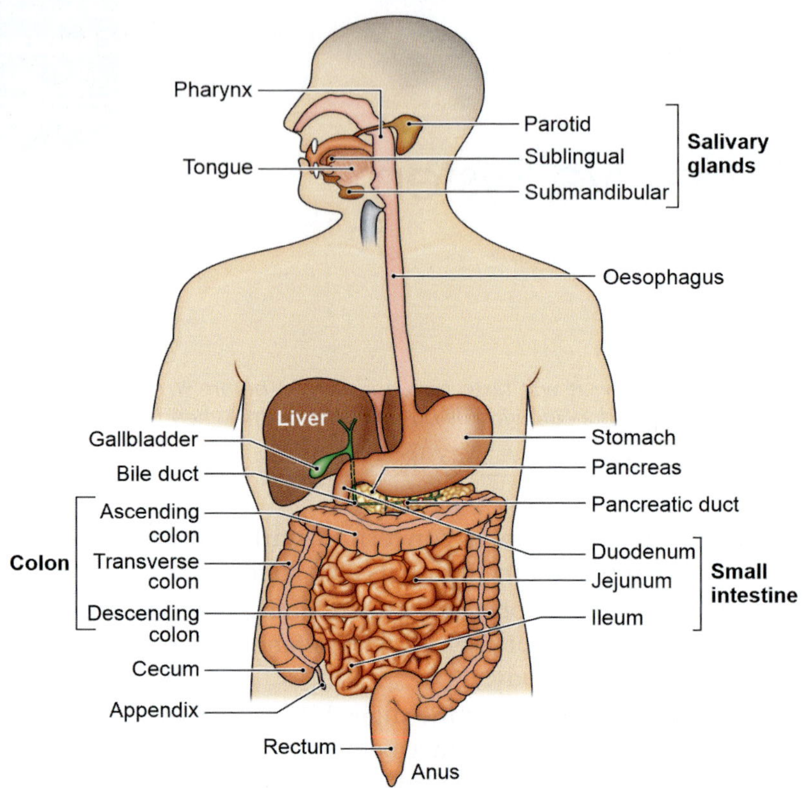

Fig. 11.1: Gastrointestinal system

LAYERS OF THE ALIMENTARY CANAL

The wall of the alimentary canal from the lower oesophagus to the anal canal has the same basic, four layered arrangement of tissue. The four layers from deep to superficial are the mucosa, submucosa, muscle layer and adventitia or serosa (Fig. 11.2).

Mucosa

It is the inner lining of the digestive tract. It is composed of three layers of tissue.

1. ***Mucous membrane:*** Composed of epithelial cells. Its function is protection, secretion and absorption. Epithelium in mouth, pharynx, oesophagus and anal canal is nonkeratinised stratified squamous epithelium (protective in function). Stomach and intestine are lined by simple columnar epithelium (function in

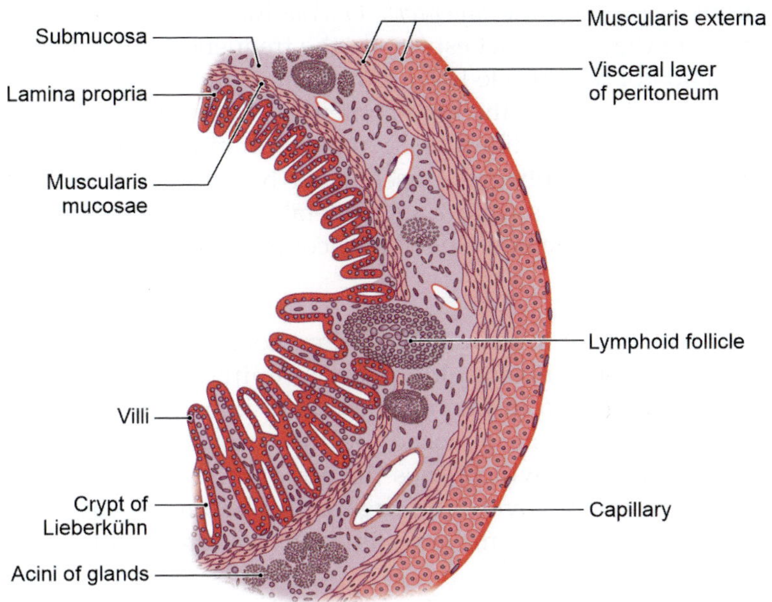

Fig. 11.2: Layers of the alimentary canal

secretion and absorption). Cells of the epithelium are replaced every 5–7 days.

2. ***Lamina propria:*** It consists of areolar connective tissue containing blood and lymphatic vessels. It also contains lymphoid tissue that has protective function. It supports the epithelium and binds it to muscularis mucosae (Fig. 11.2).
3. ***Muscularis mucosae:*** It is a thin layer of smooth muscle. It throws mucous membrane into folds, thus increasing the surface area for digestion and absorption in stomach and small intestine.

Submucosa

It consists of loose areolar connective tissue. It binds mucosa to the muscle layer. It has many blood and lymphatic vessels and lymphoid tissue. It also has a network of neurons, *submucosal plexus/plexus of Meissner*, which has sympathetic and parasympathetic nerves which supply the mucosa and submucosa.

Muscle Layer

It consists of two layers of smooth muscle—inner layer of circular fibres and outer layer of longitudinal fibres. Between two muscle layers a network of sympathetic and parasympathetic nerves and neurons is present, the *myenteric or Auerbach's plexus*. It controls motility of digestive tract especially the frequency and strength of contraction of the muscle layer. Contraction and relaxation of this layer (*peristalsis*) push the food content of digestive tract and also mixes the food with digestive secretions. In mouth, pharynx and upper part of oesophagus muscle layer has skeletal muscle that produces voluntary swallowing. Skeletal muscle is also present in external anal sphincter which allows control of defaecation.

Serosa

Serosa consists of a serous membrane consisting of an areolar connective tissue and simple squamous epithelium. It covers the organs of abdomen in membrane and is known as *peritoneum*. Peritoneum consists of a closed sac and consists of two layers—*parietal peritoneum*, which lines the abdominal wall and *visceral peritoneum*, which covers the organs in abdominal cavity. The space between two membranes is *peritoneal cavity* and contains serous fluid.

> *Competency achievement:* The student should be able to:
> AN 47.5 Describe & demonstrate major viscera of abdomen under following headings (anatomical position, external and internal features, important peritoneal and other relations, blood supply, nerve supply, lymphatic drainage and applied aspects)

DIGESTIVE TRACT/ALIMENTARY CANAL

The main parts are the mouth, pharynx, oesophagus, stomach, small intestine, large intestine. The last part of large intestine is the rectum and anal canal which ends at the anus.

Mouth

Mouth is the beginning of digestive tract and is guarded by two *lips* with the *cheeks* at the sides. It contains the *tongue* and *teeth*. It opens posteriorly into the *pharynx*. Roof of mouth is formed by palate. It is divided into anterior *hard palate* which is bony part, is longer and separates mouth cavity from the nasal cavity. The posterior part of the palate, the *soft palate*, is like a curtain. It is muscular, shorter and hangs down at the back (Fig. 11.3).

Floor of the mouth is formed by two mylohyoid muscles.

Vestibule of the mouth: It is part of mouth cavity inside the lips and cheeks and outside the gums and teeth.

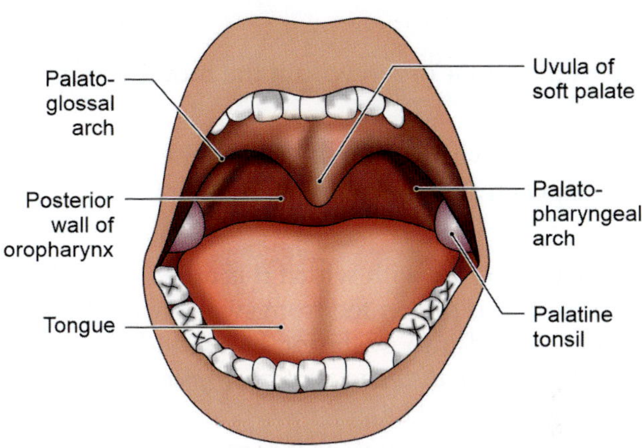

Fig. 11.3: Mouth

Mouth cavity proper: This is the cavity lying within the teeth and gums all around. It contains the mobile tongue. In the midline, the floor of front of oral cavity is a fold of mucous membrane, the *frenulum* of tongue.

Salivary Glands

Three pairs of salivary glands are parotid glands, submandibular glands and sublingual glands (Fig. 11.1).

Parotid glands are situated one on each side of face just below the external acoustic meatus. Each gland has a *parotid duct*, opening into the vestibule of mouth opposite the 2nd upper molar tooth.

Submandibular glands lie one on each side of face under the angle of jaw.

The duct of submandibular gland opens on the side of the frenulum.

Sublingual glands lie under mucous membrane of the floor of the mouth in front of submandibular glands and they open by 10–12 ducts in the floor of the mouth.

Each gland is made up of several lobules made up of small acini lined with secretory cells. The secretions are poured into ductules which join to form larger ducts leading into mouth. The saliva provides the necessary fluid for chewing and swallowing and some enzymes as well.

Nerve supply is by autonomic nervous system

- *Parasympathetic:* Increases secretion with enzymes
- *Sympathetic:* Depresses secretion

Tongue

The tongue is muscular organ within the mouth cavity proper.

Functions:

- It helps in swallowing of food. It cleans the mouth.
- It helps in speech and taste

Parts:

Tongue consists of a *root* with which it is attached to the mandible and hyoid bone and is prevented from swallowing. Its *dorsal surface* is rough and divided into posterior 1/3rd and anterior 2/3rd by V-shaped *sulcus terminalis*. The *ventral surface* is smooth and a tip pointing anteriorly (Fig. 11.4).

The dorsum of tongue is rough as it contains 3 types of papillae.

1. ***Filiform:*** Thin and pointed with no taste buds. They are present on anterior two-thirds of the tongue.
2. ***Fungiform:*** Mushroom-like structures with a few taste buds. They are present on sides and tip of tongue.
3. ***Vallate papillae:*** 10–12 in number lying in front of V-shaped sulcus. These contain maximum number of taste buds.
4. A few foliate papillae on lateral borders.

Different areas of tongue are demarcated for different papillae (Fig. 11.4).

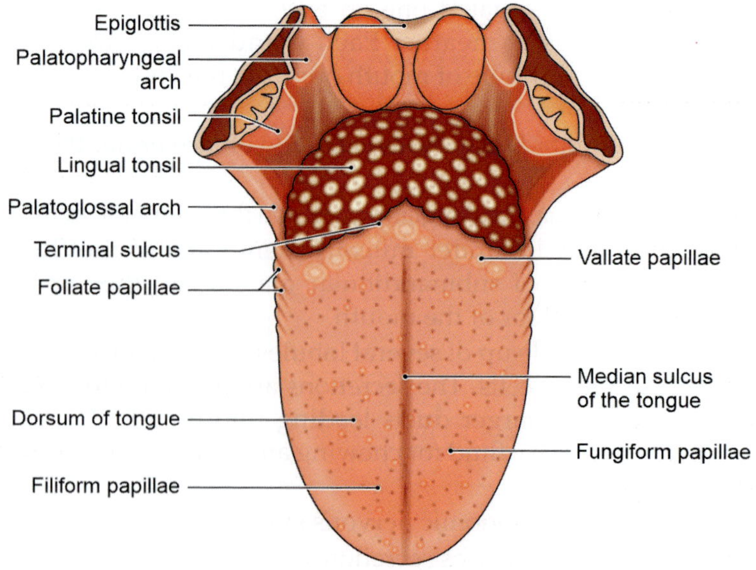

Fig. 11.4: Tongue

Muscles: Eight voluntary muscles are present in each half of the tongue. *Intrinsic* muscle change the shape of tongue. Extrinsic muscle *moves the tongue. Genioglossus* is the most important muscle as it keeps the tongue anteriorly in position and prevents it from blocking the air pathway.

Nerve supply: Most of the muscles are supplied by hypoglossal nerve (12th cranial nerve).

Arterial is derived from lingual artery, a branch of external carotid artery. *Venous drainage* is by lingual veins which join the internal jugular vein.

Teeth

There are no visible teeth in the newborn. Between 6 months and 3 years, 20 *temporary/deciduous teeth* erupt, 5 in each quarter of the jaw

Incisor	Canine	Molar
2	1	2

These are named from before backwards as *central incisor, lateral incisor, canine,* 1st molar and 2nd molar. These fall off and are replaced by permanent teeth, between 6 and 24 years of age. The *permanent teeth* are 8 in each quarter of the jaw. These are named *central incisor, lateral incisor, canine, first* and *second premolars, 1st molar, 2nd molar* and *3rd molar* (Fig. 11.5).

Incisor	Canine	Premolar	Molar
2	1	2	3

The incisors are for cutting, canine for tearing and premolars and molars for grinding the food. The tooth consists of a crown, neck and a root. The principal component is the *dentine*, a hard calcified tissue.

Crown of the tooth is best seen in the mouth and is covered by hardest calcified tissue, the *enamel. Root* is buried in the jaw and held by the *cementum* which anchors tooth to the surrounding bone. *Neck* is present at the gum margin where enamel and cementum meet. In the centre of the dentine is a *pulp cavity* with vessels and sensory nerves.

Gum or gingiva is the part of the lining of mouth, which adheres firmly to the bone of the jaw.

Nerve supply: Upper teeth are supplied by branches of maxillary division of trigeminal (V cranial nerve) while lower teeth are supplied by the mandibular division of trigeminal (V cranial nerve).

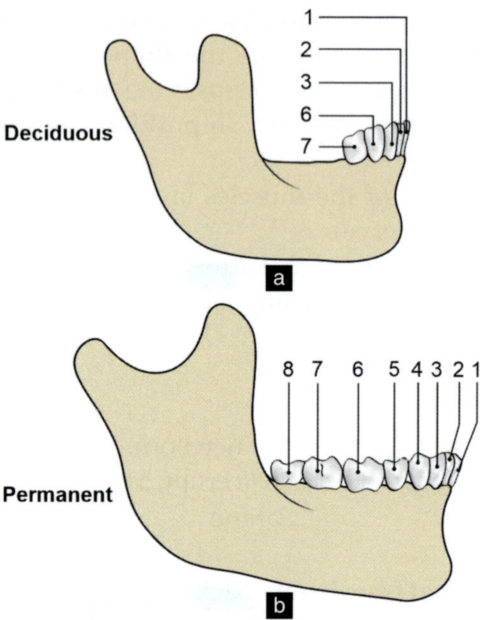

Fig. 11.5a and b: Deciduous and permanent teeth. (1) Central incisor; (2) Lateral incisor; (3) Canine; (4) 1st premolar; (5) 2nd premolar; (6) 1st molar; (7) 2nd molar; (8) 3rd molar

Pharynx

Pharynx is a 12–14 cm long tube that extends from base of skull to level of 6th cervical vertebra. It is divided into three parts—nasopharynx, oropharynx and laryngopharynx (*see* Fig. 10.2b).

Nasopharynx is nasal part of pharynx and lies behind the nose above the level of soft palate. It is important in respiration. Oropharynx and laryngopharynx are passages common to respiratory and digestive systems.

The oropharynx is the part of the pharynx between the soft palate and the upper border of epiglottis at level of third cervical vertebra. *Palatoglossal arch* on each side divides the mouth from pharynx (Fig. 11.4). Oropharynx includes two palatine tonsils. During swallowing, nasal and oral parts are separated by soft palate and the uvula.

Laryngopharynx extends from oropharynx above and continues as oesophagus below, i.e. from 3rd to 6th cervical vertebra. Food passes from oral cavity into oropharynx and laryngopharynx and then to oesophagus below.

Pharynx is composed of 3 layers of tissue—mucosa, middle layer of fibrous tissue and outer layer of three constrictor muscles. These are superior, middle and inferior constrictor muscles.

Blood supply to pharynx is by facial vessels and nerve supply is by pharyngeal plexus (X + XI nerves).

Palatine Tonsils

These are a pair of lymphoid tissue masses lying in tonsillar bed in oropharynx between anterior palatoglossal arch and posterior palatopharyngeal arch (Fig. 11.3).

Tonsil is made of lymphoid follicles embedded in connective tissue and covered on superficial surface by stratified squamous epithelium. This epithelium dips into the underlying tissue to form *crypts*, which can trap bacteria and become site of infection. Tonsils are large till puberty but regress in adulthood. These provide immunity to the body.

Oesophagus

It is muscular tube 25 cm long. It starts at level of *6th cervical vertebra*, runs the most of its part through the thoracic cavity. At the level of *10th thoracic vertebra*, it enters the diaphragm to reach abdominal cavity, where again it has a small course, to continue with the stomach. It lies behind the trachea in upper part of its course, then it passes anterior to thoracic aorta (Fig. 11.1).

Proximal one-third of oesophagus contains striated muscles and distal third smooth muscles. Oesophagus is lined by stratified squamous non-keratinised epithelium. Middle third contains a mixture of the two types of muscles.

Its function is to conduct the bolus/mass of food from the pharynx into the stomach. It is distended only during the passage of bolus, rest of the time it remains collapsed.

Arterial blood supply is by branches from thoracic aorta to the thoracic part and by branches of coeliac artery to abdominal part.

Venous drainage of thoracic part is into azygos and hemiazygos vein. Abdominal part drains into left gastric vein.

Upper end of oesophagus is guarded by *cricopharyngeal sphincter* which prevents passage of air during inspiration and aspiration of oesophageal contents. *Lower (cardiac) oesophageal sphincter* prevents reflux of acid gastric contents into the oesophagus.

Before the abdominal viscera are learnt, let us see the subdivisions of abdominal cavity.

Subdivisions of Abdominal Cavity

Two horizontal lines are drawn, one at the level of tip of 9th costal cartilage (level of first lumbar vertebra) and other at the level of tubercle of iliac crest (level of fifth lumbar vertebra).

Two vertical lines each passing through the midclavicular and midinguinal points are drawn. The upper limit of abdomen is diaphragm and lower limit is the inguinal ligament and upper border of pubic bone.

Thus, the abdominal cavity is subdivided into 9 regions:

- Right and left hypochondriac with epigastric region in centre (Fig. 11.6).
- Right and left lumbar with umbilical region in the centre.
- Right and left iliac with hypogastric region in the centre.

Various organs of abdomen are approximately placed in these nine regions.

The viscera in the abdominal cavity are related to a serous membrane, the *peritoneum*. Some are completely enveloped like the stomach and small intestine, some are partly covered and a few are only covered anteriorly. Peritoneum helps in friction free movements of the various viscera present.

Stomach

The stomach acts as a mechanical mixer, chemical digester and temporary storehouse of food. It is the most dilated part of digestive tube. Its capacity in adults is 1–1.5 litres.

Position: Left hypochondriac and epigastric regions.

Parts: The junction of oesophagus and stomach is the cardio-oesophageal junction. The stomach consists of:

- 2 ends, the proximal *cardiac end* and distal *pyloric end* (Fig. 11.7).
- 2 borders, the lesser curvature and the greater curvature.
- 2 surfaces, anterosuperior and posteroinferior surface. The latter rests on a number of organs forming the *stomach bed*.

Part of the stomach above the gastro-oesophageal junction is called the *fundus* of the stomach. The main part is the body and the distal part is the *pyloric part*. This part possesses a sphincter, the *pyloric sphincter* at its distal part.

Relations

Anterior: Anterior abdominal wall and left lobe of liver.

Posterior: Left kidney, left suprarenal, spleen and pancreas. *These form the stomach bed.*

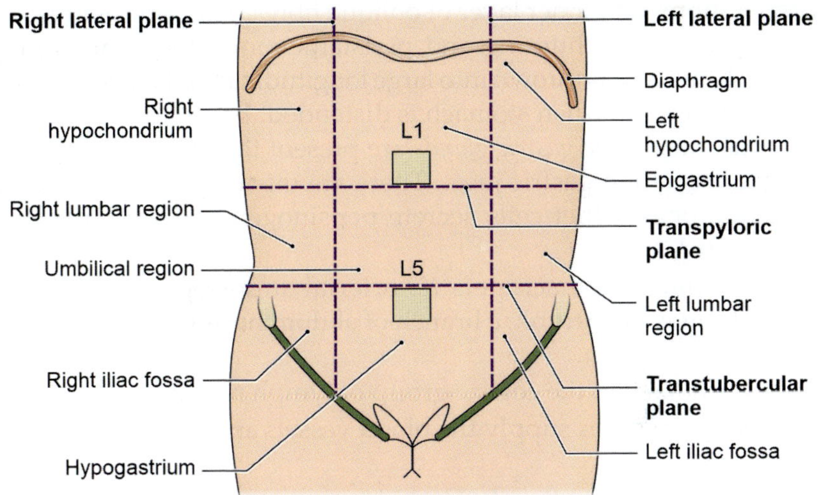

Fig. 11.6: Anterior view of abdominal regions

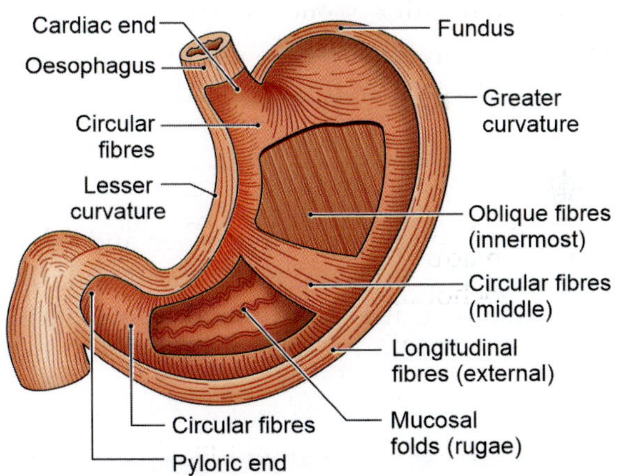

Fig. 11.7: Parts and structure of stomach

Above: Diaphragm
Below: Small intestine and transverse colon
Left: Spleen
Right: Liver

The stomach wall is composed of same four basic layers as rest of the alimentary tract but the smooth muscle layer consists of three layers—outer layer of longitudinal fibres, middle layer of circular fibres and inner layer of oblique fibres. This type of muscle arrangement has churning and peristaltic movements. In empty stomach, mucosa is thrown into large longitudinal folds called *rugae*, which disappear when stomach is distended. Below the surface of mucous membrane *gastric glands* are present that have specialised cells for secreting gastric juice. There are mucus neck cells which secrete mucus. Chief cells secrete pepsinogen and oxyntic cells secrete HCl.

Blood supply: Stomach gets its arterial supply from the three branches of coeliac trunk, a branch of abdominal aorta. Veins drain into the portal vein.

Lymph drains into the coeliac group of lymph nodes.

Sympathetic nerves supply the blood vessels and also carries pain impulses.

Vagus is secretory to the glands and causes peristalsis and inhibits the pyloric sphincter as well.

Intestines

Intestines follow the stomach. There are two parts of intestines—small intestine and large intestine. Their differences are shown in Table 11.1.

Small Intestine

It is the intestine between pylorus of stomach and ileocaecal valve. It is 5 metres long. The mucosal folds run circularly across the wall and are permanent. It is subdivided into 3 parts—proximal 25 cm is *duodenum*, middle 2/5th is *jejunum* and distal 3/5th is *ileum* (Fig. 11.1).

Table 11.1: Difference between small and large intestines

Small intestine	*Large intestine*
1. 5 metres long	1.5 metres long
2. Lies in the central part of abdomen	Lies along the periphery of abdomen
3. Has less capacity of distending	Has more capacity of distending
4. Mucosa shows villi	No villi present
5. Taenia or sacculations are absent	Taenia and sacculations both are present
6. Appendices epiploicae absent	Appendices epiploicae as tags of fat present

Duodenum

Duodenum is C-shaped with *head of pancreas* lying in its concavity. The *bile duct* and the *pancreatic duct* open by a *common opening* into the *duodenum*, 10 cm from the pylorus at *major duodenal papilla.*

Jejunum and Ileum

These two parts form most of the small intestine. These are suspended from the posterior abdominal wall by a fold of peritoneum called *the mesentery.*

The digestive process that begins in stomach is continued in the small intestine. This is also the main site of absorption of the products of digestion.

Small intestine wall is composed of same four basic layers as rest of alimentary tract. Mucosa of small intestine is thrown into permanent ridges called *circular or Kerckring's folds.* These folds enhance the absorption of nutrients by increasing the surface area and also promote mixing of chyme (digested liquid food).

The mucosa has 0.5–1 mm finger-like projections, *villi.* These vastly increase the surface area for absorption and digestion. The villi are lined by various types of cells. Absorptive cells are of simple columnar epithelium with tiny microvilli (1 µm long) on their free border, forming a fuzzy line called *brush border* along intestinal lumen. Each villus encloses a network of blood and lymph capillaries. The lymph capillaries are called *lacteals.* Nutrients absorbed by epithelial cells covering the villus pass through wall of a capillary or lacteal to enter blood or lymph, respectively.

Arterial blood supply is from the superior mesenteric artery which gives 12–15 branches for small intestine and 3 branches for large intestine as well. *Veins* drain into superior mesenteric vein which with splenvic vein forms the portal vein.

The *lymph vessels* drain into para-aortic lymph nodes and from there into the upper part of cisterna chyli, at the beginning of the thoracic duct.

Nerve supply is from vagus and sympathetic nerves. These nerves form plexuses within the wall of intestine. These are submucosal or *Meissner's plexus* and myenteric or *Auerbach's plexus* in between two coats of muscularis externa. These plexuses cause peristaltic movement for propelling the contents of small intestine towards large intestine.

Large Intestine

It is the last part of the digestive tube and follows the small intestine. It starts at ileocaecal junction. Its parts are caecum, vermiform appendix, colon, rectum and anal canal (Fig. 11.1).

Caecum

Lies in the right iliac fossa. The ileocaecal valve guards the opening of ileum into the caecum, and 2 cm below this opening is the opening of the vermiform appendix. It is continuous with the ascending colon.

Vermiform Appendix

It is the narrowest part of the digestive tube. It is usually 8 cm long and 0.5 cm wide. It has a base and a tip. The tip may occupy different positions.

Arterial supply is from appendicular artery, one of the caecal branches of superior mesenteric artery.

Colon

It forms the greatest length of large intestine, and is subdivided into *ascending colon* on right side of abdominal cavity, *transverse colon* across the abdomen, *descending colon* on the left side and *pelvic colon* in the pelvis (Fig. 11.1).

The large intestine shows the same basic layers of tissue. In colon the longitudinal muscle fibres are thickened in three thick bands called *taeniae coli*, situated at regular intervals around it. They stop at the junction of the sigmoid colon and rectum. These bands of muscle are slightly shorter than the total length of colon, they give a sacculated or puckered appearance forming a series of pouches called *haustra*. Small pouches of visceral peritoneum filled with fat are attached to taeniae coli and are called *appendices epiploicae*.

Arterial supply of ascending and most of the transverse colon is by superior mesenteric artery. Rest of the colon is supplied by inferior mesenteric artery. *Veins* drain into the portal vein. Lymph vessels drain into the para-aortic lymph nodes.

Parasympathetic nerve supply to ascending and most of transverse colon is from vagus, while to small left part of transverse colon, descending and pelvic colon is from *pelvic splanchnic nerve* (sacral 2, 3, 4 segments). *Sympathetic nerves* relax the smooth muscle and constrict ileocaecal and internal anal sphincters.

Rectum and Anal Canal

Rectum starts at the middle of sacrum and is 15 cm long. It follows forward curvature of sacrum and coccyx and ends 2.5 cm below and in front of coccyx where it continues as anal canal (Fig. 11.1). ***Anal canal*** is the last 4 cm of digestive tube. From the anorectal junction it passes downwards and backwards to the anus. In the wall of anal canal, the inner circular layer of smooth muscle becomes thickened to form *internal anal sphincter* while outside this is *external anal sphincter* of skeletal muscle. Internal sphincter is supplied by autonomic nerves while external anal sphincter by inferior rectal nerve.

Rectum and anal canal has the same basic 4 layered structure like other parts of digestive tract.

The lining membrane of anus consists of stratified squamous epithelium continuous with skin beyond external anal sphincter.

The *mucous membrane* of anal canal shows in upper part three folds which keep it mostly closed. These are due to plexus of veins. If enlarged, these form *haemorrhoids or piles* which may cause pain or bleeding or both.

Rectum and anal canal are supplied by *superior rectal artery* (continuation of inferior mesenteric artery), *middle* and *inferior rectal arteries*, branches of internal pudendal artery.

Veins draining along superior rectal artery end in portal vein, while those running along middle and inferior rectal arteries end in pudendal and systemic veins. Thus, anal canal is a site of *porto-systemic anastomosis.*

LIVER

The liver is the largest gland in the body weighing about 1500 g and receives 1500 cc of blood per minute (Fig. 11.8).

Liver lies under the diaphragm, in right hypochondriac/ epigastric and partly into left hypochondriac regions. It extends into the thoracic cavity up to 5th rib and receives protection from the costal cartilages. It may be felt below the right costal margin on deep inspiration (Fig. 11.1).

The liver is kept in position by 2–3 hepatic veins which enter the inferior vena cava, by intra-abdominal pressure and by peritoneal folds forming supporting ligaments that attach the liver to inferior surface of diaphragm. The liver has anterior, superior, posterior, right lateral surfaces which are continuous with each other.

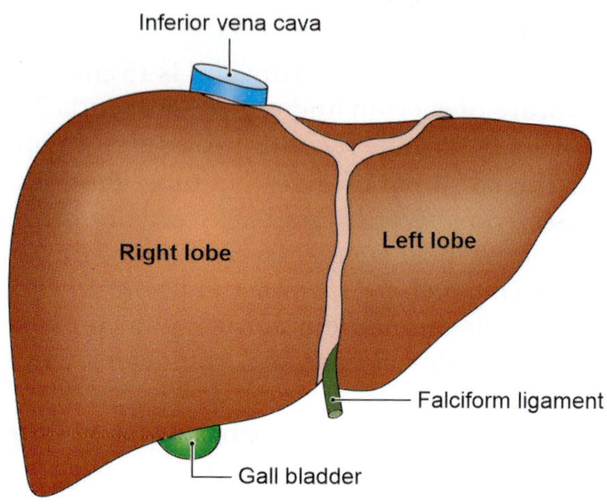

Fig. 11.8: The liver: Anterior view

Liver biopsy is done through *right 8th intercostal space* in full expiration to avoid injury to lung.

Liver also has an inferior or visceral surface which is related to various abdominal viscera. In addition, this surface shows a horizontal 5 cm fissure called the *porta hepatis*. Porta hepatis is the gateway of liver. Portal vein and hepatic artery enter the liver while hepatic ducts leave the liver. Attached to the margins of porta hepatis is a fold of peritoneum the *lesser omentum* which extends from the liver to the lesser curvature of stomach.

Liver is divided into four lobes—right lobe (largest), left lobe, caudate lobe, quadrate lobe. The caudate and quadrate lobes are seen on posterior surface and inferior surface.

Arterial supply of the liver is from common hepatic artery of coeliac trunk of the aorta (20%) while venous drainage via hepatic veins is into inferior vena cava. It receives 80% of blood from digestive tract via the portal vein.

Portal vein is formed behind the neck of pancreas by union of superior mesenteric and splenic veins. Like any artery it divides into right and left branches before entering the liver.

The liver is made up of hexagonal hepatic lobules about 1 micron in diameter. Lobules are made up of cubical cells, *hepatocytes* arranged in columns radiating from a *central vein*. Between columns of cells there are sinusoids (blood vessels with incomplete walls). Sinusoids contain a mixture of blood from branches of hepatic artery and portal vein (Fig. 11.9). Blood drains from sinusoids into central

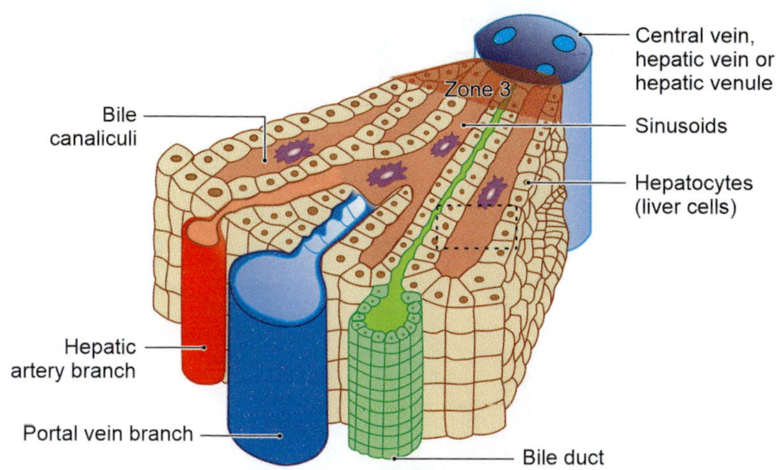

Fig. 11.9: Blood supply of liver

vein. These join with veins from other lobules, forming larger veins and eventually become *hepatic veins* which leave the liver and empty into inferior vena cava.

Bile canaliculi run between liver cells. Thus, each column of hepatocytes has a blood sinusoid on one side and a bile canaliculus on the other. The canaliculi join to form larger bile canals and eventually they form right and left *hepatic ducts* which drain bile from liver.

The combination of bile ductule, branch of hepatic artery and portal vein is known as *portal triad*. At the angles of lobule lie six portal triads. Blood flows from portal triad into hepatic sinusoid and towards the central vein. Bile flows *centrifugally* (from centre to periphery) from bile canaliculi to bile ductule.

Lymph flow from liver is large and is about 0.75 mL/minute. It drains into nodes in porta hepatis and finally reaches the thoracic duct.

Sympathetic nerves enter the liver with the hepatic artery to control the lumen of the vessels. Pain fibres are carried along the phrenic nerve (C3, 4) which supplies peritoneum over the gallbladder. Pain of gallbladder is referred to tip of right shoulder as the supraclavicular nerves also have same root value (C3, 4).

EXTRAHEPATIC BILIARY APPARATUS

Components of this apparatus are gall bladder, right and left hepatic ducts which leave porta hepatis and soon join to form *common hepatic duct*, which is 4 cm long (Fig. 11.10).

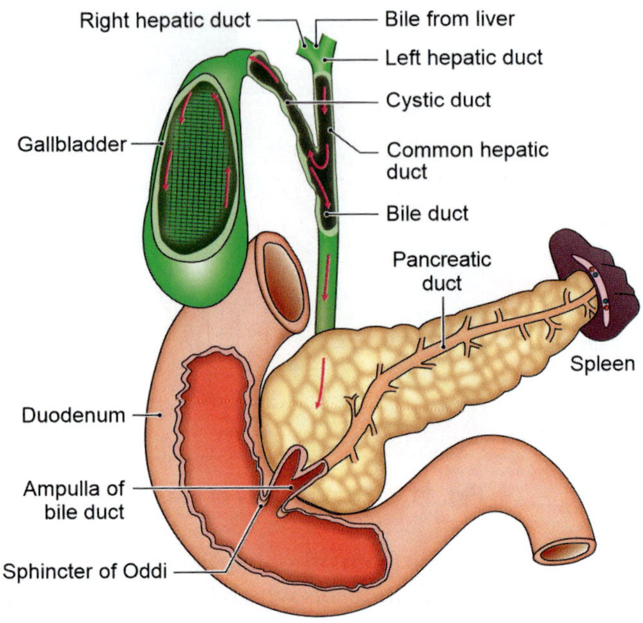

Fig. 11.10: Extrahepatic biliary apparatus and pancreas

The gallbladder is 7 cm long and lies on the under surface of liver.

Cystic duct about 3 cm long from the neck of gall bladder joins the common hepatic duct to form the bile duct.

The bile duct is 8 cm long. The bile duct and the main pancreatic duct open together at the major duodenal papilla into the second part of the duodenum.

All these components carry the bile produced in the liver. Bile runs in distinct channels and does not mix with the blood. It helps in the digestion of fats.

GallBladder

Gallbladder is pyriform organ 7 cm long with a capacity of 50 mL. It is present in a depression on the inferior surface of the liver. It acts as a storage and concentrating organ for bile. Its parts are the fundus, body, which narrows to form the neck, which continues as the cystic duct. Cystic duct allows two-way traffic to bile (Fig. 11.10).

Arterial supply of gallbladder is through the cystic artery arising from the right hepatic artery. *Cystic vein* drains into right branch of portal vein. *Lymph* from extrahepatic biliary apparatus drains into lymph nodes in the porta hepatis. *Pain fibres* from gallbladder and the ducts run with sympathetic nerves. It is referred to tip of right shoulder as the supraclavicular nerves also have same root value (C3, 4). Pain of biliary colic enters the spinal cord via 7th to 9th thoracic nerves.

Mucosa of gallbladder consists of simple columnar epithelium. Submucosa is absent. Muscular layer is of smooth muscle fibres with an additional layer of oblique fibres. Outermost layer is of peritoneum.

PANCREAS

Pancreas is a gland present across the upper part of posterior abdominal wall from right to the left side. It contains both exocrine secretion for digestion of carbohydrates, fats and proteins as well as endocrine secretion, from islets of Langerhans, which act on the carbohydrate metabolism (Fig. 11.10).

Pancreas is 15 cm long, and consists of a *head, neck, body* and *tail.* It lies behind the peritoneum. Head of pancreas lies in the 'C' of the duodenum. Bile duct runs behind head of pancreas. An *uncinate process* from the lowest part of head passes to left behind superior mesenteric vessels. *Neck* is small segment behind which superior mesenteric vein and splenic vein join to form the portal vein.

Body is triangular in shape and is related to the splenic artery along the upper border, transverse mesocolon along the anterior border. The *tail* is the part lying anterior to left kidney reaching up to the hilum of spleen.

Exocrine secretions of pancreas are secreted by secretory cells present in the lobules (acini). Each lobule is drained by a tiny duct and these eventually unite to form pancreatic duct. Secretions are delivered to duodenum by the *main* and *accessory pancreatic ducts.*

Main pancreatic duct and common bile duct open in the *hepatopancreatic ampulla,* which enters the duodenum at major duodenal papilla situated at a distance of 10 cm from the pylorus. Duodenal opening of ampulla is controlled by *sphincter of Oddi.*
Blood supply to pancreas is by splenic and mesenteric vessels.

SPLEEN

The spleen is the largest lymphoid organ of the body. It is purplish red, highly vascular organ lying at the back of left hypochondriac region (Fig. 11.10).

It is situated well under cover of the costal margin, between the diaphragm on one side and kidney, stomach, colon and tail of pancreas on the other side. These four viscera make impressions on the visceral surface of spleen. This surface also has a deep fissure, the **hilum**, for the passage of splenic vessels. Spleen is 2.5 cm thick, 7.5 cm broad, 12.5 cm long, weighs 200 g and lies between 9th and 11th ribs. According to 42nd edition of Gray's Anatomy, spleen lies between 10th and 12th ribs. The spleen is supported by peritoneal ligaments, i.e. gastrosplenic and lienorenal ligaments.

Spleen is supplied by the tortuous *splenic artery* from coeliac trunk, which runs along the upper border of pancreas to the hilum.

Splenic vein runs behind the pancreas to join superior mesenteric vein and so forms the portal vein.

Lymph vessels leave the hilum and drain into coeliac nodes.

Spleen is covered by a dense connective tissue *capsule*. *Trabeculae* extend inwards from capsule. Cellular material of spleen is divided into *white pulp* and *red pulp*. Red pulp consists of blood filled venous sinuses and white pulp is of lymphatic tissue, comprise lymphocytes and macrophages.

Spleen is part of the lymphatic system and its functions are:

1. ***Phagocytosis:*** Leukocytes and platelets are phagocytosed in spleen. Old and abnormal RBCs are destroyed in spleen and breakdown products (bilirubin and iron) are passed to the liver.
2. ***Storage of blood:*** Spleen contains up to 350 mL blood. In shock, sympathetic stimulation can return a large part of this volume to circulation.
3. ***Immunity:*** Spleen contains B- and T-lymphocytes which are important in immune response to infections.
4. ***Erythropoiesis:*** RBC production occurs in spleen and liver in fetal life and in adults also in times of great need.
5. ***Storage of platelets***.

Clinical Anatomy of Digestive System

Mouth

Angular stomatitis: The angles of mouth show painful cracks due to vitamin B deficiency or infection by herpes simplex virus. It usually occurs after an attack of common cold or influenza.

Aphthous stomatitis: Recurrent painful oral ulcers develop inside the mouth. They are often associated with vitamin B complex deficiency.

Fungal infection of mouth: It occurs in bottle fed babies and in elderly people with low immunity. It is usually caused by *Candida albicans*.

Cancer of mouth: This mostly occurs in people who keep betel nut in their mouth for long periods. Chronic irritation of delicate mucous membrane of mouth and tongue results in squamous cell carcinoma.

Glossitis: Inflammation of the tongue causes areas of redness on the tongue, which are quite painful. The tongue becomes smooth in deficiency of vitamin B. In anaemia, the undersurface of tongue looks pale. Chronic irritation due to sharp edge of the tooth or betel nut may cause cancer which spreads fast and is usually fatal.

Tumours of salivary glands: Pleomorphic adenoma is benign tumour consisting of epithelial and connective tissue cells and it usually occurs in parotid gland. Malignant tumour may also develop in any salivary gland.

During embryonic development, roof of mouth (hard palate) develops as two separate halves (right and left) and a median premaxilla part. Before birth these fuse with each other. The upper lip/hard palate may show a developmental defect due to incomplete fusion in the form of *cleft lip or cleft palate* (partial or complete or both).

In the newborn baby with cleft palate, there is communication between mouth and nasal cavity. These children when fed with milk, get choked as the milk enters the nasal cavity, pharynx, larynx and there is defective speech.

Teeth: Teeth are the hardest tissues of our body. They are used in medicolegal practice for identification and age determination.

In *caries*, the enamel gets removed and the nerves get exposed, causing severe pain.

The gums may get inflamed. The condition is called *gingivitis*. Teeth provide proper shape to the face and must be maintained well.

1. ***Mumps:*** Viral infection of the parotid (especially), submandibular and sublingual glands, is called mumps. The virus may also spread to the testis, ovary, brain and pancreas.
2. ***Tonsillitis and adenoids*** occur at the oropharyngeal junction.

Oesophagus

1. *Oesophagus* may get partly fibrosed if caustic materials are taken accidently leading to narrowing *(stricture)* and difficulty in swallowing.

2. The lower end of oesophagus may develop dilatation of veins in liver fibrosis *(cirrhosis)*. These veins may rupture to cause haematemesis (vomiting of blood).

Stomach

Gastritis

It occurs when there is imbalance between corrosive action of gastric juice and protective effect of mucus on gastric mucosa. The insufficient amount of mucus in stomach leads to damage of surface epithelium from hydrochloric acid.

Acute gastritis develops due to regular, prolonged use of aspirin and other non-steroidal anti-inflammatory drugs (NSAIDs); excessive intake of alcohol, heavy cigarette smoking, food poisoning, ingestion of corrosive acids and alkalis.

Chronic gastritis is a milder form. It may follow acute attacks or autoimmune disease.

Vomiting

Vomiting/emesis is the forcible expulsion of contents of upper gastrointestinal (GI) tract (stomach and sometimes duodenum) through the mouth. It usually occurs due to irritation of stomach. Nurses have to observe, record and report about the vomiting of the patient for treatment.

An ulcer is crater-like lesion in membrane. Ulcers that develop in areas of the GI tract exposed to acidic gastric juice are called peptic ulcers.

Helicobacter pylori is the most frequently seen in cases of peptic ulcer. This bacterium produces ammonia which damages the protective layer of the stomach.

The stomach bears the brunt of all wrong types of food including too hot/too cold food or fluids. The ulcers in the stomach occur along its lesser curvature and in first few centimetres of duodenum in alcoholics and heavy smokers. People with erratic eating habits with erratic timings are also subjects of peptic ulcers. The ulcers may cause bleeding or perforation. If untreated, the chronic ulcers may become cancerous.

Small Intestine

1. ***Typhoid fever*** is caused by *Salmonella typhi*. It occurs due to intake of contaminated water. It causes ulcers in the small intestine. It may affect the liver, spleen and gallbladder.

2. ***Tuberculosis*** also affects the intestine. The most common site is ileocaecal junction. TB intestine causes intestinal obstruction.
3. ***Food poisoning*** by *E. coli* causes vomiting and diarrhoea.
4. ***Cholera*** is caused by *Vibrio cholerae* and causes severe vomiting, diarrhoea and dehydration. It needs urgent attention and transfusion of intravenous fluids to correct dehydration.

Large Intestine

1. ***Caecum*** is the beginning of large intestine. It is a common site of *intestinal tuberculosis*.
2. ***Appendicitis:*** Inflammation of vermiform appendix results in appendicitis. In its early stages, there is pain around umbilicus while in later stage, it gets localised in the right iliac fossa. The removal of appendix is called *appendicectomy*.
3. ***Dysentery*** is either bacterial or amoebic according to the nature of causative agent. *Bacterial dysentery* is caused by *Shigella* while the *amoebic dysentery* is caused by *Entamoeba histolytica* with mucus.
4. ***Cancer of the colon*** is a common entity in people who eat less of fibre in their diet. It is less common in India as Indians eat vegetables, which contain good amount of fibres.

Glands

Pancreas

Inflammation of pancreas is called *pancreatitis*. It may be acute or chronic leading to damage to pancreas. Most commonly it is caused by gallstones and alcoholism. Lack of insulin causes diabetes.

Liver

Liver is like the 'reserve bank' of our body. Most of the nutrients are deposited here to be used if and when necessary.

1. ***Cirrhosis*** results from long-term inflammation caused by a variety of agents in which liver tissue is destroyed and replaced by fibrous tissue. Various causes of cirrhosis are alcoholism, hepatitis B and C virus infection, parasitic infections of liver, chemicals that destroy hepatocytes. Symptoms include jaundice, oedema in legs and uncontrolled bleeding due to oesophageal varices, ascites (collection fluid in peritoneal cavity).

2. ***Hepatitis*** is inflammation of liver that can be caused by viruses, drugs and chemicals including alcohol. Viral infections are the most common cause and include types A, B, C and E.
3. ***Jaundice*** results from abnormal bilirubin metabolism and excretion. The bilirubin level in the blood rises and it gets deposited in various tissues, e.g. skin, conjunctiva and brain.

Gallbladder

Since it stores bile, it is subjected to inflammation, called *cholecystitis*. The pain may radiate to the tip of right shoulder.

The bile gets concentrated in gallbladder. At times the salts may precipitate to cause multiple gallstones. This condition is called *cholelithiasis*. Surgical removal of gallbladder is called *cholecystectomy*.

Obesity

When the weight is more than 20–25% of normal weight, the person is said to be obese. Obesity itself is a disease as it leads to diabetes, hypertension, arthritis and heart disease. Weight reduction should be slow and sustained. It must not be too fast, as the weight lost tends to come back.

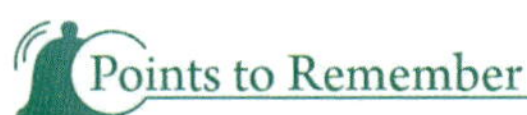

1. In human, teeth erupt two times only. These are called milk teeth and permanent teeth.
2. There are nine regions in the anterior abdominal wall.
3. Most dilated part of digestive system is the stomach.
4. Liver is the largest gland of the body.
5. Pancreas secretes insulin. Lack of insulin results in diabetes.

Multiple Choice Questions

1. Parts of pharynx from above downwards are:

a. Nasopharynx, laryngopharynx, oropharynx
b. Oropharynx, laryngopharynx, nasopharynx
c. Nasopharynx, oropharynx, laryngopharynx

2. Subdivisions of abdominal cavity are:

a. Eight b. Seven c. Nine d. Ten

3. Synthesis of bile occurs in:

a. Liver b. Gallbladder
c. Pancreas d. Duodenum

4. Part of large intestine that is joined to rectum is called:

a. Ascending colon b. Transverse colon
c. Descending colon d. Sigmoid colon

Answers

1. c **2.** c **3.** a **4.** d

Chapter 12

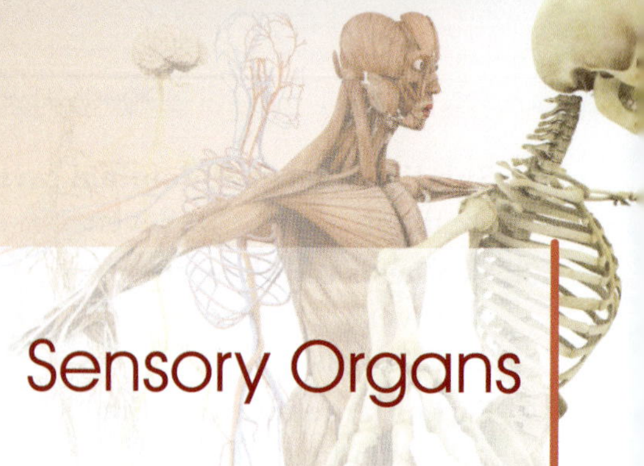

Sensory Organs

Control your thought process when you are alone. Control your speech process when you are together.

The sensory organs of taste (tongue), smell (nose), hearing (ear), sight (eye) and touch (skin) have specialised receptors present outside the brain. These sense receptors are in close vicinity of brain and are governed by cranial nerves. Special senses work in harmony with each other and also with various muscles and glands.

Competency achievement: The student should be able to:
AN 39.1 Describe and demonstrate the morphology, nerve supply, embryological basis of nerve supply, blood supply, lymphatic drainage and actions of extrinsic and intrinsic muscles of tongue

TONGUE

It is a voluntary muscular organ situated in the oral cavity. It has following functions:

1. Helps in speech
2. Helps in swallowing
3. Contains *taste buds* which make us aware of various tastes. The multitude of eating shops like Pizza Huts, etc. are to please the taste buds. Stomach has none at all.

Musculature of tongue is comprised of intrinsic muscles (lying within tongue) and extrinsic muscles (one attachment is outside the tongue and other within it). Most of these are supplied by XII or hypoglossal nerve.

The sensation of taste is carried by branch of VII (facial) from most of the anterior two-thirds; by branch of IX (glossopharyngeal) from vallate papillae and posterior one-third of tongue; by branch of X (vagus) from posterior most part of tongue.

General sensation from anterior two-thirds is carried by lingual branch of V3 (mandibular branch of trigeminal nerve); from posterior one-third by IX; from posterior most part by X.

There are three types of papillae according to their shape.

1. ***Filiform***, which make the dorsal surface of tongue rough.
2. ***Fungiform*** seen on the sides, contain a few taste buds.
3. ***Vallate*** present in posterior part of anterior two-thirds of tongue. Contain maximum taste buds (Fig. 12.1a and b).

The basic tastes are sweet, salt, sour and bitter (Fig. 12.2).

1. ***Sweet:*** Mainly on tip of tongue
2. ***Sour:*** Mainly on edges of tongue
3. ***Salt:*** Mainly on dorsum anteriorly
4. ***Bitter:*** Mainly at back of tongue.

Arterial supply of tongue is by lingual artery, a branch of external carotid artery.

Veins unite to form lingual veins which drains into internal jugular vein.

Lymph drains to submandibular and deep cervical nodes. Lymph vessels cross within tongue from one side to the other.

Cancer of the tongue may involve lymph nodes of both sides. Cancer is common in people who keep betel nuts with lime for hours in their mouth.

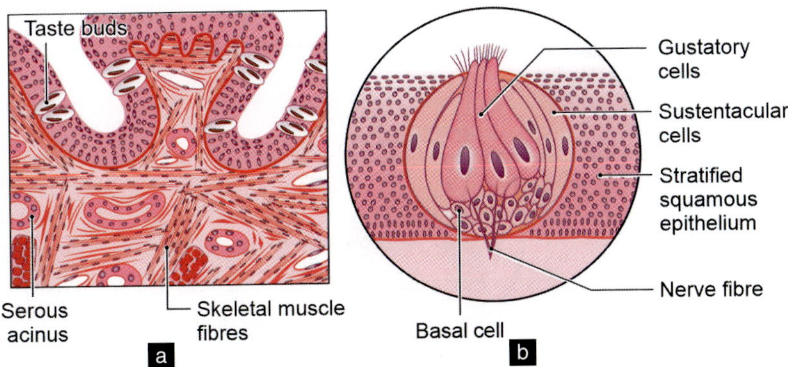

Fig. 12.1a and b: Circumvallate papilla of tongue. Taste buds contain receptors on papillae of tongue. These are stimulated by chemicals that enter the pores dissolved in saliva

12

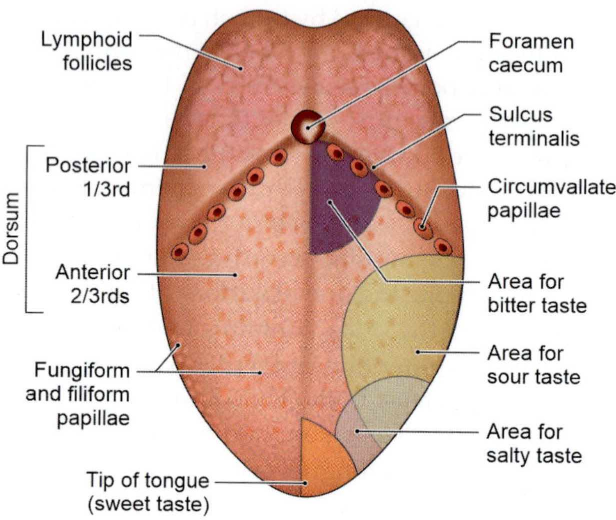

Fig. 12.2: Tongue with areas for taste

Taste pathway: It is carried VII, IX and X cranial nerves to nucleus of tractus solitarius for a relay. These fibres then pass up to thalamus for another relay and finally reach postcentral gyrus of the cerebrum (Fig. 12.3).

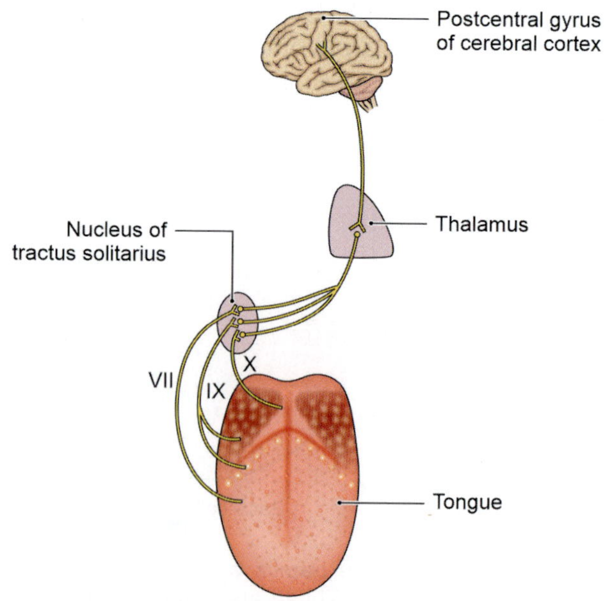

Fig. 12.3: Taste pathway

Competency achievement: The student should be able to:
AN 37.1 Describe and demonstrate features of nasal septum, lateral wall of nose, their blood supply and nerve supply

NOSE

The nose is for breathing and the uppermost part of its lining contains olfactory nerve cells for smell. The nose consists of external nose and nasal cavity. The *external nose* is made of only two bones, the nasal bones, the rest is cartilage. The two openings on the face are the *anterior nares*.

Nasal cavity is divided into right and left halves by a median *nasal septum*. The septum is formed by thin bones and cartilage and is covered by mucoperiosteum or mucoperichondrium. At times, the septum may be deviated to one side.

Nasal cavity opens at the back into the nasopharynx through the posterior nares.

The lateral wall of nasal cavity shows three projections: (1) Superior, (2) middle and (3) inferior conchae to increase the surface area. Below each concha is the respective meatus (Fig. 12.4). ***The paranasal air sinuses*** open into these meatuses. These are sphenoidal, ethmoidal, frontal and maxillary. These sinuses make the skull lighter, give resonance to the voice and humidify the inspired air.

The main *artery* of the nasal septum is sphenopalatine artery, the continuation of maxillary artery. Veins drain into maxillary vein.

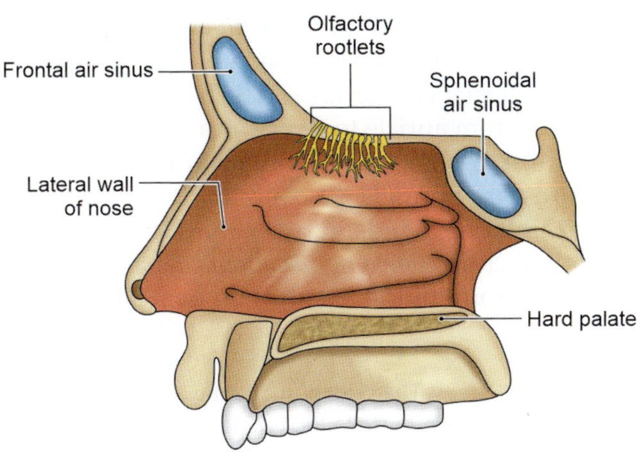

Fig. 12.4: Olfactory rootlets for sense of smell

Lymph drains into pharyngeal and deep cervical nodes.

The nerve supply to nasal cavity is of two types, *general sensation* like pain, touch, temperature carried by branches of V1 (ophthalmic) and V2 (maxillary) divisions of V or trigeminal nerve. The uppermost part of septum and lateral wall (1 cm) contains olfactory cells for carrying sense of smell.

The nerve rootlets pass through holes (cribriform plate) in the ethmoid bone and reach lower aspect of frontal lobe. These join the olfactory bulb, which continues into olfactory tract to end in the uncus of temporal lobe.

Sense of smell is related to sense of taste. Sense of smell is also connected to X or vagus nerve which secretes the gastric juice in relation to good smell. Human beings can distinguish 2,000 to 4,000 different odours. Highly lipid and water-soluble substances produce strong odours.

> *Competency achievement:* The student should be able to:
> AN 40.1 Describe and identify the parts, blood supply and nerve supply of external ear

EAR

The ear is an important organ. Its functions are hearing and maintenance of the balance of body.

Ear consists of three parts: (1) External ear, (2) middle ear and (3) internal ear.

External Ear

Made up of *pinna or auricle and external auditory meatus*. *Auricle* projects from the side of head and is composed of elastic cartilage covered with skin. *External auditory meatus* is a S-shaped tube about 2.5 cm long and extends from auricle to tympanic membrane (Fig. 12.5).

Outer one-third of external auditory meatus is cartilaginous and inner two-thirds are bony. It is covered with skin, that contains numerous ceruminous glands in outer third, that secrete ear wax and has hair follicles. *Tympanic membrane* separates the external auditory meatus from middle ear. It is an oval-shaped membrane placed obliquely.

> *Competency achievement:* The student should be able to:
> AN 40.2 Describe and demonstrate the boundaries, contents, relations and functional anatomy of middle ear and auditory tube

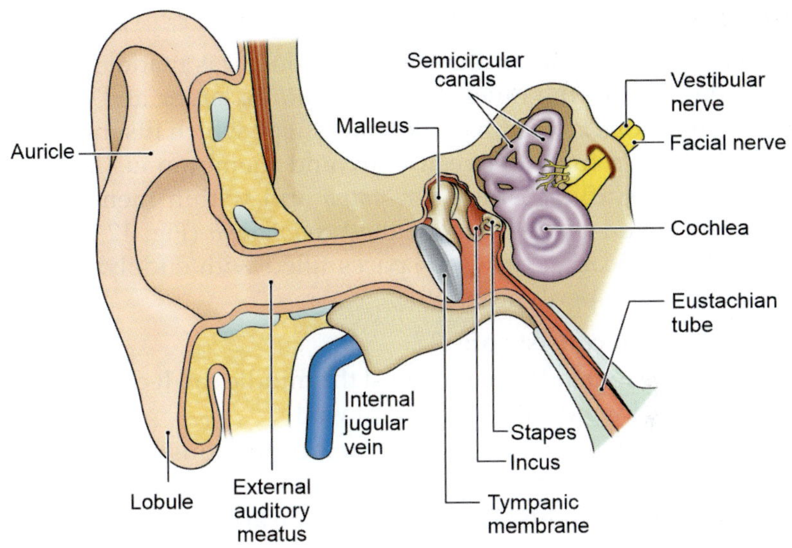

Fig. 12.5: Components of ear

Middle Ear

A box-like small cavity with six walls, having a *chain of ossicles, malleus, incus* and *stapes* from lateral wall towards the medial wall (Fig. 12.5). The ossicles transmit the sound vibrations of tympanic membrane to internal ear.

Its *roof* is thin plate of bone in the middle cranial fossa.

Floor is small piece of bone near carotid canal.

Anterior wall contains auditory tube which equalises the pressure outside the ear and within the ear. It opens into the nasopharynx. Opening of auditory tube usually remains closed but opens during chewing, swallowing, yawning. Anterior wall also contains a canal for tensor tympani muscle.

Posterior wall consists of mastoid antrum, facial canal, pyramid containing stapedius muscle.

Lateral wall is formed by tympanic membrane (Fig. 12.5).

Medial wall has an oval window, a round window and promontory between the two windows formed by the basal turn of cochlea. The oval window is occluded by part of stapes and round window by a fine sheet of fibrous tissues.

Competency achievement: The student should be able to:
AN 40.3 Describe the features of internal ear

Internal Ear

Internal ear is a cavity in the temporal bone. It is made up of two parts, one within the other. *Bony labyrinth* is larger and encloses the membranous labyrinth of the same shape which fits into it, like a tube within a tube. Between bony and membranous labyrinth there is watery fluid called *perilymph* and within membranous labyrinth there is watery fluid called *endolymph* (Fig. 12.6). There is no communication between spaces filled with endolymph and those filled with perilymph.

Bony labyrinth consists of:

1. ***Vestibule:*** Expanded part nearest the middle ear. It contains oval and round windows in its lateral wall.
2. ***Cochlea:*** It has broad base where it is continuous with vestibule and a narrow apex.
3. ***Semicircular canals:*** The three tubes are arranged so that one is situated in each of the three planes of space. They are continuous with the vestibule.

Membranous labyrinth comprises same three parts but the vestibule contains utricle and saccule.

The membranous labyrinth comprises the cochlea which functions as a hearing unit and a vestibular part which functions for proper balancing of the body and maintenance of posture of the body.

Cochlea

There is a bony cochlea like a shell which forms two and three-fourths circle. It contains perilymph and inside it is the membranous cochlea or cochlear duct.

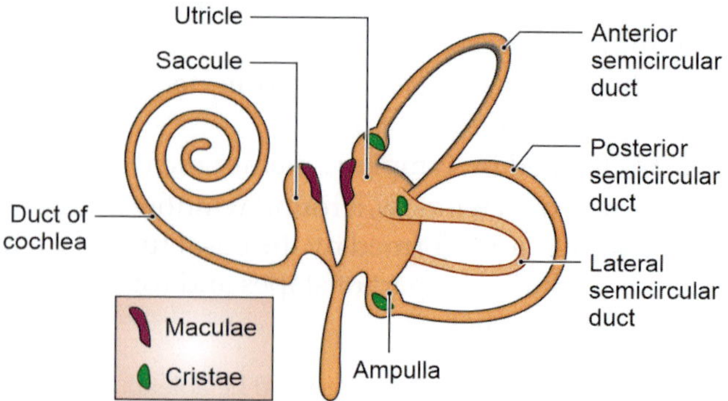

Fig. 12.6: Membranous labyrinth

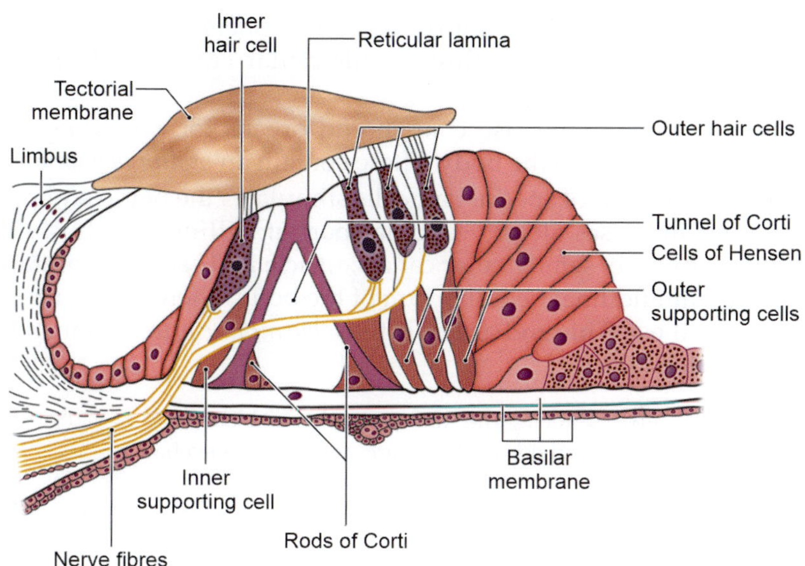

Fig. 12.7: Cochlea

The cochlear duct or scala media consists of basilar membrane on which phalangeal cells and rods of Corti are resting (Fig. 12.7).

The phalangeal cells support the hair cells.

Movement of perilymph through bony cochlea causes vibrations in the basilar membrane, to stimulate the hair cells.

Nerve fibres from hair cells reach the spiral ganglion from where the impulses travel along auditory (cochlear) nerve to reach cochlear nuclei. Then, through medial geniculate body the impulses reach the auditory area in the upper part of temporal lobe of the cerebrum.

Vestibular Part

Vestibular part is comprised of three bony semicircular canals: (1) Lateral, (2) posterior and (3) superior bony canal.

Each contains a membranous semicircular canal. There is a dilatation at one end of membranous canal. This is called the ampulla (Fig. 12.6). Ampulla has a gelatinous mass called cupola. Its lining contains special cells with nerve endings. Any deformation of these cells send impulses to vestibular division of VIII nerve, to reach the vestibular nuclei. These are connected to cerebellum of brain. The semicircular canals maintain the angular equilibrium of the body.

Vestibular part is also comprised of *bony vestibule*, which contains the utricle connected to three semicircular canals and *saccule* connected to the cochlea.

Utricle and saccule also contain end organs for providing the linear equilibrium to the body. These contain an *otolith membrane*.

The movement of special hair cells stimulates the nerve endings and send impulses along vestibular part of VIII nerve. Thus, the vestibular nerve, semicircular canals, utricle and saccule maintain the angular and linear equilibrium of the body. There is one artery for internal ear. This end artery is the *labyrinthine artery*, branch of basilar artery.

Competency achievement: The student should be able to:
AN 41.1 Describe and demonstrate parts and layers of eyeball

EYE

Eye is the sense organ for the sense of sight. It is situated in the orbital cavity and sense of sight is carried by optic nerve.

Each eye is almost spherical in shape and has a diameter of about 2.5 cm. The space between the eye and orbital cavity is occupied by adipose tissue. Activities of both the eyes are coordinated so they function as a pair. It is possible to see with one eye but the judgement of depth and distance is impaired when only one eye is used.

Eye consists of the *eyeball* (partly seen when the eyelids are open) including muscles and nerves related to the eyeball and *lacrimal apparatus*.

Eyeball consists of the following three layers:

1. ***Outermost is the sclera***, which is tough and white in colour forms 5/6th of the eyeball. Muscles of eyeball are inserted into it. Anterior 1/6th of eyeball is formed by the transparent *cornea* (Fig. 12.8).
2. ***Middle coat is the uveal tract***. It is comprised of pigmented vascular *choroid*, anterolaterally *ciliary body* with ciliary muscles and anteriorly curtain like iris with a circular aperture, the *pupil*. The size of pupil can change according to the amount of light entering the eye (Fig. 12.8).

   Ciliary body consists of *ciliary muscle* (smooth muscle) and secretory epithelial cells. It is attached to suspensory ligament which, at its other end, is attached to capsule of lens. Contraction

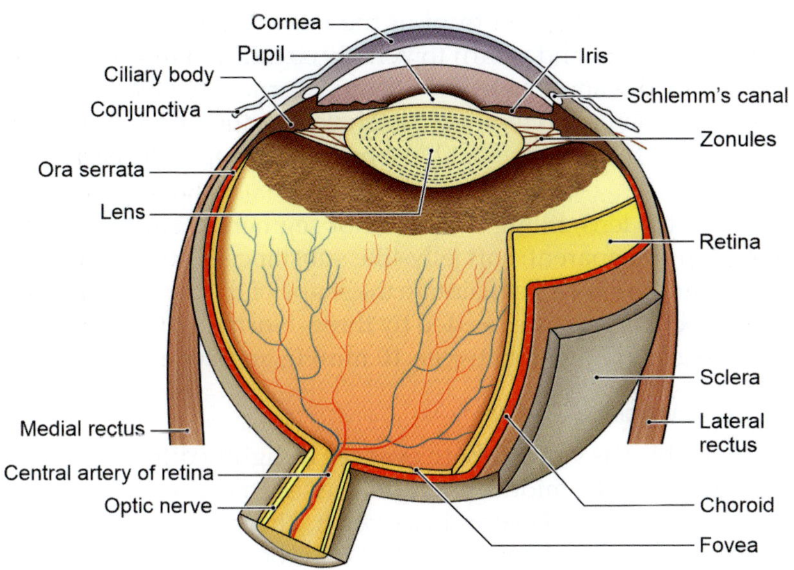

Fig. 12.8: Horizontal section of the eye

and relaxation of ciliary muscles changes the thickness of lens and helps to focus the light rays on retina. Epithelial cells secrete aqueous fluid into anterior segment of the eye, i.e. anterior and posterior chambers. Ciliary muscles are supplied by 3rd cranial (oculomotor) nerve. Stimulation causes contraction of smooth muscle and accommodation of eye.

Iris is visible coloured part of eye, lying behind cornea in front of lens. It consists of two layers of smooth muscle fibres.

Lens is circular biconvex structure lying behind the pupil. It is enclosed in a capsule and suspended from ciliary body by suspensory ligament.

3. ***The innermost layer is the photosensitive retina***, comprising of layers of numerous *rods* (for night vision) and *cones* (for day vision, colour vision and brightness of vision), bipolar cell layer and ganglionic cell layer.

Axons of ganglionic cell layer form the optic nerve (II), which courses through the optic canal, forms optic chiasma, optic tract, synapses in the lateral geniculate body to end in the occipital lobe of the cerebral cortex.

Anterior segment of eye, i.e. anterior and posterior chambers contain *aqueous humour*. It is secreted into posterior chamber by ciliary processes. It circulates in front of the lens, through pupil into the anterior chamber and return to venous circulation through *canal of Schlemm* in the angle between iris and cornea. Aqueous humour supplies nutrients and removes metabolic products from transparent structures in front of eye that have no blood supply, i.e. cornea and lens.

Behind the lens, filling the posterior segment is *vitreous humour*, which is a transparent, soft jelly-like substance. Both aqueous and vitreous humour help to maintain the shape of the eyeball because of the intraocular pressure exerted by these. Normally, the intraocular pressure is maintained between 10 mmHg and 20 mmHg.

Binocular Vision

When an object is viewed, both eyes see it slightly differently. There is an overlap in the middle but right eye sees more on the right than can be seen by the left eye and vice versa. The images from two eyes are fused in cerebral cortex so that only one image is perceived. Binocular vision is important to perceive the depth and proportion of the object.

Lacrimal Apparatus

These are the components in relation to anterior part of eyeball which secrete lacrimal fluid for lubrication between the eyelids and the eyeball. These are the laterally situated *lacrimal gland* and its ducts which open into the conjunctival sac (Fig. 12.9).

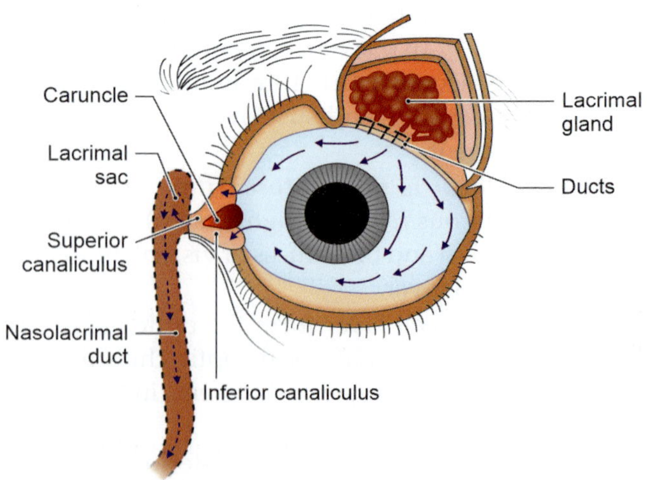

Fig. 12.9: Lacrimal apparatus

At the medial end of the conjunctival sac are the two *lacrimal canaliculi*. They join together to open into *lacrimal sac*, which is connected by *nasolacrimal duct* to the inferior meatus of the nose.

The secretions *(lacrimal fluid)* flows in the sac and is drained into the nasal cavity. If excessive amount is secreted, these are called the *tears*.

Eyes are very important to a person, as one views the external world through his/her eyes. The clinician can see retina, central artery and vein of retina through an instrument called *ophthalmoscope*, put opposite the cornea with dilated pupil.

Clinical Anatomy of Sensory Organs

Tongue

1. ***Ulcers:*** The sides of the tongue may show small/big ulcers. These are mostly due to deficiency of vitamin B complex. Eating food containing chillies is very painful in such times. If the ulcer does not heal, it must be followed closely, as the chronic ulcers may change into cancer of tongue.
2. ***Ageusia*** is the term used for absence of sense of taste. *Hypogeusia* is diminished sense of taste. *Dysgeusia* is distorted sense of taste.

Nose

The nose and nasal cavity are affected by the following maladies:

1. Forceful hit on the nose may cause fracture of nasal bones. Nasal bone is the most common facial bone to be fractured.
2. The nasal septum may be deviated to one or the other side.
3. The anteroinferior area of nasal septum can bleed, if it is picked too often. It is called 'Little's area'.
4. All paranasal sinuses open into each side of the nasal cavity. In *sinusitis*, there is mucus or watery discharge from the nose.
5. Common cold affects the nose. It is a viral infection and takes about 1 week for the person to become alright.
6. Loss of sense of smell is known as *anosmia*. *Hyposmia* is decreased sense of smell and *dysosmia* is distorted sense of smell.

Diseases of the Ear

1. ***Otitis externa:*** Occurs due to infection of the external auditory meatus by a boil. It is painful, as there is very limited space.

2. ***Otitis media:*** This is the inflammation of the narrow middle ear cavity. Mostly, the infection reaches from the throat via the auditory tube. If not treated completely, acute otitis media may become chronic and cause meningitis, mastoiditis, labyrinthitis and other complications.
3. ***Otosclerosis:*** If the foot plate of stapes get fused to the oval window, the condition is called 'otosclerosis'. The sound waves cannot be transmitted to the internal ear and the person develops conductive hearing loss.
4. ***Deafness:*** Inability to hear properly is called deafness. It may be *conductive deafness* (due to impaired transmission of sound waves from outside to oval window) or *nerve deafness* (due to diseases of cochlea, cochlear nerve) or mixed, i.e. both conductive and nerve deafness.

Meniere's disease: Excessive accumulation of endolymph leads to increased pressure and distension within the membranous labyrinth. Patient presents with recurrent attacks of dizziness, nausea, vomiting, ringing in the ear and gradually nerve deafness develops.

Presbycusis is gradual hearing loss associated with ageing. It is due to gradual loss of hair cells and neurons.

Diseases of the Eye

1. ***Congenital:*** There may be abnormalities in the eye. There may be 'congenital cataract'. This is usually due to rubella or Down syndrome. There may be non-formation of lacrimal gland, absence of nasolacrimal duct.
2. ***Inflammatory diseases***
   - ***Blepharitis*** is an inflammation of margin of the eyelid.
   - ***Hordeolum:*** It is infection of tarsal glands of the margin of eyelid. The hordeolum or stye occurs repeatedly.
   - ***Conjunctivitis:*** This is inflammation of the conjunctiva, due to infection or allergy.
   - ***Trachoma*** is a chronic inflammation of the conjunctiva caused by *Chlamydia trachomatis*. It is an important cause of preventable blindness in developing tropical countries.
   - ***Corneal ulcers:*** These ulcers develop due to infection of cornea following any injury even by edge of newspaper or infection.

- ***Uveitis:*** It is the inflammation of the uveal tract, i.e. inflammation of iris, ciliary body or choroid.
- ***Glaucoma:*** There is increased intraocular pressure due to lack of drainage of aqueous humour through the canal of Schlemm. Glaucoma leads to pressure on optic nerve fibres and blindness.

3. ***Cataract:*** The lens gets opaque, interfering with the passage of light. The cataract causes blurring of vision and the lens needs to be removed. This is replaced by an artificial lens (intraocular lens implant).
4. ***Retinal detachment:*** In this condition, there is partial or complete separation of the inner nine layers of retina from the outer pigmented layer. It needs surgery for its correction.
5. ***Retinitis pigmentosa:*** It is a hereditary disease in which there is degeneration of retina, mainly affecting the rods. There is defective vision in the dim light *(night blindness)*.
6. ***Dacryocystitis:*** There is inflammation of the lacrimal sac. It is associated with partial or complete blockage of the lacrimal duct.
7. ***Squint:*** Normally, the movements of the two eyes are synchronous, so that the same image falls on corresponding parts of the retina in both eyes. In weakness or paralysis of one muscle, the images fall on different parts of the two retinae, leading to two images for the brain and *diplopia* (double vision).
8. ***Myopia (near sightedness):*** The image of distant objects falls in front of the retina because eyeball is too long. So, concave lens is given to diverge the image, so that these fall on the retina. Near objects are seen in focus.
9. ***Hypermetropia (far sightedness):*** The near image falls behind the retina because eyeball is too short. Convex lens is required to correct the defect. Distant objects are focused normally.
10. ***Astigmatism:*** The curvature of the part of the cornea is abnormal. The light rays are refracted to a different focus causing a blurred image. It is corrected by a cylindrical lens.

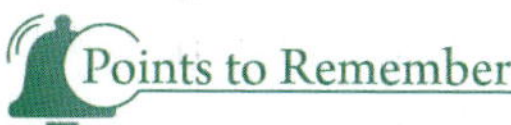

1. The basic tastes are sweet, sour, salt and bitter.
2. Anything to be smell has to be in form of vapour.

3. Only uppermost part of nasal cavity has olfactory epithelium.
4. Eyeball comprises three layers. These are—sclera with cornea; choroid, ciliary body, iris and retina.
5. Internal ear functions both for hearing and balance.
6. Fingerprints are unique to each and every person.
7. Acne occurs due to blockage of duct of the sebaceous gland.

Multiple Choice Questions

1. Appendages of skin are all *except*:
   a. Hair
   b. Nail
   c. Sebaceous gland
   d. Arrector pilorum muscle

2. Full nail grows in:
   a. 30–60 days
   b. 60–90 days
   c. 90–120 days
   d. 120–160 days

3. Circumvallate papillae are present at:
   a. Tip of tongue
   b. Lateral border of tongue
   c. Anterior to sulcus terminates
   d. Posterior to sulcus terminates

4. Order of bony ossicles from lateral to medial side is:
   a. Malleus, stapes, incus
   b. Stapes, incus, malleus
   c. Malleus, incus, stapes

Answers

1. d **2.** c **3.** c **4.** c

Chapter 13

Endocrine System

Everything is easy, when you are crazy about it and nothing is easy, when you are lazy about it.

Most of the functions in the human body are regulated by two main systems—autonomic nervous system, and endocrine system.

These two systems mostly work independently to maintain the homeostasis of the internal environment. The autonomic nervous system is concerned with rapid changes while the endocrine system is involved in slower and more precise adjustments.

Endocrine system consists of widely separated endocrine glands. Each endocrine gland is composed of specialised secretory cells, which secrete a chemical substance called hormone and release it into the blood stream directly. These glands do not have a duct system, so are also known as ductless glands. The hormone released is carried by the bloodstream to another (target) organ or tissue where it exerts its effects by affecting cellular growth and metabolism. Endocrine glands though work independently, their balanced action is necessary to maintain body homeostasis (Fig. 13.1).

Most hormones released are either derived from amino acids or steroids.

All endocrine glands have different embryologic origin, differ histologically and are located in different parts of the body. The various endocrine glands are:

1. Hypothalamus, pituitary gland and pineal gland
2. Thyroid gland (Fig. 13.2)
3. Parathyroid glands

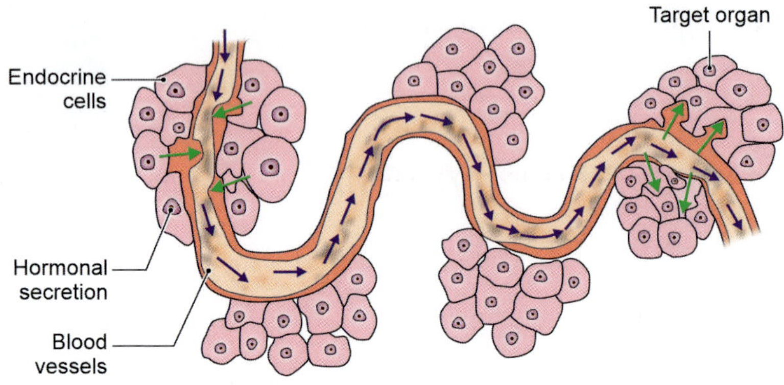

Fig. 13.1: Endocrine gland

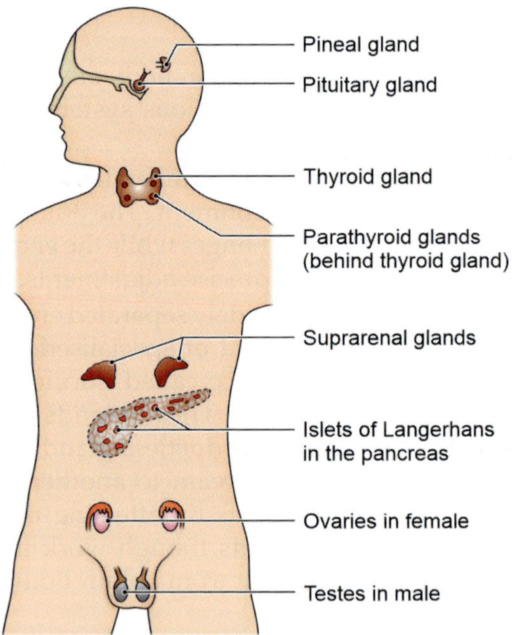

Fig. 13.2: Various endocrine glands

4. Adrenal/suprarenal glands
5. Islets of Langerhans in pancreas
6. Pineal gland
7. Ovaries (in female)
8. Testes (in male)
9. Placenta
10. Juxtaglomerular apparatus in kidney.

HYPOTHALAMUS AND PITUITARY GLAND

Hypothalamus is present in the floor of the third ventricle of brain. It is the *master gland* of the endocrine system. It secretes two true hormones, i.e. *oxytocin* and *antidiuretic hormone (ADH)*. It also secretes the releasing and inhibiting factors to control the trophic hormones released from the anterior pituitary and thereby control the activity of most of the endocrine glands.

Pituitary gland (hypophysis cerebri) is a small ovoid structure attached to the base of the brain. It lies in the hypophyseal fossa located on the superior surface of the body of sphenoid bone. It lies below the hypothalamus to which it is attached by a stalk. It weighs about 500 mg and has three distinct parts (Fig. 13.3).

1. ***Anterior pituitary (adenohypophysis):*** It constitutes 80% of pituitary gland. It contains five different types of glandular cells. It is richly supplied by blood vessels and is linked with hypothalamus through the blood vessels. This link is called *hypothalamohypophyseal portal vessels* through which products of hypothalamus are brought to the anterior pituitary.
2. ***Posterior pituitary (neurohypophysis):*** It constitutes 20% of pituitary gland. It consists of nervous tissue and blood vessels.

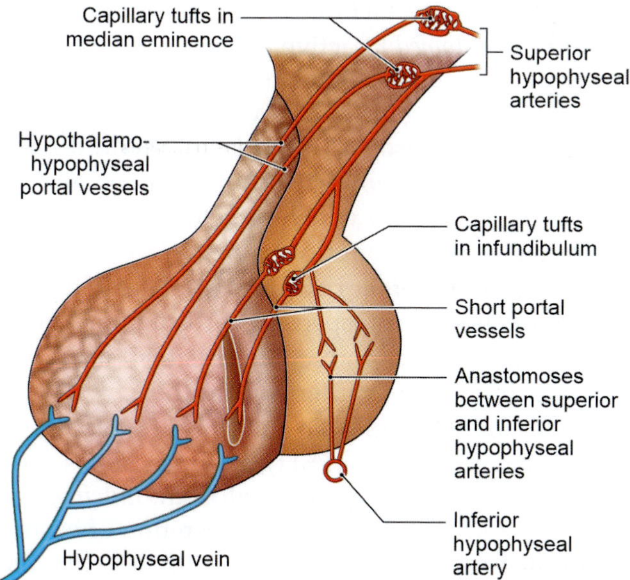

Fig. 13.3: The lobes of the pituitary gland and their relationship with the hypothalamus

13

There are *no glandular cells*. It does not synthesise any hormone. It is linked with hypothalamus by a *neural hypothalamohypophyseal tract*. The hormones, ADH and oxytocin, are synthesised in hypothalamus and transported by neural tracts to posterior pituitary and are released from there.

3. ***Intermediate lobe:*** It is a thin strip of tissue between anterior and posterior lobes. Its function in humans is not well known.

Anterior Pituitary

Some of the hormones secreted by the anterior pituitary stimulate or inhibit secretion by other endocrine glands while others have a direct affect on target tissues. The various releasing/inhibiting hormones released by the hypothalamus release/inhibit specific hormones from anterior pituitary. The trophic hormone released from the anterior pituitary in turn stimulates the target gland to produce and release its hormone. Rise in blood level of that hormone inhibits the secretion of releasing factor by hypothalamus *(negative feedback mechanism)*. Low level of hormone in blood stimulates the release of appropriate releasing hormone from hypothalamus.

Growth hormone (GH) is the most abundant hormone synthesised by the anterior pituitary. It is important for the growth and development in the body. GH does not act itself but it stimulates the synthesis of *somatomedin* (active principle of GH). It promotes linear growth of bones and skeletal muscles. It helps in growth and maturation of genital organs and development of secondary sex characters. It also affects protein, fat and carbohydrate metabolism.

Thyroid stimulating hormone (TSH) stimulates and regulates the activity of thyroid gland which secretes hormones T4 and T3 (tetraiodothyronine and triiodothyronine).

Adrenocorticotrophic hormone (ACTH) stimulates and regulates the secretion of steroid hormones especially cortisol from adrenal cortex.

Prolactin stimulates milk production *(lactation)* and has a direct effect on breasts immediately after childbirth.

Gonadotrophins are released from anterior pituitary after puberty. *Follicle stimulating hormone* (FSH), in both sexes, stimulates production of gametes (ova or spermatozoa). *Luteinising hormone* (LH) and FSH in females stimulate the secretion of oestrogen and progesterone during menstrual cycle. In males, LH also called *interstitial cell stimulating hormone* (ICSH) stimulates interstitial cells of testes to produce the hormone testosterone.

Posterior Pituitary

It releases oxytocin and ADH hormone. These hormones act directly on target tissues.

1. ***Oxytocin*** acts on uterine smooth muscle and muscle cells of the lactating breast. During childbirth it stimulates the uterine contractions and causes expulsion of fetus. It stimulates contraction of myoepithelial cells surrounding the mammary ducts to facilitate ejection of milk.
2. ***Antidiuretic hormone*** (ADH) reduces the urine output. It causes an increase in the permeability to water of the distal convoluted and collecting tubules of nephrons of the kidney. It is responsible for 20% reabsorption of total volume reabsorbed in kidneys. Thus, it is responsible for maintaining water and acid–base balance of the body. In high concentration, it causes contraction of smooth cells of blood vessels of skin and abdominal organs, thus raising the blood pressure. So, it is also called vasopressin.

Intermediate Lobe

It probably produces *melanocyte stimulating hormone* (MSH). MSH stimulates melanocyte cells in deeper layers of epidermis to synthesise *melanin*. This hormone is more important in lower animals for increasing/decreasing the amount of melanin in the skin for safety reasons.

> *Competency achievement:* The student should be able to:
> AN 35.2 Describe and demonstrate location, parts, borders, surfaces, relations and blood supply of thyroid gland

THYROID GLAND

Thyroid is an endocrine gland, which pours its secretion directly into the blood. There is no duct in this gland. The gland lies in front of the trachea and larynx in neck, and is enclosed in deep cervical fascia. So, the gland moves during swallowing (Fig. 13.4).

It weighs about 25 g. It comprises two lobes and median isthmus. The two lobes are joined by a narrow isthmus, lying in front of trachea. The lobes are roughly cone shaped, about 5 cm long and 3 cm wide. It is related to two tubes—trachea, oesophagus; two nerves—external laryngeal and recurrent laryngeal and their accompanying arteries. Superior thyroid artery runs with external

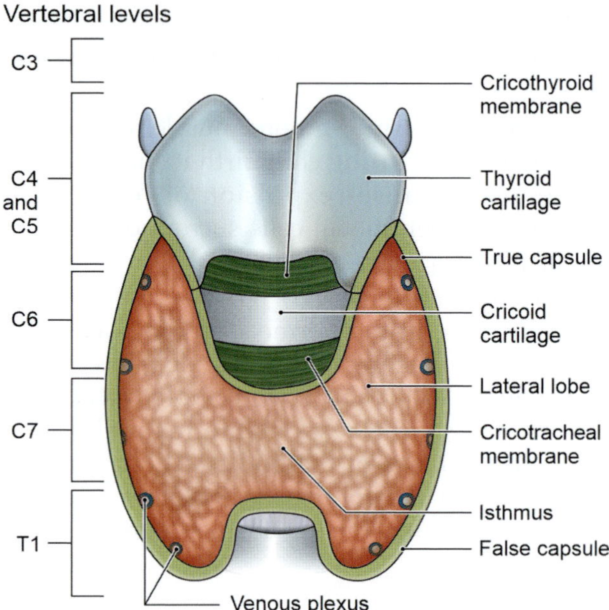

Fig. 13.4: Thyroid gland from front

laryngeal nerve and inferior thyroid artery runs with recurrent laryngeal nerve.

Arterial blood supply is through superior and inferior thyroid arteries. The *venous drainage* is by thyroid veins, which drain into internal jugular veins.

Thyroid gland is made of numerous *follicles* lined by cuboidal to columnar epithelial cells. The cells selectively take up iodine from blood. Iodine plus tyrosine amino acid synthesise triiodothyronine (T3) and tetraiodothyronine/thyroxine (T4). These two hormones are kept in combination with globulin to form *thyroglobulin* in the lumen of the follicle to be released, if and when required. Thyroglobulin is broken to active hormones according to the need of the body.

Between the follicles are cells called *parafollicular cells (C cells)*, which secrete the hormone calcitonin.

PARATHYROID GLANDS

Parathyroid glands are four pea-shaped glands situated two each on the posterior surface of the each lobe of thyroid gland. These are supplied by branches of inferior thyroid artery (Fig. 13.2).

The gland secretes a hormone, *parathormone/parathyroid hormone (PTH)*, which maintains blood calcium level.

Secretion of this hormone increases the level of serum calcium. It acts by increasing the amount of calcium absorbed from small intestine and reabsorbed from renal tubules. It also stimulates resorption of calcium from bones by stimulating osteoclasts (bone destroying cells). Thus, it regulates blood calcium level which is important for muscle contraction and blood clotting.

SUPRARENAL/ADRENAL GLANDS

This pair of endocrine gland lies above the kidneys (Fig. 13.5). Each gland is made up of peripheral cortex and a central medulla. They are about 4 cm long and 3 cm thick.

The cortex and medulla are structurally and functionally different from each other. Both of these function to combat stress.

Cortex has three zones each with different secretions:

1. ***Outermost zone*** is *zona glomerulosa* which secretes mineralocorticoids. Aldosterone is the main mineralocorticoid. It is concerned with regulation of water and electrolyte balance in the body.
2. ***Middle zone*** is *zona fasciculata* which secretes glucocorticoids. These are essential for life. They regulate metabolism and responses to stress. Main glucocorticoids are cortisol, corticosterone and cortisone.
3. ***Innermost zone*** is *zona reticularis*. It secretes sex hormones [androgens, dehydroepiandrostenedione (DHEA)] are

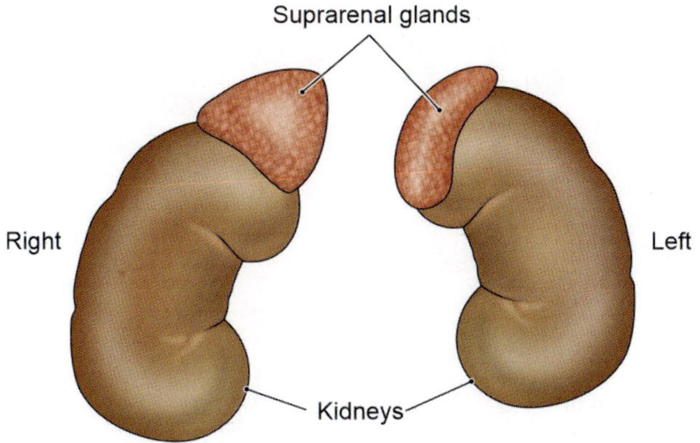

Fig. 13.5: Kidneys with suprarenal glands

synthesized in adrenal cortex. These are converted into testosterone in peripheral tissues and exert their effect.

Medulla secretes epinephrine/adrenaline and norepinephrine/noradrenaline (Fig. 13.5).

Both epinephrine and norepinephrine are synthesised from amino acid tyrosine. *Epinephrine* is a hormone of emergency though it is not absolutely essential for life. *Norepinephrine* is released from postganglionic neurotransmitter at sympathetic division of autonomic nervous system. They are hormones of emergency, together they help the body during the conditions of *fight or flight* after sympathetic stimulation by increasing the heart rate and blood pressure, increasing metabolic rate, dilating the pupils and diverting the blood to essential organs, e.g. heart, brain and skeletal muscles.

PANCREAS—ISLETS OF LANGERHANS

Pancreas is unique as it is both an exocrine and endocrine gland. The *pancreatic acini* secreting *pancreatic juice* form the exocrine part as it is carried by the pancreatic duct to the duodenum. The endocrine part is islets of Langerhans, whose cells secrete glucagon (by α cells), insulin (by β cells) and somatostatin (by δ cells) (Fig. 13.6). Normal blood glucose level is 80–120 mg%. Blood glucose level is maintained by the opposing actions of insulin and glucagon—insulin decreases blood glucose levels while glucagon increases it.

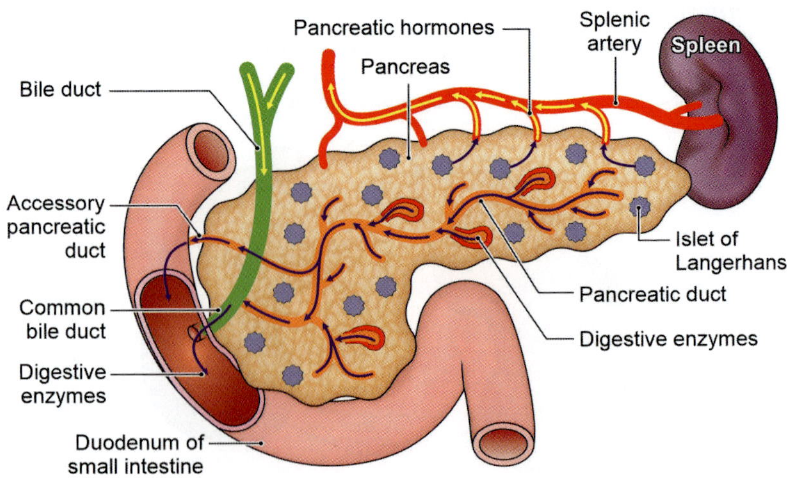

Fig. 13.6: Duodenum, pancreas with islets of Langerhans and spleen

13

PINEAL GLAND

It is about 1 cm long and found attached to the roof of third ventricle of brain.

Melatonin hormone is secreted by the pineal gland. It causes:

1. Inhibition of growth and development of sex organs before puberty.
2. Because of its neural connection with hypothalamus it coordinates *circadian* (events that occur at approximately 24 hours interval) and *diurnal* (events that occur during daytime) rhythm of many tissues.

OVARIES, TESTES

Described in, 'Reproductive System'.

JUXTAGLOMERULAR APPARATUS IN KIDNEYS

Described in Chapter 14, 'Urinary System'.

Local Hormones

Histamine: It is synthesised by the mast cells. It increases capillary permeability.

Serotonin: Present in brain and platelets. It causes contraction of smooth muscles.

Prostaglandins: These cause vasoconstriction, bronchospasm, etc.

Clinical Anatomy of Endocrines

Endocrine diseases result from either overproduction (hypersecretion) or underproduction (hyposecretion) of hormones.

Diseases of Pituitary Gland

Gigantism and Acromegaly

It is a result of prolonged hypersecretion of GH from anterior pituitary. Usually, it results from a tumour of GH secreting cells.

Excess of GH during childhood before fusion of metaphysis and epiphysis results in *gigantism*. The individual has abnormal increase in stature due to skeletal overgrowth but body proportions are normal.

Acromegaly results when there is hypersecretion of GH after puberty and ossification is complete, i.e. epiphysis and metaphysis have fused. The person develops abnormal thickening of bones and soft tissues leading to prominent mandible, enlargement of hands and feet. The person also develops enlarged tongue and liver.

Hypopituitarism

Deficient secretion of various hormones of pituitary leads to hypopituitarism. If all the hormones of pituitary are absent, it is known as *panhypopituitarism*.

Deficient secretion of GH in childhoods leads to short stature with normal body proportion *(pituitary dwarfism)*. There will also be lack of sexual development.

Diabetes insipidus results from hyposecretion of ADH. There is excretion of excessive amounts of dilute urine causing dehydration, extreme thirst.

Diseases of Thyroid Gland

Goitre

There is enlargement of the thyroid gland without signs of hyperthyroidism. Secretion of T4 and T3 is reduced and their low levels stimulate TSH secretion resulting in enlargement of thyroid gland. Enlarged gland may cause pressure on adjacent tissues leading to difficulty in swallowing and breathing, hoarseness of voice. It is usually due to iodine deficiency.

Hypothyroidism

It results from insufficient secretion of T4 and T3.

Cretinism develops when deficiency of thyroxine (T4) occurs in fetal life or early childhood. It leads to decreased (retarded) physical and mental development, coarse dry skin, enlarged tongue and prominent abdomen.

Myxoedema develops when thyroid hormone deficiency occurs in adults. It is more common in females. Clinical features are weight gain, constipation, depression, dry skin, broad bloated face, tiredness, intolerance to cold. Body hair is sparse and short. Heart rate is slow (bradycardia).

Hyperthyroidism

It results from excessive levels of T4 and T3 hormones. The clinical features are due to increased metabolic rate. The patient presents with weight loss, warm sweaty skin, heat intolerance, tachycardia, hair loss. There is enlargement of thyroid gland and *exophthalmos* (eyeballs appear protruded out).

Diseases of Parathyroid Glands

Hyperparathyroidism

Excessive secretion of PTH causes resorption of calcium from bones, raising the blood calcium level (hypercalcaemia). There is formation of renal stones, calcification in soft tissues, muscle fatigue, polyuria and extreme thirst. The condition is called osteitis fibrosa cystica.

Hypoparathyroidism

Deficiency of PTH causes abnormally low levels of blood calcium (hypocalcaemia). There is tetany, seizures, premature cataract and mental disturbances. "Tetany" results in painful spasms of skeletal muscle.

Diseases of Adrenal Gland

Diseases of Adrenal Cortex

Deficiency of glucocorticoids leads to low blood glucose, muscle weakness and decreased gluconeogenesis. Hyposecretion of both glucocorticoids and mineralocorticoids leads to *Addison's disease*. Clinical features of Addison's disease are muscle weakness and wasting, loss of appetite, increased pigmentation of skin, tiredness, mental confusion, hypotension, menstrual disturbances and electrolyte imbalance.

Hypersecretion of glucocorticoids leads to *Cushing's syndrome*. Clinical features include painful adiposity of face *(moon face)*, neck and abdomen, excessive protein catabolism leading to muscle wasting, osteoporosis, hyperglycaemia, susceptibility to infection due to depressed immune response, mental disturbances.

Diseases of Adrenal Medulla

The disorders affecting the adrenal medulla (pheochromocytoma) usually result in excessive secretion of epinephrine and norepinephrine. Clinical features are hypertension, hyperglycaemia, excessive sweating and increased metabolic rate.

Diseases of Islets of Langerhans

Diabetes Mellitus

It is usually due to deficiency or absence of insulin or to insulin resistance, i.e. impaired insulin activity. Deficiency of insulin leads to disruption of carbohydrate and fat metabolism. Diabetes is classified into:

1. ***Type I, insulin-dependent diabetes mellitus (IDDM):*** Seen in children and young adults. It is of sudden onset. Deficiency of insulin is due to destruction of β islet cells.
2. ***Type II, non-insulin-dependent diabetes mellitus (NIDDM):*** This type involves 80% of cases and tends to develop in persons over 45 years. In this type, the insulin secretion may be below or above normal. It is due to insulin resistance, i.e. there is change in cell membrane which blocks the insulin assisted movement of glucose into cells.
3. ***Secondary diabetes:*** It develops secondary to drug intake, pregnancy or other endocrinal disturbances.

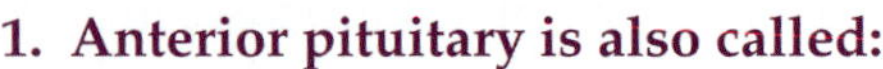

Multiple Choice Questions

1. Anterior pituitary is also called:
   a. Adenohypophysis
   b. Neurohypophysis
   c. Corpus callosum
   d. Arachnoid villi

2. Pineal gland is located at:
   a. Epithalamus
   b. Thalamus
   c. Hypothalamus
   d. Subthalamus

3. All the following hormones are secreted by anterior pituitary *except*:
   a. Growth hormone
   b. FSH
   c. Prolactin
   d. Insulin

4. Milk ejecting hormone is:
   a. Progesterone
   b. Oestrogen
   c. Melatonin
   d. Oxytocin

Answers

1. a **2.** a **3.** a **4.** d

Chapter 14

Urinary System

See yourself in every situation and in every shape. But most important, "find your own ways to flow".

Competency achievement: The student should be able to:

AN 47.5 Describe and demonstrate major viscera of abdomen under following headings (anatomical position, external and internal features, important peritoneal and other relations, blood supply, nerve supply, lymphatic drainage and applied aspects)

Waste products are products not required by the body. These have to be eliminated. Gases like carbon dioxide and nitrogen are expelled through expiration. Solid waste products of food including fibres are expelled through the anal canal. Some amount of water and a few salts are removed as sweat from the skin.

The various metabolic waste products, salts, urea, uric acid and water are expelled as urine by the urinary system.

COMPONENTS OF URINARY SYSTEM

Urinary system comprises various organs. These are 2 kidneys, 2 ureters, one urinary bladder and single urethra (Fig. 14.1).

Urinary system plays a vital part in maintaining homeostasis of water and electrolyte concentrations within the body. The kidneys produce urine that contains metabolic waste products.

Kidneys

The two bean-shaped kidneys lie behind the peritoneum on each side of posterior abdominal wall from 12th thoracic vertebra to

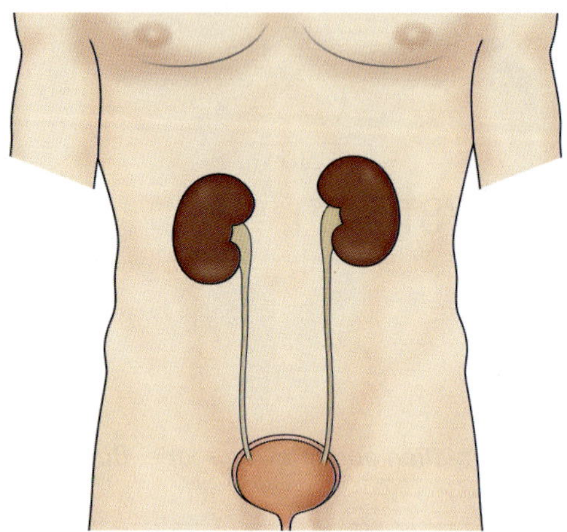

Fig. 14.1: Urinary system

3rd lumbar vertebra. Each kidney is about 11 cm long, 6 cm wide, 3 cm thick and weighs 150 g.

Hilum lies at level of 1st lumbar vertebra. Upper ends are medial while lower ends are lateral. Hilum is present in the middle of the medial border. Structures present at the hilum are renal vein, renal artery and pelvis of ureter from before backwards (Fig. 14.2).

Right kidney is little lower, because of the huge liver present on the right side.

Supports of the Kidney

These are (from within outwards) renal capsule, perirenal fat, renal fascia, pararenal fat and vessels at the hilum. These support the kidney and keep it in position.

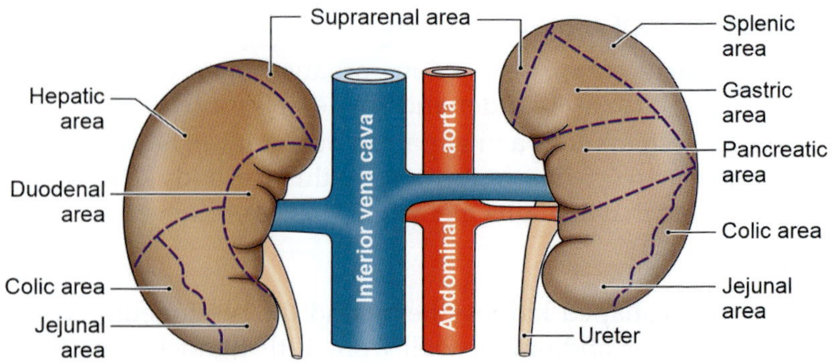

Fig. 14.2: Anterior relations of kidneys

Relations

Posterior relations are similar on two sides except that left kidney is related to 11th and 12th ribs, and right kidney only to 12th rib. Diaphragm is related in the *upper part*. The *lower part* is related to muscles of the posterior abdominal wall.

Anterior relations are different on the two sides.

1. Right kidney is related to suprarenal on its upper pole, to duodenum at its hilum, liver on the upper part, ascending colon along lateral border and coils of intestine.

   The *left kidney* is related to suprarenal on the upper pole, spleen along upper lateral border, pancreas across the kidney and stomach between pancreas and spleen. Along the lateral border is the descending colon and at the lower pole and adjacent area are the coils of intestine.
2. Renal pelvis emerges from the hilum. This is a reservoir for urine and soon narrows and changes its name to ureter. Anterior to renal pelvis is renal artery and anteriormost is the renal vein. VAP (vein, artery, pelvis) from before backwards.

Blood Supply and Lymphatic Drainage

The paired *renal arteries* arise from abdominal aorta at right angles at the level of second lumbar vertebra. Each artery divides into 5 segmental arteries which after repeated divisions reach the glomeruli.

The single renal vein lies in front of the artery and drains into inferior vena cava.

The right vein is 2.5 cm long while the left one is 7.5 cm long.

Into the left renal vein, the left gonadal and left suprarenal veins also drain. Same veins of right side drain directly into inferior vena cava.

Lymphatics drain into para-aortic lymph nodes.

GROSS STRUCTURE OF KIDNEY

Longitudinal section of kidney reveals the following structures:

1. The *fibrous capsule* surrounding the kidney.
2. The peripheral reddish brown *cortex* between the capsule and the 8–15 pyramids.
3. The inner *medulla* comprised of triangular renal pyramids. *Lobe* of the kidney is comprised of a pyramid and the cortical tissue capping it.

4. The *renal pelvis* containing the expanded end of the ureter (pelvis of ureter) which divides into 2–3 major calyces. Each major calyx further divides into 2–3 minor calyces. Each minor calyx is indented by the apex of the pyramid of the renal medulla.

Urine formed in the kidney passes through a papilla at the apex of a pyramid into a minor calyx, then into a major calyx before passing through the pelvis into the ureter. Peristalsis of the smooth muscle in the walls of the calyces propels urine through the pelvis and ureters to the bladder.

BLOOD SUPPLY OF THE KIDNEY

The renal artery, a branch of abdominal aorta is the only artery to the kidney. Each renal artery divides into 5 segmental arteries after entering the hilum. These segments are apical, upper, middle, lower and posterior segments.

Course of renal artery and vein is shown in Flowchart 14.1.

NEPHRON

It is the structural and functional unit of kidney. There are 1–1.3 million nephrons in each kidney (Fig. 14.3).

Flowchart 14.1: Course of renal artery and renal vein

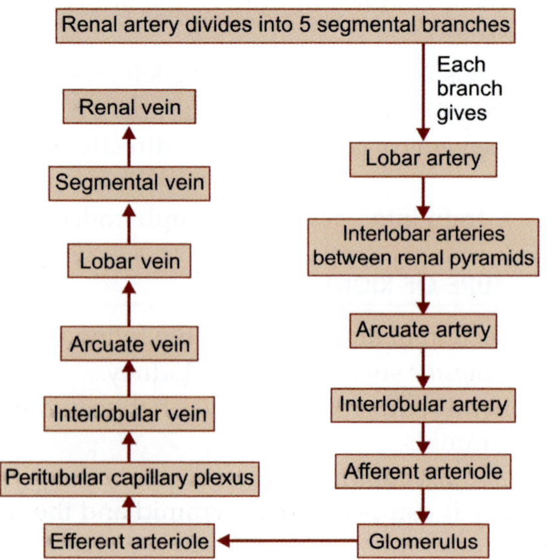

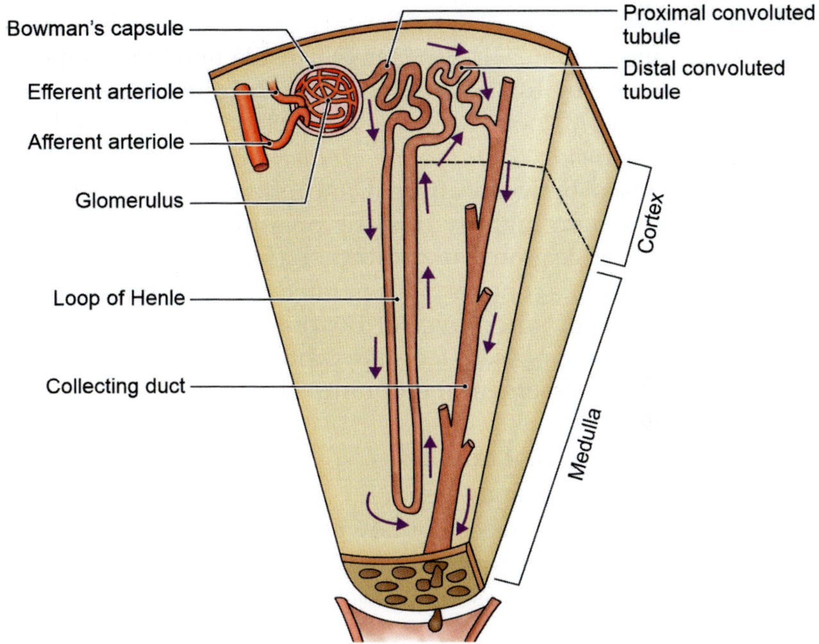

Fig. 14.3: Nephron

Structure and Functions of Nephron

There are two types of nephrons in each kidney: (1) Cortical and (2) juxtamedullary. Their differences are as follows.

Cortical Nephron

1. 85% are located in cortex.
2. Short loop of Henle and rate of filtration is slow.
3. Less concentrated urine is formed.

Juxtamedullary Nephron

1. 15% located at the junction of cortex and medulla.
2. Long loop of Henle and rate of filtration is high.
3. Highly concentrated urine is formed.

Approximately 2 million nephrons present in both the kidneys filter blood plasma in their glomeruli. The ultrafiltrate which is formed is free from blood cells and proteins but contains all the other constituents present in blood plasma. This tubular fluid passes through various portions of renal tubule. It is greatly modified and urine is formed.

Parts of the Nephron

Parts of the nephron are: (1) Bowman's capsule lined by epithelial cells and indented by tuft of capillaries (glomerulus), (2) proximal convoluted tubule, (3) loop of Henle and (4) distal convoluted tubule.

1. ***Bowman's capsule contains the glomerular capillaries***. These are interposed between afferent and efferent arterioles. This helps to maintain high hydrostatic pressure in the capillaries required for huge glomerular filtration (Fig. 14.3).

   The glomerulus consists of fenestrated type of capillaries. The epithelial cells of inner layer of Bowman's capsule are called *podocytes* as these possess feet-like processes which rest on the outer aspect of basement membrane. The *glomerular membrane* consists of:

   - Endothelial cells of capillaries.
   - Basement membranes fused.
   - Podocyte epithelial cells of Bowman's capsule.

   From the blood in the capillaries the fluid passes through fenestra of endothelial cells, basement membranes and slits between network of podocytes.

2. ***Proximal convoluted tubule*** (PCT) constitutes major portion of the nephron and bulk of renal parenchyma. The tubule is lined by single layer of epithelial cells that show prominent brush border at the luminal surface and a large number of mitochondria in the cytoplasm.

   Because of brush border the cells are able to reabsorb 70% water and electrolytes including 100% reabsorption of glucose and amino acids from the filtrate. The necessary energy is provided by large number of mitochondria.

3. ***Loop of Henle:*** It consists of thick descending segment followed by a thin descending segment. The latter forms a loop with a thin ascending segment in the medulla and a thick ascending segment that enters back in the cortex.

   The thin segment of loop of Henle is lined with squamous epithelial cells with a few microvilli and mitochondria. The thick descending segment of loop of Henle resembles PCT structurally and functionally. In the same way, the thick ascending segment of loop of Henle resembles distal convoluted tubule (DCT). Each thick ascending segment of loop of Henle returns to the cortex and comes in contact with the glomerulus between the afferent and efferent arterioles. The epithelial cells of this part of tubule are close together with crowded nuclei and are named *macula densa*.

The loop of Henle penetrates the medulla to a varying degree. The loops arising from the glomeruli in the deeper part of the cortex (juxtamedullary glomeruli) descend deeper into the medulla than the superficially placed glomeruli. By the time the filtrate enters the descending limb of loop of Henle, its water content has been reduced by 70%. At this point, the filtrate contains high amount of sodium. As the filtrate moves along the loop of Henle, osmosis draws even more water into extracellular spaces, thus the filtrate is further concentrated.

4. ***Distal convoluted tubule*** (DCT) is lined by epithelial cells. These cells contain large number of mitochondria only and the brush border is absent. 10–20% water and electrolytes are reabsorbed from DCT.

DCT reabsorption is affected by anti-diuretic hormone (ADH) of posterior lobe of pituitary gland.

Collecting tubule is lined by cuboidal cells and it joins the collecting duct. Many collecting ducts pass through the pyramid and open into the minor calyx.

Juxtaglomerular Apparatus (JGA)

It is composed of modified cells at the junction of distal convoluted tubule, where it comes in close contact with afferent arteriole of glomerulus in that region. It consists of three types of cells:

1. ***Juxtaglomerular (JG) cells:*** These are myoepitheloid cells formed due to proliferation of vascular smooth muscle cells of afferent arteriole at the junction where it comes in contact with DCT. These JG cells release a proteolytic enzyme *renin* in response to low blood volume, hypoxia and low blood pressure and help to regulate blood pressure (Fig. 14.4).
2. ***Macula densa cells:*** These are crowded large columnar cells in the inner lining of DCT at the point where it comes in contact with the afferent arteriole. These are sensitized due to low sodium in tubular fluid and stimulate the JG cells to release renin.
3. ***Supporting cells:*** These are present between JG cells and macula densa cells. These cells may contract and regulate the glomerular filtration.

Ureters

Each ureter is a smooth muscle tube about 25 cm long, lined by transitional epithelium or urothelium. It does not allow absorption of urine.

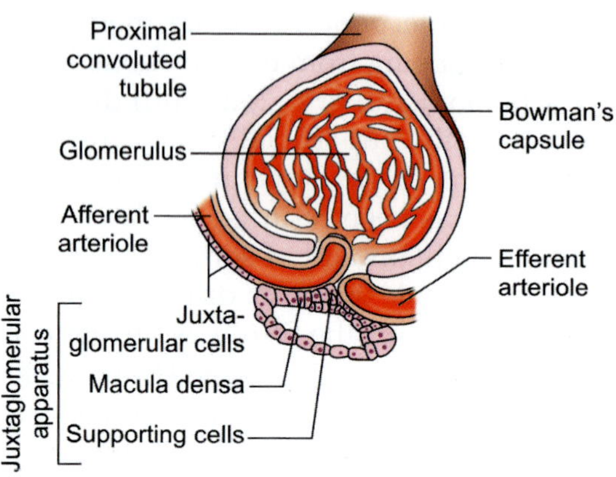

Fig. 14.4 Juxtaglomerular apparatus

Ureter passes behind the peritoneum of posterior abdominal wall over the psoas major muscle. It lies opposite the transverse processes of lumbar vertebrae.

At the division of common iliac artery into internal and external iliac arteries, the ureter enters the pelvis and lies on the side wall of pelvis in front of the internal iliac artery. On reaching the pelvic floor, it turns medially and forwards to enter the urinary bladder (Fig. 14.5).

Ureter shows *three main constrictions*, at pelvi-ureteric junction, while crossing the pelvic brim and at the entry into the bladder. Ureteric stones are more liable to get impacted at these sites of constriction.

Ureter is supplied by blood through small branches of renal, gonadal and iliac arteries. Veins follow the arteries and drain into respective veins.

Lymph vessels drain into adjacent abdominal and pelvic lymph nodes.

Nerve supply is from both sympathetic and parasympathetic fibres. Pain is carried along sympathetic nerves. These enter spinal cord via T11–12 and L1–2 nerves.

The ureters consist of three layers of tissue: (1) Fibrous tissue (outer), (2) muscular layer (middle) of smooth muscle, and (3) mucosa (inner) lined by transitional epithelium. The ureters convey urine from the kidneys into the bladder by peristaltic contraction of the smooth muscle layer.

Urinary Bladder

Urinary bladder is the temporary storehouse for urine. Its capacity is 250–500 mL. Its mucous membrane is lined by urineproof transitional epithelium.

Situation and Surfaces

It is situated in front part of the pelvis, behind the pubic symphysis. In adult, it is entirely a pelvic organ, but a distended bladder is an abdominal organ. In a child, up to 2–3 years due to small size of pelvis, bladder is an abdominal organ.

It consists of a superior surface, two inferolateral surfaces and a posterior surface or base (Fig. 14.5).

The base is related posteriorly to rectum in male and to vagina in female.

The lower part of the base is trigone of the bladder. At its upper part, the two orifices are the openings of ureters, and at the lowest part of trigone lies the *internal urethral orifice*. The region of internal urethral meatus at the lowest part of trigone is called the neck of the bladder.

The superior surface and inferolateral surfaces are related to coils of intestine. In female, body of uterus normally lies on top of the bladder.

The *arterial supply* is from superior and inferior vesical branches of internal iliac artery. *Veins* drain into internal iliac veins. *Lymphatics* run with the blood vessels to internal iliac and para-aortic lymph nodes. The bladder wall consists of three layers:

1. An outer layer of loose connective tissue
2. Middle layer of smooth muscle and elastic tissue. The smooth muscle is known as detrusor muscle. The inner layer is lined with transitional epithelium.

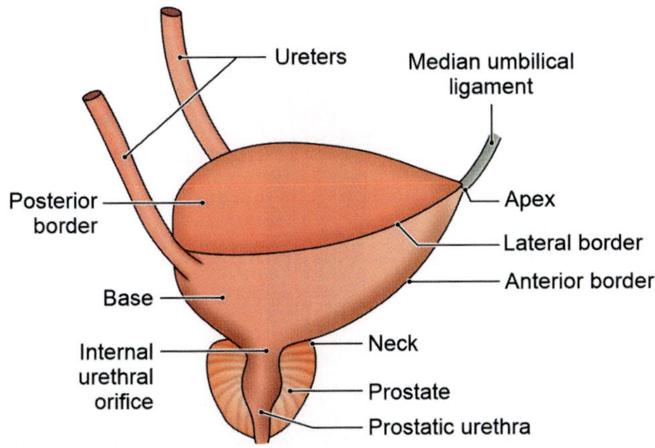

Fig. 14.5: Urinary bladder

Female Urethra

It is a straight tube 4 cm long, lying in front of vagina between the internal urethral meatus and the external urethral meatus. Urethra is lined by urineproof transitional epithelium. Almost the whole length of urethra is surrounded by sphincter urethrae, which maintains urinary continence. Catheter can be easily passed in females.

Male Urethra: Posterior and Anterior Parts

Male urethra is 15–20 cm long and has 2 parts.

I. Posterior part is comprised of:
   1. *Preprostatic*
   2. *Prostatic* which is 3 cm long when it courses through the prostate gland.
   3. *Membranous* (narrowest and shortest part).

II. Anterior part is comprising of:
   1. Perineal part present in perineum.
   2. Penile or spongy part passing through corpus spongiosum of penis to open at external urethral orifice at the tip of the glans penis.

The male urethra provides a common pathway for the flow of urine and semen, the combined secretions of the male reproductive organs (Fig. 14.6).

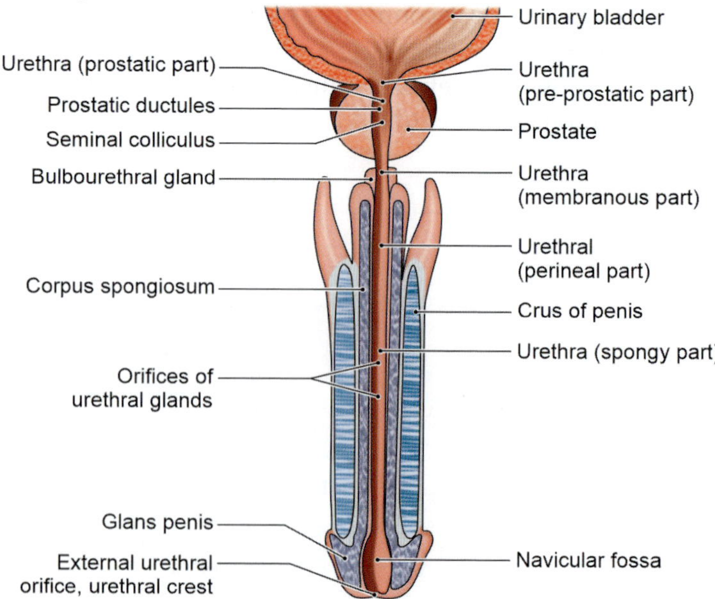

Fig. 14.6: Parts of male urethra

Clinical Anatomy of Urinary System

Congenital Anomalies

1. ***Pelvic kidney:*** Kidney develops in the pelvic region and then ascends to lumbar region. If it does not ascend, the condition is called pelvic kidney. Such a kidney may cause problem during pregnancy as the renal vessels or ureter may get pressed by the enlarging uterus.
2. ***Polycystic kidney:*** If the excretory and collecting parts of kidney do not join each other properly, multiple cysts are formed in the kidneys. These cysts are present at the junction of distal convoluted and collecting tubules. These cysts gradually enlarge and cause destruction of nephrons due to pressure. Chronic renal failure usually develops.

Infective Disorders

1. ***Acute glomerulonephritis:*** This is an inflammatory condition of the glomerulus. This is either due to bacterial infection or immune reaction to toxins of bacteria, especially *Streptococcus haemolyticus*. It may become a chronic condition if untreated. It may affect all the glomeruli (diffuse) or some glomeruli (focal). The patient presents with haematuria (passage of blood in urine), proteinuria (passage of proteins in urine), hypertension, fluid retention, anuria or oliguria. There may be chronic renal failure due to irreversible destruction of nephrons.
2. ***Cystitis:*** Inflammation of urinary bladder is called *'cystitis'* and that of urethra is known as *'urethritis'*.

Renal Dialysis and Renal Transplant

If both kidneys are not functioning, renal dialysis is done repeatedly before the kidney can be transplanted. Dialysis can be done by two ways: (1) *Haemodialysis* and (2) *peritoneal dialysis*. Kidney from blood relation is accepted better. Life is prolonged by some years if the grafted kidney is taken up well by the host.

Renal Calculi

When some components of urine get precipitated to form crystals, the condition is called 'renal calculus'. If the calculus is small, these pass down into the ureter, as ureteric calculi. Sometimes, renal calculus may become big to become one large stone in the renal pelvis. Pain in renal stone is present in 'renal angle' between the 12th rib and the lateral border of erector spinae muscle. In ureteric stone pain extends from 'loin to the groin'. Drinking more water is the key to prevent calculi formation.

Tumours

1. Hypernephroma is a malignant tumour of tubular epithelium.
2. Nephroblastoma is highly malignant tumour in children.
3. Papilloma arises from the transitional epithelium of urinary bladder.

Urinary Incontinence

There is involuntary passage of urine due to defective voluntary control of external urethral sphincter.

Acute Renal Failure

There is sudden and severe reduction in glomerular filtration rate and kidney function. It is reversible over days or weeks when treated.

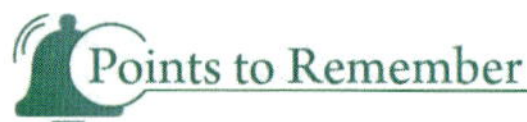

1. Right kidney is lower than the left as bulky liver pushes it down.
2. Structures in hilum of kidney from before backwards are renal vein, renal artery and pelvis of ureter
3. Kidney is supported by perirenal fat, renal fascia and pararenal fat.
4. Adequate water intake will prevent formation of renal stone.

Multiple Choice Questions

1. Blood vessels entering the glomerulus is known as:

a. Afferent b. Efferent
c. Renal artery d. Renal vein

2. Length of female urethra is:

a. 2 cm b. 3 cm
c. 4 cm d. 6 cm

3. Order of structures of hilum of kidney from before backwards is:

a. Renal artery, renal vein, pelvis of ureter
b. Pelvis of ureter, renal vein, renal artery
c. Renal vein, renal artery, pelvis of ureter
d. Renal vein, pelvis, renal artery

4. Functional unit of kidney is:

a. Bowman's capsule
b. Malpighian corpuscles
c. Pyramid
d. Nephron

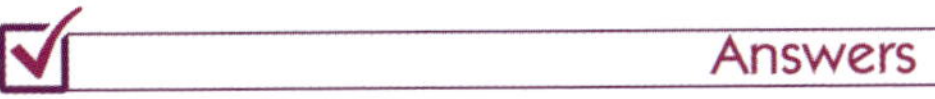

Answers

1. a **2.** c **3.** c **4.** d

Chapter 15

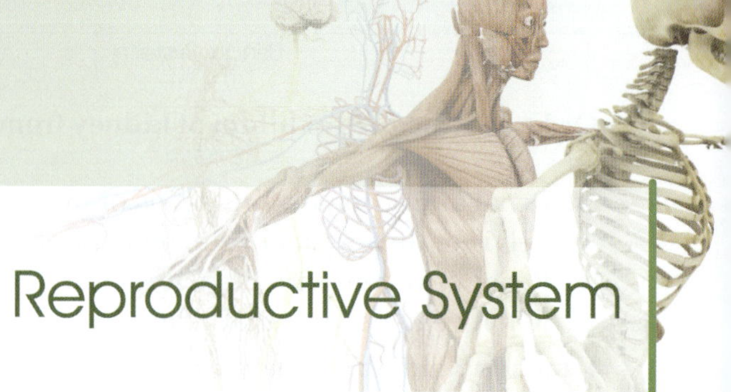

Reproductive System

Let us do our best in all circumstances, leaving the result to the divine's decision.

The living beings have the property of reproduction by which they give rise to offsprings. In human beings, both males and females produce specialised germ cells called *gametes*. The male gametes are called *spermatozoa* (produced by testes) and the female gametes are called ova (produced by ovaries). These contain the genetic material/genes, on chromosomes, which pass inherited characteristics to the next generation.

Competency achievement: The student should be able to:
AN 48.2 Describe and demonstrate the (position, features, important peritoneal and other relations, blood supply, nerve supply, lymphatic drainage and clinical aspects of) important male and female pelvic viscera

FEMALE REPRODUCTIVE SYSTEM

Reproductive system in female comprises internal pelvic genital organs and external genital or perineal genital organs.

Internal genital organs are a pair of ovaries, pair of fallopian or uterine tubes, a single uterus and vagina (Fig. 15.1a and b).

External genital organs include:

- Mons pubis
- Labia majora
- Labia minora
- Clitoris
- Bulb of the vestibule, greater vestibular glands and the vestibule of the vagina.

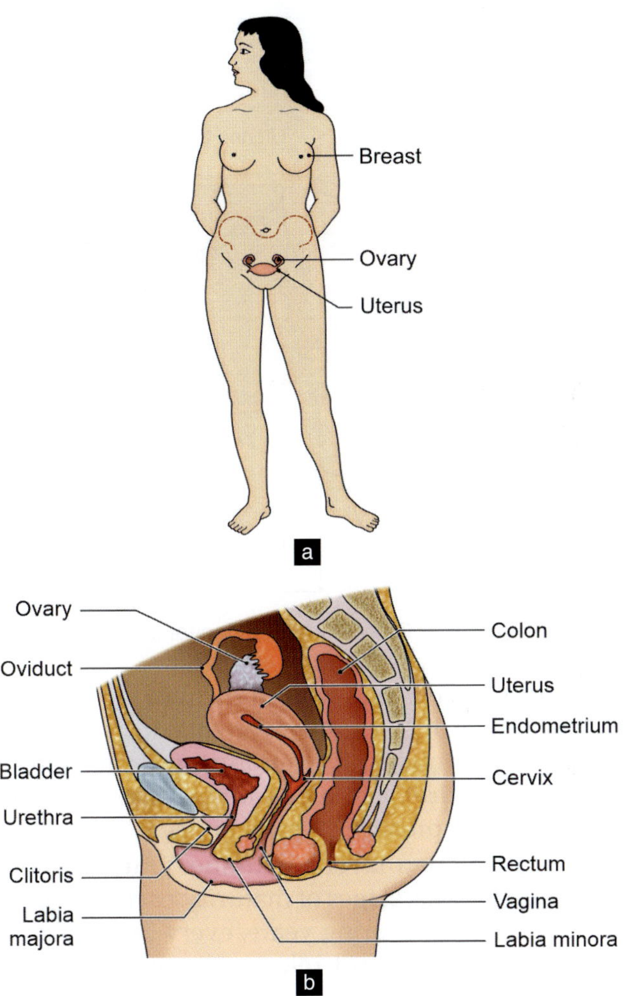

Fig. 15.1a and b: (a) Organs of female reproductive system; (b) sagittal section of female pelvis

Internal Genital Organs

Ovary

Each ovary is an almond-shaped structure, 3 cm long, 2 cm wide and 1 cm thick, lying near the side wall of pelvis. It is suspended by a fold of peritoneum from the back of broad ligament. Fallopian tube almost embraces the ovary all over except the lateral surface. The ovary has a *hilum* for the entry and exit of vessels, nerves and lymphatics (Fig. 15.2).

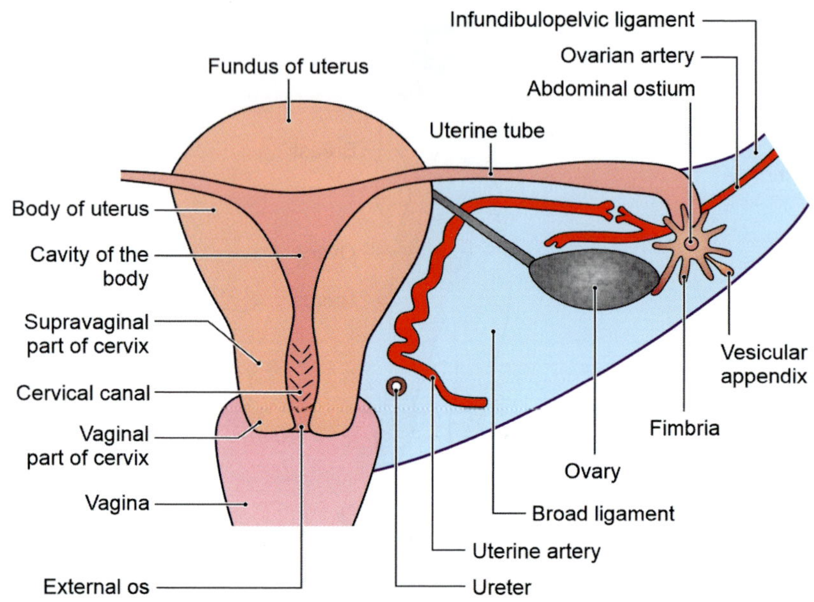

Fig. 15.2: Female internal genital organs

Ovary receives *arterial supply* from ovarian artery which arises from aorta at the level of 2nd lumbar vertebra. It also supplies lateral part of the fallopian tube. Left ovarian vein drains into left renal vein while right one drains into inferior vena cava. Lymph drains into lateral aortic and preaortic lymph nodes.

Ovary consists of two layers of tissue. Outer *cortex* contains *ovarian follicles*, in various stages of maturity, each of which contains an oocyte. During child bearing years, every 28 days, one ovarian follicle matures, ruptures and releases its ovum into peritoneal cavity. This is called ovulation. *Medulla* lies in centre and consists of fibrous tissue, blood vessels and nerves. Ovary also produces hormones like oestrogen and progesterone (Fig. 15.3a and b).

The oestrogen and progesterone along with prolactin, follicle-stimulating hormone (FSH) and luteinising hormone (LH) from the anterior pituitary regulate the menstrual cycle, maintain pregnancy and prepare the mammary glands for lactation. They also promote development and maintenance of feminine secondary sex characters (development and enlargement of breasts, feminine pattern of growth of pubic and axillary hair).

Menopause: This stage occurs between 45 years and 55 years and is the end of child bearing period. Oestrogen and progesterone become

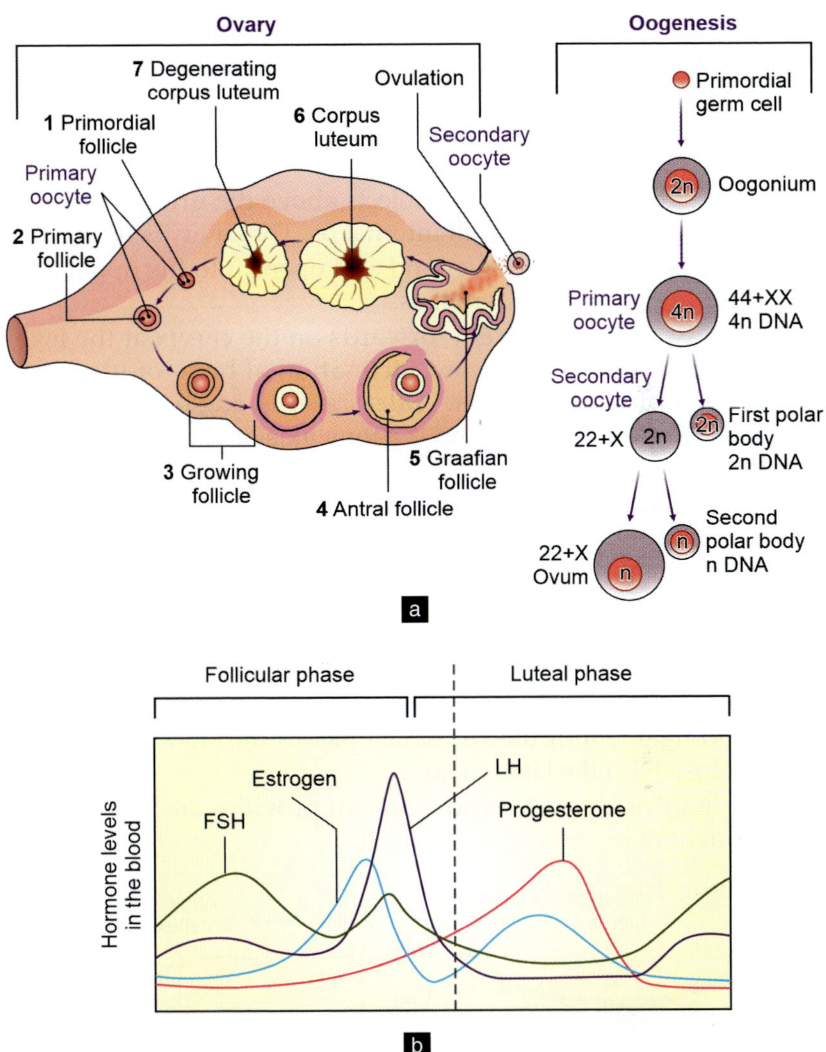

Fig. 15.3a and b: (a) Follicles in ovary and oogenesis; (b) Effects of hormones leading to ovarian cycle including phases of endometrium in menstrual cycle

less and less and menstruation stops. Ovaries do not respond to LH and FSH of the hypophysis cerebri.

Uterus

The uterus (womb) is a muscular organ composed of smooth muscle fibres. It is flattened pear-shaped organ 7.5 cm long, 5.0 wide and

2.5 cm thick (3″ × 2″ × 1″). It is present between urinary bladder and rectum. It is divided into three parts: (1) Fundus, (2) body and (3) cervix.

1. ***Fundus*** is the part which projects above the opening of fallopian tubes.
2. ***Body*** is the main part and projects above the urinary bladder. It is narrowest inferiorly at internal os. The cavity is triangular.
3. ***Cervix*** is the narrow lower end and opens into the upper part of the vagina at the external os.

The body of uterus is bent forwards on the cervix at the level of internal os and this forward inclination of body of uterus on cervix constitutes *anteflexion. Anteversion* is angle between the long axis of body of uterus and the long axis of vagina (Fig. 15.4a and b).

Peritoneal relations: Uterus is suspended from each side of the pelvis by a double-fold of peritoneum, the *broad ligament*. In its upper free margin lies the *fallopian tube* which is 10 cm long. The lateral end of *fallopian tube* has a number of *fimbriae*. These fimbriae lie near the side wall of pelvis below the ovary so that the ovum at ovulation can easily be picked up (taken) by the tube.

The anterior layer of broad ligament provides a fold in which runs the round ligament of uterus, which passes through the inguinal canal to fuse with the labia majora.

The posterior layer of broad ligament provides another fold for the ligament of ovary and ovary itself.

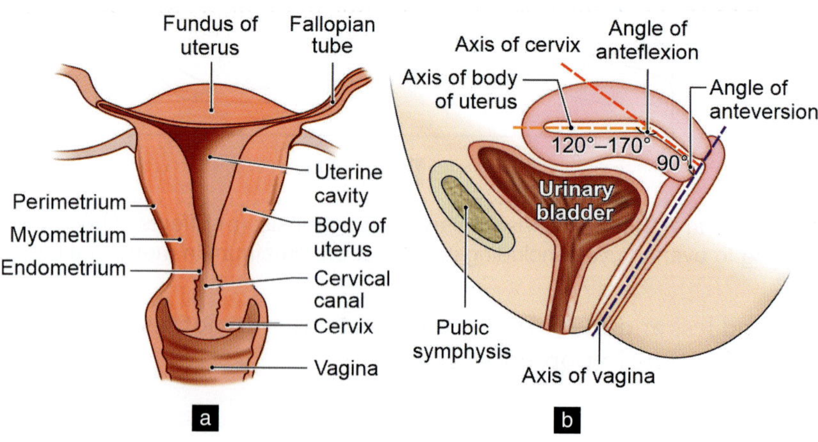

Fig. 15.4a and b: (a) Parts and structure of uterus; (b) Angulation of uterus and vagina

Supports of the uterus:

1. ***Muscular supports:*** *Levator ani, urogenital diaphragm* and *perineal body* with number of perineal and pelvic floor muscles attached to it.
2. ***Ligaments:***
   a. *Lateral ligaments* or *cervical ligaments* pass from cervix of uterus and vagina laterally to the lateral pelvic wall (Fig. 15.5).
   b. *Uterosacral ligaments* pass from the cervix and vagina backwards to the sacrum.
   c. *Pubocervical ligaments* pass from the pubic bone to the cervix. These ligaments support the uterus.
3. Angulation of uterus, angle of anteversion.
4. Peritoneal folds like broad ligaments.
5. Round ligaments.

Structure:

1. ***Walls of uterus are composed of three layers of tissue:*** (1) perimetrium, (2) myometrium and (3) endometrium. *Perimetrium* consists of peritoneal covering. Bulk of uterine wall consists of smooth muscle called the *myometrium*. The mucous membrane lining myometrium internally is called *endometrium*. It is composed of columnar epithelium, tubular glands and stroma.
2. ***Arterial supply*** to uterus is by uterine arteries (branches of internal iliac arteries). Uterine artery crosses the ureter and runs on the side of the uterus in a tortuous manner. It supplies cervix, body, fundus of uterus and medial part of fallopian tube. *Venous drainage* occurs into internal iliac veins. *Lymphatic drainage* occurs to aortic lymph nodes and lymph nodes associated with iliac blood vessels. Some lymphatics pass to the superficial inguinal nodes.

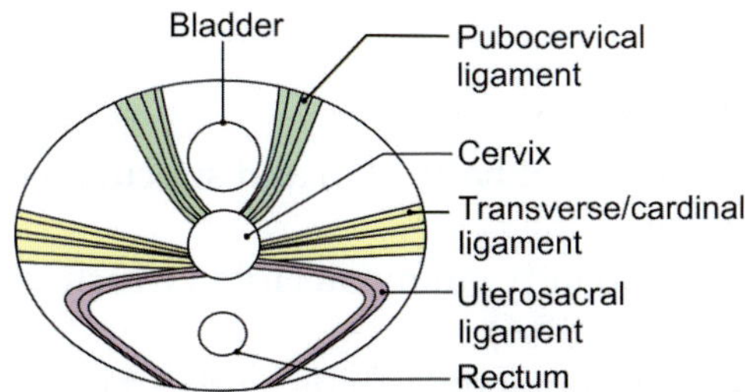

Fig. 15.5: Ligaments supporting the uterus

Vagina

It is female organ of copulation. It is a muscular tube 10 cm long—lying obliquely behind pubic symphysis and in front of rectum and anal canal (Figs 15.2 and 15.4a).

The menstrual products are discharged from it. It is lined by stratified squamous epithelium and an underlying connective tissue stroma with no glands. In reproductive age group (15–49 years), pH of vagina is maintained between 3.5 and 4.9 by *Lactobacillus acidophilus* (Doderlein's bacilli) bacteria.

Hymen: It is a thin layer of mucous membrane which covers the opening of vagina. It gets perforated at menarche due to menstrual flow. It gets torn at the time of intercourse or by strenuous exercises. The condition of the hymen is not a reliable sign of virginity.

Around the upper end of vagina, into which the cervix of the uterus projects, are the *fornices*. They are the right, left, anterior and posterior fornices. The posterior fornix is the deepest. Lower end of vagina opens into the perineum.

It is supplied by uterine and vaginal branches of internal iliac vessels. Lymphatic drainage is through deep and superficial iliac glands.

It functions as a copulatory organ and also provides an elastic passage through which baby passes out during childbirth. It connects the external and internal organs of reproduction.

Fallopian Tube/Oviduct

These are two muscular tubes one on each side of the uterus and each is 10 cm long. It is subdivided into four parts. From medial to lateral the parts are intramural, isthmus, ampulla and infundibulum. The end of each tube has the finger-like projections called fimbriae. The fertilisation occurs normally in the ampulla of the tube (Fig. 15.2). If implantation occurs in the tube itself, it is known as ectopic pregnancy. Such tube mostly ruptures, leading to severe bleeding.

External Genital Organs

Mons pubis is a mound of hairy skin and subcutaneous fat in front of pubic symphysis.

Labia majora are two fatty cutaneous folds which pass backwards from mons pubis (Fig. 15.6).

Labia minora are two cutaneous folds, without fat lying internal to labia majora. These form the boundary of vestibule of the vagina.

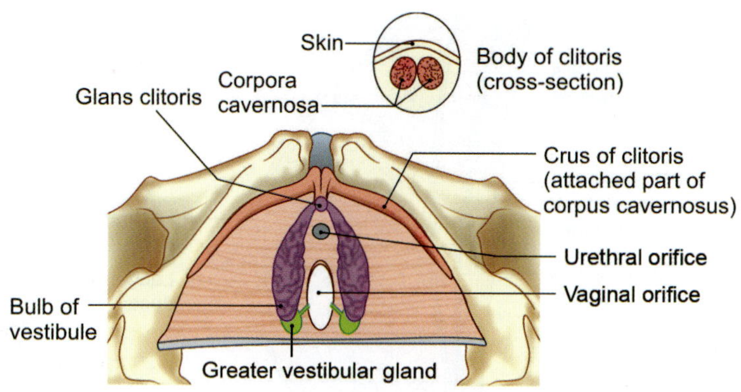

Fig. 15.6: Structure of clitoris

Vagina, urethra and ducts of greater vestibular glands open into the vestibule. Just inside the vaginal orifice, a fold of mucous membrane, the hymen obstructs the opening.

Clitoris lies at the anterior end of labia minora. It is formed by two small *corpora cavernosa* and two bulbs of the vestibule. It corresponds to penis in the male but clitoris has no corpus spongiosum and is not traversed by the urethra. It has no reproductive significance.

Greater vestibular glands lie under cover of the back part of bulb of vestibule. Their duct, 2 cm long, opens into the vagina.

Ovulation

It takes place between 12–14 days prior to the next menstrual cycle. Graafian follicle ruptures to release secondary oocyte in a process called ovulation (Fig. 15.3a).

During ovulation, the body temperature rises by 0.5–1.0°C.

BREAST/MAMMARY GLAND

The breast is present both in males and females, but is rudimentary in males and children. It is well-developed in the female after puberty (Fig. 15.7).

The breast is a modified sweat gland. It is an important accessory organ of female reproductive system and provides nutrition to the newborn in the form of milk.

The breast lies in the superficial fascia of the pectoral region. A small extension of the breast called the *axillary tail of Spence*, pierces the deep fascia and lies in the axilla.

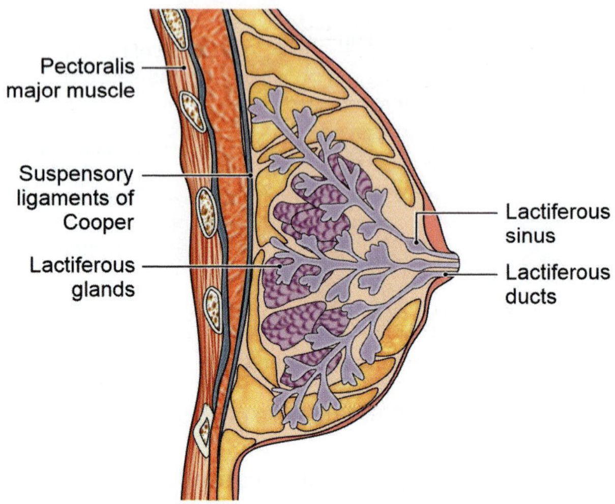

Fig. 15.7: Structure of the breast

It extends vertically from the second to the sixth ribs. Horizontally, it extends from lateral border of sternum till the mid-axillary line.

The deep surface of the breast is related to pectoralis major and serratus anterior muscles.

Structure of the Breast

The structure of the breast is divided into skin, parenchyma and stroma. The skin covers the gland and presents a conical projection called the *nipple,* situated at the level of 4th intercostal space. Nipple is pierced by 15–20 lactiferous ducts.

The skin around the base of the nipple is pigmented, circular and is known as the *areola.*

The parenchyma is made up of glandular tissue. The gland comprises 15–20 *lobes*. Each lobe is made up of lobules which are formed by various acini. The glands drain into lactiferous sinuses which open onto the nipple (Fig. 15.7).

The stroma is the supporting framework of the gland. It is made up of fibrous as well as fatty tissue.

Blood supply: The breast is supplied by branches of axillary and internal thoracic arteries. Venous drainage occurs into axillary and internal thoracic veins.

Nerve supply: Breasts are supplied by branches from 4th, 5th and 6th intercostal nerves.

Lymphatic drainage: Lymphatic drainage is important as cancer of breast spreads through lymphatics. 75% of lymph from breast drains into various groups of axillary lymph nodes, 20% into the internal mammary nodes and 5% into the posterior intercostal nodes.

Cancer of the breast may spread to the same side axillary lymph nodes. It may also spread to opposite breast and opposite side axillary lymph nodes.

For early diagnosis every female must palpate her both breasts every month to note any growth.

The essential function of breast is the synthesis, secretion and ejection of milk. These functions called *lactation* are associated with pregnancy and childbirth. *Milk secretion* is stimulated by hormone *prolactin* from anterior pituitary with contributions from progesterone and oestrogen. The *ejection* of milk is stimulated by *oxytocin* released from posterior pituitary in response to the sucking of an infant on the mother's nipple (suckling).

MALE REPRODUCTIVE SYSTEM

Male reproductive system consists of following internal and external genital organs.

External genital organs are:

- Testis
- Epididymis
- Ductus deferens (partly)
- Spermatic cord
- Penis (Fig. 15.8)

Internal Genital Organs

Internal genital organs are ductus deferens (partly), seminal vesicle, ejaculatory duct, prostate gland (Fig. 15.8).

External Genital Organs

Scrotum: It is a pouch in the perineum and is divided into two compartments by a raphe. Each compartment contains one testis, one epididymis and part of ductus deferens. Scrotum lies below symphysis pubis and behind the penis.

> *Competency achievement:* The student should be able to:
> AN 46.1 Describe and demonstrate coverings, internal structure, side determination, blood supply, nerve supply, lymphatic drainage and descent of testis with its applied anatomy

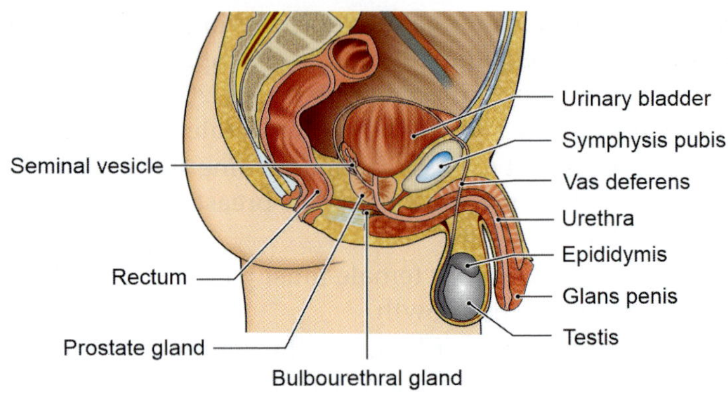

Fig. 15.8: Sagittal section of male pelvis

Testis

The testis is an oval egg-shaped structure 4 cm long, 2.5 cm wide and 3 cm thick, suspended by the *spermatic cord* into the *scrotum.*

Each testis is covered by three layers of tissue. Outermost is a sac of peritoneum called the *tunica vaginalis*. Testis during foetal life descends from the upper part of posterior abdominal wall through lower part of anterior abdominal wall into the scrotum taking peritoneal covering and blood vessels with it.

Tunica albuginea lies outside the tunica vaginalis and fibrous septa from it divide the testis into lobules.

Innermost is *tunica vasculosa* consisting of a network of capillaries supported by delicate connective tissue.

Each testis is made up of 200–300 lobules. Each *lobule* has 1–4 convoluted loops called *seminiferous tubules*. Each tubule is composed of *germinal epithelial cells* (spermatogenic cells) and *Sertoli cells*. Between tubules are *interstitial cells of Leydig* that secrete hormone testosterone after puberty (Fig. 15.9a).

At upper pole of testis tubules combine to form a single tubule. This single tubule is about 6 metres long. It is repeatedly folded and tightly packed into a mass called epididymis. It leaves the scrotum as *ductus deferens* in spermatic cord.

Testis lies outside the abdominal cavity as lower temperature by 2–4°C is required for spermatogenesis. Testis produce spermatozoa in seminiferous tubules and are stored in epididymis.

Spermatozoa (sperm) are produced in the seminiferous tubules by spermatogenic cells of testis and mature as they pass through epididymis. The production of sperms in testis is controlled by anterior pituitary hormone FSH. Sertoli cells support and protect developing sperms.

Spermatozoa: Each spermatozoon is made up of a head, middle piece and a tail (Fig. 15.9b). The head contains a nucleus. Anterior to nucleus is the acrosome with enzymes, which help in penetration of sperm into secondary oocyte. Middle piece contains mitochondria. The tail pushes the sperm along its way.

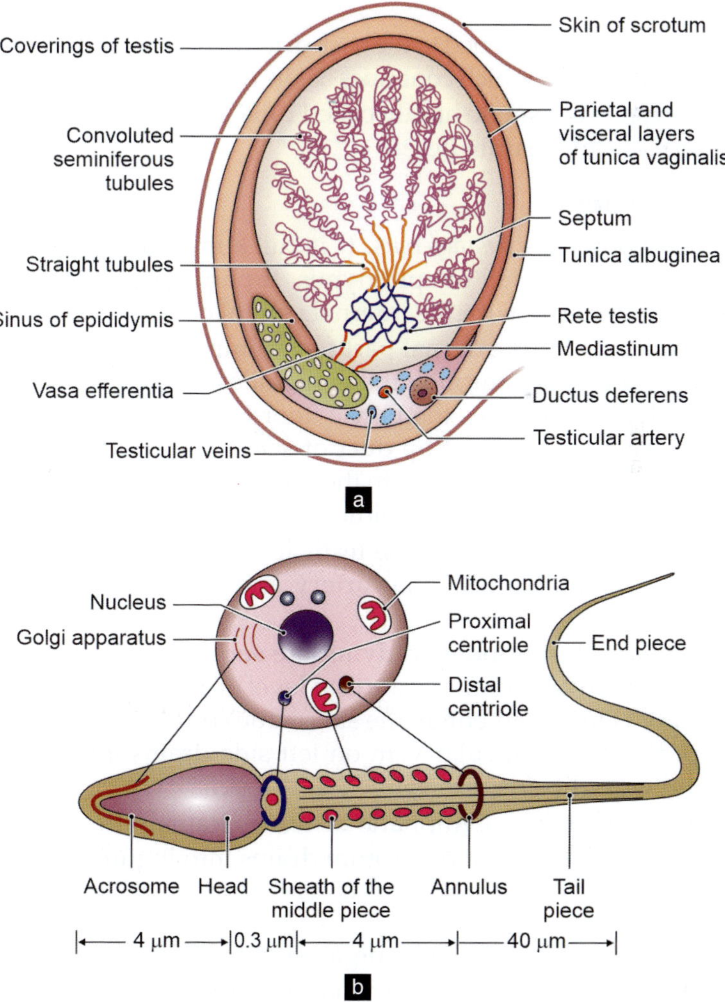

Fig. 15.9a and b: Longitudinal section of a testis and ductus deferens and parts of spermatozoa

The main hormone produced by testis is *testosterone*, a male sex hormone/androgen. Testosterone regulates the production of sperms, stimulates the development and maintenance of masculine secondary sex characteristics.

> *Competency achievement:* The student should be able to:
> AN 46.2 Describe parts of epididymis

Epididymis

Each epididymis is attached to the back of its own testis, and comprises head, body and tail which continues as the ductus deferens.

Epididymis is a single highly coiled tube. It stores the sperms. In addition, sperms mature here.

Ductus Deferens

It is also known as *vas deferens*. It is thick muscular tube and is the continuation of tail of epididymis. It partly lies with external genitalia and partly with the internal genital organs.

Vas deferens in its external part forms important component of spermatic cord, runs through the inguinal canal, and the side wall of the pelvis and crosses the pelvic floor to reach back of urinary bladder. There it is joined by duct of seminal vesicle to form the *ejaculatory duct*, which opens into the prostatic urethra. It carries the maturing spermatozoa from epididymis till the prostatic urethra.

Spermatic cord suspends the testis in the scrotum. Besides vas deferens, it contains testicular artery and vein, lymphatics and autonomic nerves.

Blood supply: Testis and epididymis are supplied by the testicular artery, a branch of abdominal aorta at level of 2nd lumbar vertebra. The artery is long and enters the spermatic cord to reach the testis and epididymis. Testicular vein on left side drains into left renal vein and on right side drains into inferior vena cava.

Lymphatic drainage: Lymphatic of testis drains into para-aortic nodes, while that of skin of scrotum drains into inguinal nodes.

Prostate

It is a fibromuscular glandular organ situated in the lowest part of pelvis, below the bladder, surrounding first 3 cm of urethra. It is 4 cm wide, 3 cm long and 2 cm deep. It lies in front of rectum and rests on the levator ani muscles.

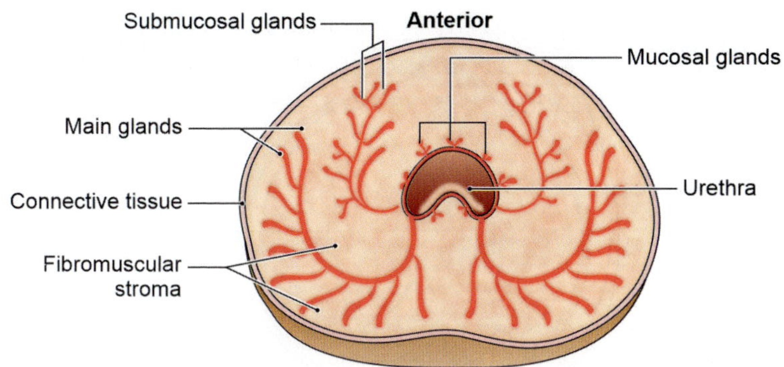

Fig. 15.10: Glands of the prostate gland

Prostate contains glands present within the mixture of fibrous and smooth muscles (Fig. 15.10). The secretion of glands forms 30% of the seminal fluid.

Prostate is small till puberty. Testosterone secreted by the testis enlarges the size of prostate. The secretion of prostatic gland is discharged into the prostatic urethra through its 10–12 ducts. It helps in maturation of spermatozoa.

Its arterial supply is from branches of inferior vesical and from middle rectal artery. Veins drain finally into the internal iliac veins.

Seminal Vesicle and Ejaculatory Duct

The *seminal vesicles* are a pair of pouch-like structures with smooth muscle. It is 4–5 cm long. Each vesicle lies against the back of bladder. The duct of seminal vesicle joins with vas deferens to form *ejaculatory duct*. This duct is 2 cm long and runs through the prostate to open into prostatic urethra. The genital ducts of both sides drain into the urinary tract, so the urethra serves as a common channel for semen and urine.

Secretions of the seminal vesicles add to the volume of semen and help in maturation of spermatozoa.

> *Competency achievement:* The student should be able to:
> AN 46.3 Describe penis under the following headings: Parts, components, blood supply and lymphatic drainage

Urethra and Penis

Male urethra provides a common passage for the flow of urine and semen. It is about 19–20 cm long (*see* Fig. 14.6).

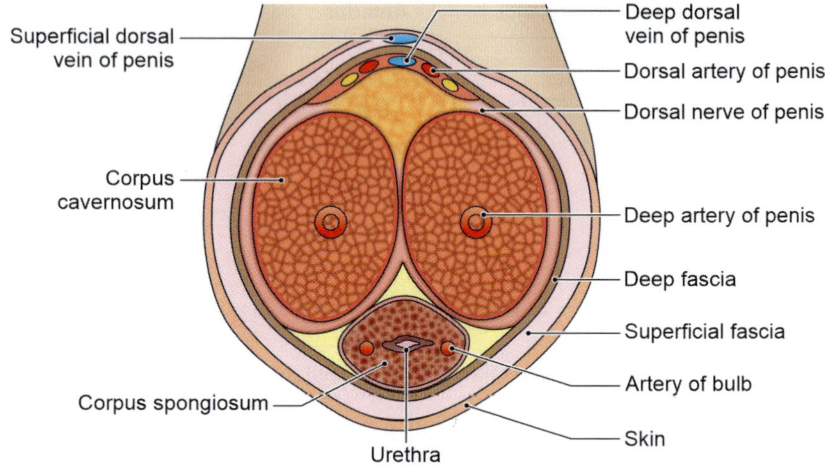

Fig. 15.11: Transverse section through body of penis

Penis is the male organ of copulation and contains the longest, spongy part of the urethra. Penis is made of three spongy erectile tissue: (1) One central, (2) the *corpus spongiosum* with urethra and (3) on each two *corpus cavernosum* (Fig. 15.11). Urethra opens on the glans penis, the expanded end of corpus spongiosum. Just above the glans, the skin is folded upon itself and forms a movable double layer, the *prepuce*.

Blood supply of penis is by internal pudendal vessels.

Nerve supply is by autonomic and somatic nerves.

Penis functions as a tube for the passage of urine most of the time, and for passage of semen whenever required.

Clinical Anatomy of Reproductive System

Syphilis

Syphilis is caused by spirochaete *Treponema pallidum*. The organism after penetrating the genital mucosa produces local as well as distant lesions.

Primary syphilis occurs approximately 3 weeks after sexual contact with an infected individual. A single, firm, non-tender, raised lesion (chancre) forms at the site of organism invasion on penis, cervix, anus or vaginal wall. It ulcerates and heals spontaneously in 2–8 weeks.

Secondary syphilis occurs 2–10 weeks after primary stage. It consists of skin rash, lesions on mucous membrane, fever, lymph node enlargement. These lesions resolve spontaneously.

Female Reproductive System

Pelvic Inflammatory Disease

It is inflammatory condition of female pelvic organs, usually caused by bacterial infection. It usually begins as vulvovaginitis (inflammation of vulva and vagina) and spreads to cervix, uterus, uterine tubes and ovaries. Clinical features are fever, foul smelling vaginal discharge, pain in lower abdomen, abnormal uterine bleeding. Complications include infertility intestinal obstruction due to adhesions.

Imperforate hymen: Hymen is a membrane close to lower end of vagina. It allows the menstrual flow to come out. If hymen is so complete and does not even allow the menstrual flow to come out, the condition is called 'imperforate hymen'.

Rape

Sexual intercourse with a female without consent, i.e. forced penetration of penis into vagina is called rape.

Ovary

Ovary is subjected to tumours, which may be benign or malignant. Benign tumours are more common and dermoid cysts are the most common type.

Malignant ones are epithelial cell tumours or luteal cell tumours. Ovary is also a common site of metastases from the tumour of stomach, pancreas or breast.

Uterus

1. ***Fibroid*** is a very common clinical entity. These are benign tumours of myometrium (smooth muscle). They are of variable size and are usually multiple. They are common in reproductive period (15–49 years). Clinical features are discomfort, frequency of micturition, irregular periods, painful periods (dysmenorrhoea) and reduced fertility.
2. ***Endometrial cancer:*** Uterus may also be the site of *endometrial cancer*. It is seen in women 50–60 years of age, who are obese,

hypertensive or diabetic. It may spread to liver, lungs and bones via blood or lymph.

3. ***Cancer of the cervix*** is extremely common. It starts from the cervical epithelium, involving its whole thickness. It may spread locally to body of uterus, vagina, bladder or rectum. It occurs most commonly between 35 and 50 years of age. It is more frequent in women who have started sexual activity at an early age, who have many partners or who have many pregnancies. Human papillomavirus infection is also associated with this cancer. There may be metastases in the bones, liver or lungs.
4. ***Prolapse uterus*** is supported by muscles of pelvic diaphragm and also by urogenital diaphragm. Many strong ligaments also provide support. If these muscles get injured (during delivery) or ligaments get overstretched, the uterus descends downwards. This condition is known as *prolapse of the uterus*.

Fallopian Tubes

1. ***Salpingitis:*** Inflammation of fallopian tube is called *'salpingitis'*. It is usually due to spread of infection from uterus. If not completely treated, the tube may get blocked, leading to infertility.
2. ***For female sterilisation***, 1.5–2 cm of lateral part of fallopian tube is removed bilaterally and their ends are ligated separately. This prevents the oocyte being fertilized by the spermatozoa.
3. ***Ectopic pregnancy:*** The fertilisation of oocyte takes place in the lateral part of the fallopian tube. Then, it migrates to the uterine cavity. In some cases, the zygote stays in the fallopian tube and cells multiply. Such a pregnancy is called 'ectopic pregnancy'. Such pregnancy ends within 2–3 months by rupture of tube and it can cause severe haemorrhage.

Mammary Gland (Breast)

Gynaecomastia

There is a proliferation of breast tissue in men. It is usually benign and affects one breast only. It is common in a young adult and older men. Common causes are drug intake, e.g. digoxin, cirrhosis of liver and endocrine disorders leading to high oestrogen levels.

Mastitis

Inflammation of the breast can be non-suppurative (during lactation due to congestion of breast) or suppurative (due to pyogenic bacteria). Suppurative mastitis is due to infection by *Staphylococcus aureus* and *Streptococcus pyogenes*. The infection enters through the nipple abrasion and spreads along the mammary ducts of lobe causing pus formation in one or more lobes of the gland.

Tumours

Most breast tumours (90%) are benign. *Fibroadenoma* is the most common type. They usually occur after puberty. Malignant tumours are usually found in upper outer quadrant of the breast. It is commonly seen after 35 years of age. These are painless nodules in one of the breasts only. Early spread via lymphatic vessels is common to axillary and internal mammary nodes. It can spread even to opposite breast and opposite axillary lymph nodes. Local spread may occur to skin, muscle and pleura. Factors predisposing to it are genetic component, disorders leading to high oestrogen levels, early menarche, late menopause and no pregnancies. Early diagnosis and treatment can prevent its spread. Every adult woman must palpate both her breasts with the palm of her hands, to detect any nodule at an early stage.

Male Reproductive System

1. ***Phimosis:*** When the skin of prepuce cannot be retracted, leading to narrowing of urethral orifice, the condition is called phimosis.
2. ***Urethritis:*** Urethra may get infected by infection descending from urinary bladder. Urethra may also get infected during catheterization, and infection may ascend up to other organs like seminal vesicles, prostate, testis and epididymis.

Testis

1. ***Orchitis:*** Inflammation of testis is called orchitis. It may be an ascending infection from the urethra or occur secondary to mumps.
2. ***Undescended testis:*** Testis develops in the lumbar region and then descends down via the inguinal canal. If it does not descend and remain in lumbar or inguinal region, the condition is called undescended testis. There is increased risk of infertility and testicular cancer in undescended testis.

3. ***Hydrocele:*** There is collection of fluid in the tunica vaginalis (extension of peritoneal cavity) surrounding the testis.
4. ***Testicular tumour:*** The testicular tumours are mostly malignant. These are common in undescended or ectopic testis.

Prostate

Prostatitis: Acute or chronic inflammation of prostate is called prostatitis.

Benign enlargement of prostate: Median lobe of prostate gland enlarges to cause obstruction to the internal urethral orifice. This causes back pressure to cause hydronephrosis of kidney. It is common in men over 50 years of age. In benign enlargement, the prostate gland needs to be removed.

Malignant tumours of prostate: The peripheral glands of prostate are affected by cancer. The cancer spreads by venous plexus into bones especially the vertebral column. It also spreads to neighbouring organs. It is common in men over 50 years of age.

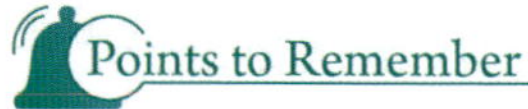

1. Male gonad (testis) lies outside the abdominal cavity as spermatogenesis needs lower temperature by 2–3°C.
2. Male urethra carries urine and seminal fluid at different time.
3. Clitoris does not contain urethra.
4. Vasectomy and tubectomy are important family welfare methods.

Multiple Choice Questions

1. Angle of anteversion between uterus and vagina is:

a. 80 b. 120

c. 90 d. 60

2. Most important ligamentous support of uterus is:

a. Pubocervical ligament

b. Uterosacral ligament

c. Transverse cervical ligament

d. Rectouterine fold of peritoneum

3. Hormones required for ovulation are:

a. Oestrogen
b. LH
c. FSH
d. FSH and LH

4. Narrowest part of male urethra is:

a. Prostatic part
b. Membranous part
c. Internal urethral orifice
d. External urethral meatus

5. Structure of penis is:

a. Two corpora cavernosa, one corpus spongiosum
b. Two corpora cavernosa, two corpus spongiosum
c. One corpus spongiosum, two corpora cavernosa
d. Only two corpus cavernosa

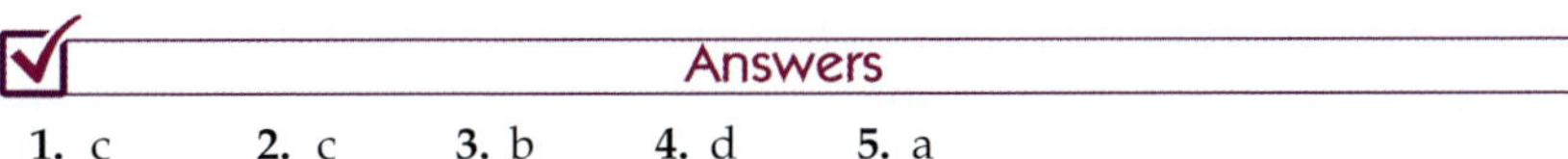

Answers

1. c **2.** c **3.** b **4.** d **5.** a

Chapter 16

Principles of Radiography

"The tragedy of human history is decreasing happiness in the midst of increasing comfort."
—Swami Chinmayananda

The spectrum composing electromagnetic radiation includes gamma rays, UV rays, infra red and electric waves. X-rays are a part of this gamma ray spectrum emitted by the cosmic system.

Medical X-rays, which are used routinely for diagnostic purposes, are not emitted from any radioactive material. Instead, they are produced by heating a tungsten or molybdenum cathode in a vacuumized tube at high temperatures, such that electrons having short wave emit radiation from the surface of these materials. This radiation is then raced towards a tungsten anode by a strong electrical current, which results in abrupt stopping of the X-ray beam and a change in its direction, thereby focusing the rays on to the part of the body under examination. Thereafter upon penetrating the body, they cast an impression on the X-ray plate kept under the area of study. This plate is subsequently processed and an image is generated for medical evaluation.

Since the X-rays have a short wavelength, they are invisible to human eyes. Hence the need to be conscious about the dangerous side effects of X-rays. The X-rays are composed of particles of energy called photons, which have no mass, no charge and travel at the speed of light. These photons are called X-ray photons.

HISTORY OF X-RAYS

X-rays were discovered accidentally on the 8th of November 1895, by Wilhelm Conrad Roentgen.

Roentgen was a German physicist from the University of Wurzburg. He was engaged in studying the behavior of an electron beam as it passed through a vacuumized tube to strike a tungsten plate. To his surprise, he observed that, in addition to electrons, certain unknown rays were also produced, which could penetrate the glass envelope of his apparatus and produce a glow on a distant fluorescent screen. He was able to photograph the bones of the hand of his wife by placing it over a photographic plate and then shining the rays on it.

Since no name had been given to this kind of radiation, the name X-ray was given by him. For his unique discovery, Roentgen was awarded the Nobel Prize in Physics in the year, 1901.

The discovery of X-rays provided a new dimension to the advancement of medical and other sciences.

The medical use of X-rays are for both diagnostic and therapeutic purposes. The technique of using X-rays for imaging body parts is called radiography, for diagnosing disease, radio-diagnosis and for treatment of disease, radiotherapy.

As a diagnostic tool radiography has proved of immense value in detection of the diseases, fractures and many other problems in the human body.

Therapeutically, X-rays are used in the treatment of many types of cancers because, the rays can destroy cancer cell, though the adjacent normal cells also get affected.

PROPERTIES OF X-RAYS

The relevant properties of X-rays are as follows.

1. Penetrating Power

X-rays closely resemble visible light rays in having a similar photographic effect. But they differ from the light rays in being invisible and in having a shorter wavelength. The wavelength of X-rays is 0.01 to 10 nanometers. It is this property of short wavelength which gives them the power of penetration through different materials.

When X-rays pass through matter, they are absorbed to varying extent. The degree of absorption depends on the density (atomic weight) of the matter. Radiography is based on the differential absorption of the X-rays. Dense tissues such as bones, metals and materials having high atomic numbers absorb X-rays far more readily than do the soft tissues of the body. These cast a white shadow on the image plate as no X-rays can reach the imaging plate. Structures which are easily penetrated by X-rays such as air and fat allow the X-rays to reach the image plate, thereby casting a black to grey impression, identical to the physical appearance of the intervening structure. These are described as radiolucent shadows and the structures which are penetrated with difficulty or are not penetrated at all are described as radiopaque.

Different density structures, therefore, can be arranged in a scale of increasing radiopacity.

a. Air, in the respiratory passages, stomach and intestines is black.
b. Fat is greyish black and relatively less dark than air.
c. Soft tissue, e.g. muscles, vessels, nerves, and viscera cast an impression by virtue of the adjoining fat or air outlining them or else they would not be visible on X-rays.
d. Bones, due to their calcium content appear grayish white.
e. Enamel of teeth, and metallic foreign bodies, e.g. metallic filling of the teeth, and radiopaque contrast media also appear white, the brightness being much more than the bone.

2. Photographic Effect

When X-ray photons strike a photosensitive film, the image of the object under examination gets imprinted on the film. When such a film is developed and fixed chemically, a radiography image becomes visible.

The X-ray film has a base made up of cellulose acetate, which is coated on either side with silver bromide (photosensitive) emulsion 0.001 inch thick. The film is blue tinted and transparent.

An X-ray image (picture) is called skiagram (skia = shadow), radiograph, or roentgenogram.

Computed and Digital Radiography

The conventional X-ray cassette containing the X-ray film is now replaced by a novel imaging system. The imprint of the body part made by exposing it to X-rays, can either be directly read off by a digital radiographic system and displayed straight on the monitor screen or visualized through an indirect computed radiographic system. These technologies are called direct digital radiographic system—DR system or, if indirect, they are called CR system. An image of the exposed part can be obtained in these systems on an imaging film by processing it through an image printer.

Alternatively, the image can simply be stored on the computer, e-mailed or burnt on a CD and given to the patient. These systems have several advantages over the conventional film screen method.

The images can be manipulated and improved so that unnecessary repetitions of radiographs due to quality concerns can be avoided. The films can be stored in the computer, retrieved, mailed or even printed on paper. This saves money, time, storage space and even reduce the cost of silver which is needed to make the conventional X-ray films. Hence as of today, most institutions have switched over to either CR or DR system.

3. Fluorescent Effect

When X-rays strike certain metallic salts (phosphorous, zinc, cadmium, sulphide), the rays cause them to light up, that is, light rays are produced and the image of the object becomes visible to the naked eye during the period of the exposure. This property of X-rays is utilized in live screening of objects such as bowel loops, bones, blood vessels, heart and spinal cord to name a few structures.

4. Biological Effect

X-rays can destroy both normal and abnormal cells. This effect is utilized in the treatment of various cancers but at the costs of destroying adjacent normal cells as well.

Hence, X-rays are potentially dangerous. On repeated exposures, they can cause burns, hair loss, brittle nails, development of cancers and even genetic mutations. Therefore, adequate protective measures must be taken against repeated exposures to X-rays. Wherever and whenever possible they should be avoided, particularly in children, young people and pregnant women. However, should the need arise, they must be used with adequate precautions to reduce morbidity and mortality.

Radiography

The method of obtaining X-rays of different body parts is called radiography. Radiographs are generally obtained from a single direction if it is the chest or abdomen or from two directions at right angles to each, if it is the extremities and spine. This gives complete information about the area in question. The term used by radiologist for this is "views".

The 'view' expresses the direction of flow of the X-ray beam. In AP (anteroposterior) view, the rays pass from the front to back, the latter resting against the X-ray plate. In PA (posteroanterior) view the X-rays pass from the back to front, the front surface resting against the X-rays plate. The part of the body touching the X-ray plate (i.e. near the X-ray plate) casts a sharper shadow than the part facing the X-ray tube.

The views can be anteroposterior (AP), lateral or oblique depending on the relationship of the body part with the X-ray beam. Chest X-rays are usually posteroanterior (PA) views. For visualizing the thoracic spine, AP view is preferred.

RADIOGRAPHIC PROCEDURES

1. Fluoroscopy

Fluoroscopy is visualizing the body part in real time using X-rays. It is of special advantage in observing the movements of the organs (lungs, gastrointestinal tract, diaphragm), flow of administered contrast through blood vessels and bowel and in positioning the subject during the examination.

Fluoroscopy in earlier days was done in a dark room. But now image intensifiers and television monitors are used which have eliminated the need for darkening the room.

The fluoroscopic image is visualized directly on the fluorescent screen which is covered with a sheet of lead glass to absorb unwanted X-rays and to protect the fluoroscopist. Nowadays the conventional fluoroscopic screen has been replaced by an image intensifier system with the image being projected on an accompanying television monitor.

The sharpness of the fluoroscopic image is inferior to that of a radiograph but it provides information about motion and flow which a static X-ray cannot do.

2. Plain Radiography

An X-ray image, obtained directly without using any contrast medium, is called a plain X-ray. It is useful in the study of normal bones, lungs, normal joints, paranasal air sinuses and gaseous shadows in the abdomen.

Strength: Covers a large area quickly, relatively low X-ray exposure and low cost. Easy accessibility (Figs 16.1 to 16.3).

Weakness: Relatively low resolution and low soft tissue contrast as compared to CT scans.

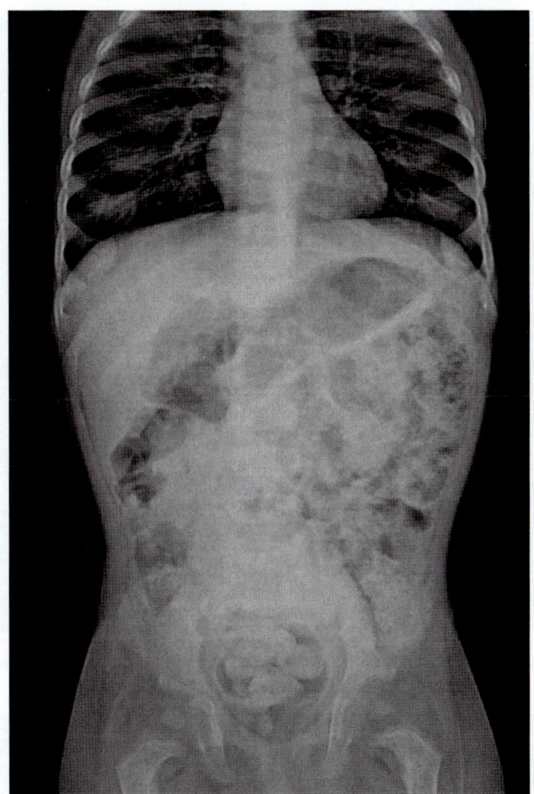

Fig. 16.1: Plain X-ray of the abdomen AP view showing part of the lower chest as well as the entire abdomen

3. Contrast Radiography

The hollow viscera and solid organs cannot be visualized in plain radiography due to their having similar soft tissue densities. However, their differences or contrast can be accentuated by filling such organs or cavities with either a radiopaque or a radiolucent substance.

Radiography done after artificial accentuation of the contrast density is called contrast radiography.

The radiopaque compounds used in contrast radiography are:

1. Barium sulphate suspension (emulsion) in water for gastrointestinal tract (Figs 16.4 to 16.6).
2. Aqueous solution of appropriate iodine compounds, for urinary and biliary passages and vascular system.

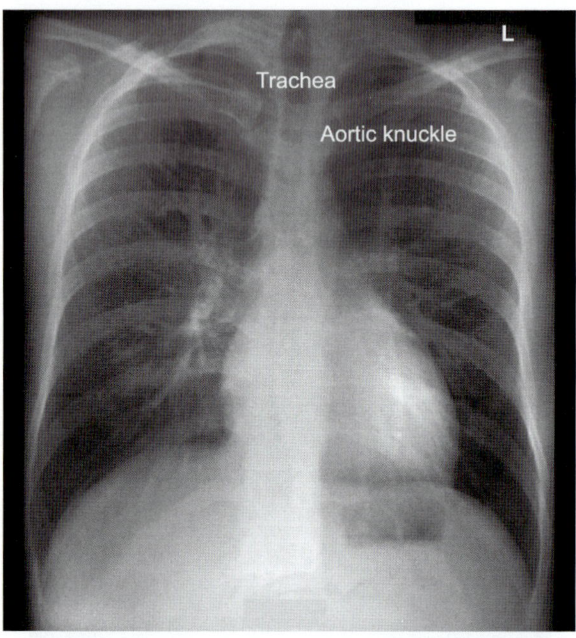

Fig. 16.2: Chest X-ray PA view showing lungs, cardiac shadow and bones

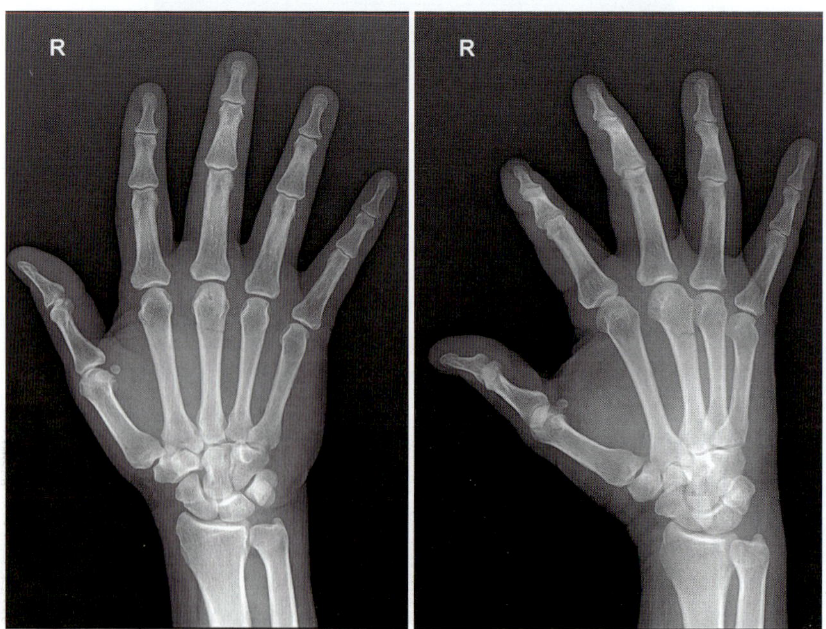

Fig. 16.3: X-ray of the hand PA and oblique view

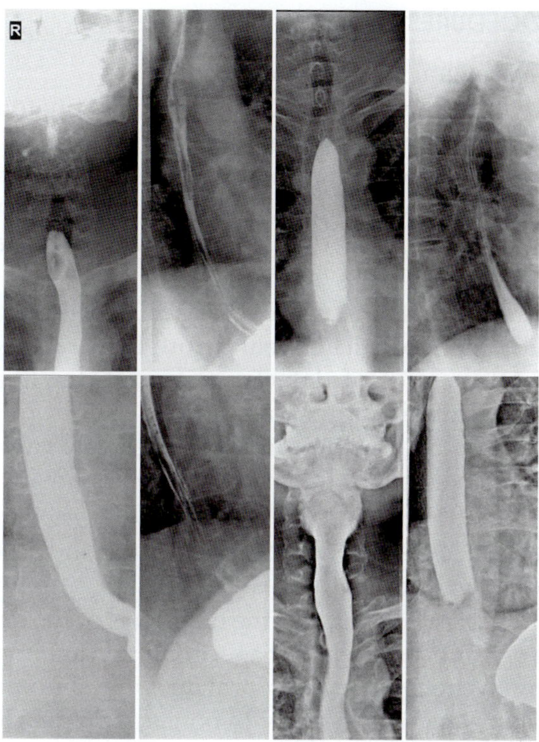

Fig. 16.4: Barium swallow. High density barium given by mouth is seen outlining the esophagus

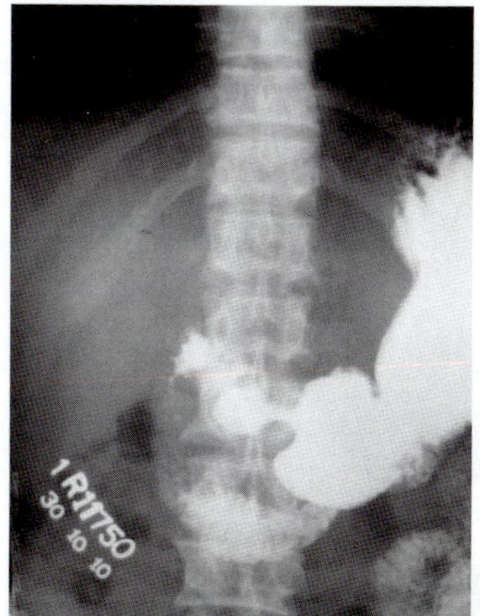

Fig. 16.5: Barium meal upper gastrointestinal tract showing stomach and part of the duodenum

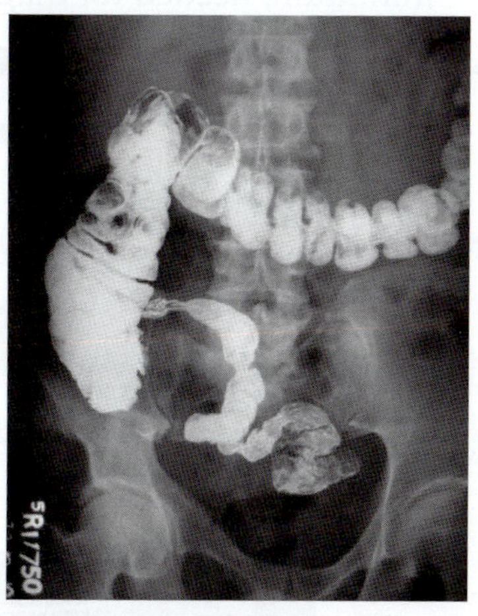

Fig. 16.6: Barium meal follow through showing ascending colon and part of transverse colon

SPECIAL PROCEDURES

These include several newer technologies.

CT scans, ultrasound and MRI are primarily anatomic studies. PET scan is the study of metabolism. PET-CT or PET-MRI is a combination of metabolic and anatomic study. Nuclear medicine is a metabolic study with capability of concentrating into specific body parts depending upon the composition of the radioisotope and the tissue specific atom used.

1. ***Computed tomography (CT scanning):*** Computed tomography is a major technological breakthrough in radiology. Using X-rays and a series of detectors, it provides images of the body comparable to gross anatomical slices ranging from 0.25 to 10 mm and even more, by which one can distinguish tissues with even slight differences in their density.

   Differentiation between vascular and avascular areas can be enhanced by simultaneous scanning and injection of a radiopaque medium in the vessels.

   Thus CT scanning helps in the diagnosis of the exact location and size of tumours, haemorrhage, infarction and malformation, including hydrocephalus, cerebral atrophy, abdominal lesions, chest lesions, and in the study of bones and joints lesions.

   This technique must be used sparingly, if at all, in pregnant women and children. The radiation must be regulated to bare minimum, needed for diagnostic quality images (Fig. 16.7).

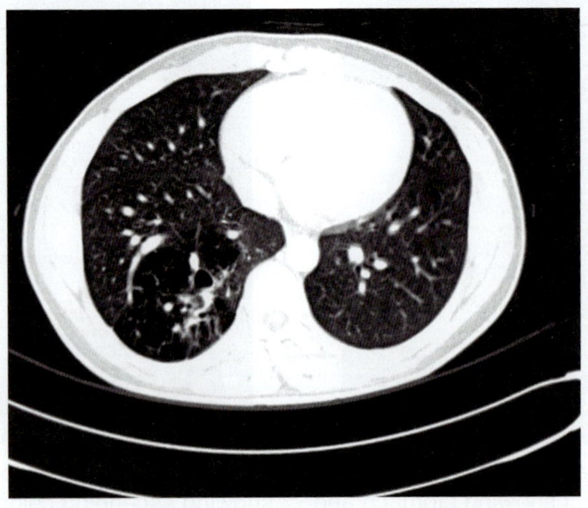

Fig. 16.7: High resolution CT chest

Strength: Excellent resolution.

Weakness: Relatively high radiation exposure.

2. ***Ultrasonography:*** Ultrasonography is a process using high frequency sound waves to create images of soft tissue structures of the body. It is a safe procedure because instead of X-rays, sounds waves are used. These sound waves are sent into the body by an electrically stimulated piezoelectric crystal, housed in an ultrasound probe. They are then reflected back to the crystal from the interfaces formed by tissues having different densities. In this process, their character undergoes a change. Using a computer, the data is reconstructed into an image which one can see on the accompanying display system of the machine (Fig. 16.8).

   The sound waves used are above the range of human hearing, i.e. above 20,000 cycles per second, or 20 kilohertz (1 hertz = 1 cycle per second). As the technique is quite safe, it is especially valuable in obstetric and gynecological problem.

   Strength: Non-invasive.

   Safe, as it does not involve electromagnetic radiation

   Soft tissue contrast enables study of the soft tissues of the body.

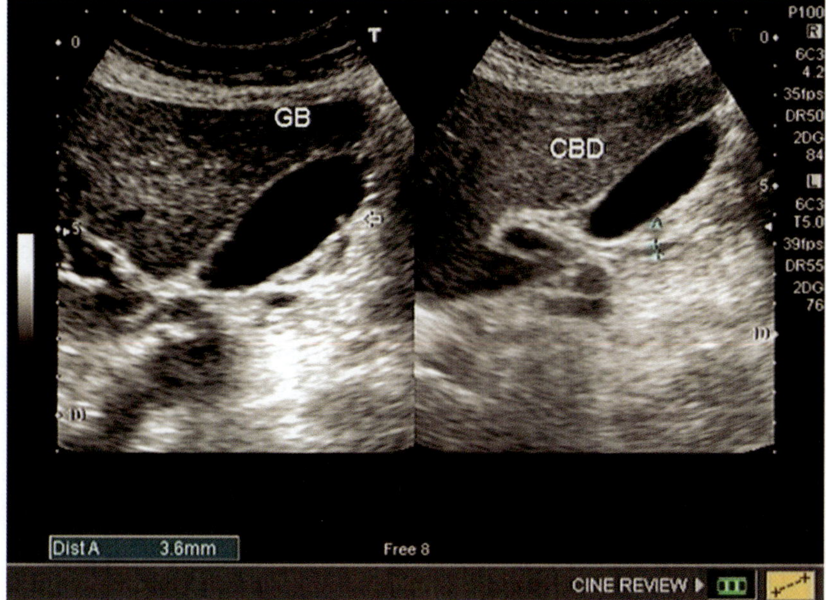

Fig. 16.8: Ultrasound showing gall bladder and common bile duct

High accessibility and low cost.

Extremely versatile, can be used in studying blood flow, heart, brain, abdomen, musculoskeletal system, pregnancy and many more areas.

No radiation.

Weakness: Operator dependent.

Air and bones cannot be penetrated.

MAGNETIC RESONANCE IMAGING (MRI)

MRI is an imaging technique, which, unlike CT, does not use X-rays to produce images. Instead, using a strong magnet which creates an external magnetic field and radiofrequency pulses, it first disturbs hydrogen atoms in the body from their resting position and then allows them to revert to their original state. The resultant energy deposited in the atoms, is released in the form of radiofrequency signals which are picked up by antennas. These signals are then evaluated by a computer, which through a series of complex mathematics, locates the position and number of hydrogen atoms which had send them the signals, thereby accurately identifying their location and quantity in the part under investigation. Thereafter, the computer converts this data into an anatomical image which is displayed on the computer screen.

There are various pulse sequences used in MRI for creating images. These are T1, T2 and proton density sequences. These sequences produce different appearances of the images which help in identifying the nature of the disease process.

Additionally, by using signal characteristics of various structures, such as water, fat, calcium, bones, minerals, it can give an exquisite detail of the composition of the part under examination. Since several atoms besides hydrogen, produce MR signals, this capability can be used in studying blood flow, vascularity of various diseases and organs. These agents—called contrast agents, enhance the diagnostic capability of MRI. Further, MRI can produce images in axial, coronal and sagittal planes. This helps in examining diseases from different angles and planning treatment (Figs 16.9 and 16.10).

Strength: It is the investigation of choice to study brain and spinal cord. It is also used for abdominal, musculoskeletal and cardiac imaging and in studying blood flow (Fig. 16.11).

No radiation is used. Multiplanar images can be obtained for further evaluation of organs.

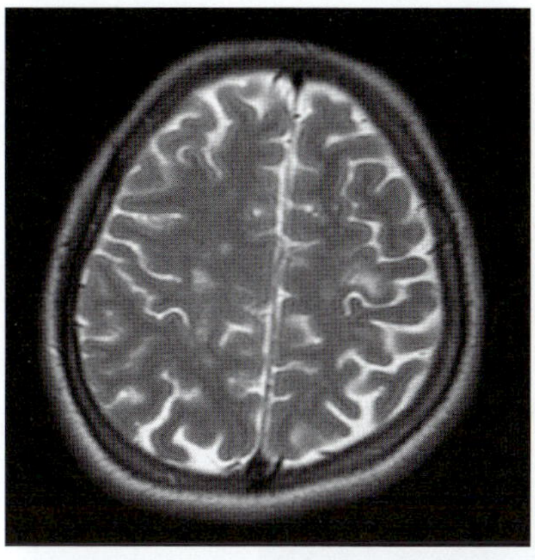

Fig. 16.9: Brain MRI T2 W image

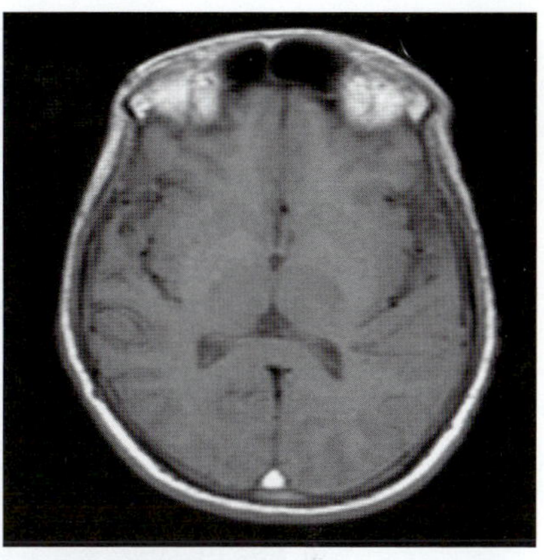

Fig. 16.10: Brain MRI T1 W image

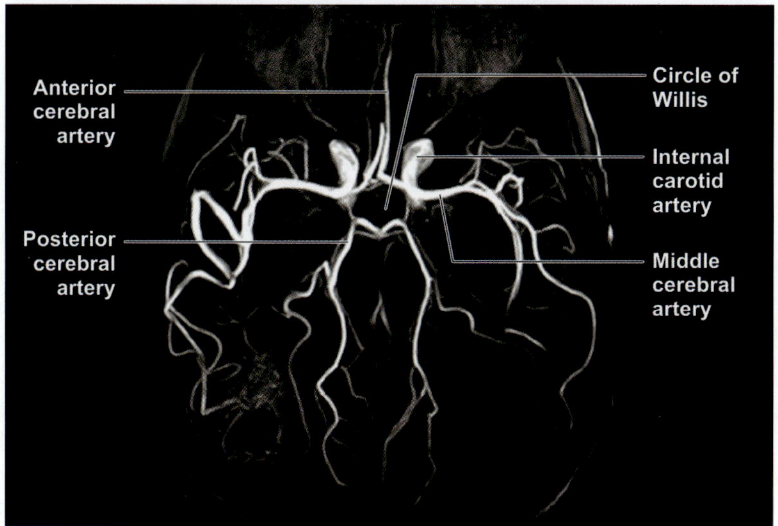

Fig. 16.11: Brain MR angiography

High soft tissue contrast is seen in the images obtained on MRI.

Weakness: Claustrophobia

Long examination times

High cost.

POSITRON EMISSION TOMOGRAPHY (PET)

A PET scan uses radioisotopes which are combined with a carrier such as FDG and injected into the body. The FDG is fluorodeoxygluconate

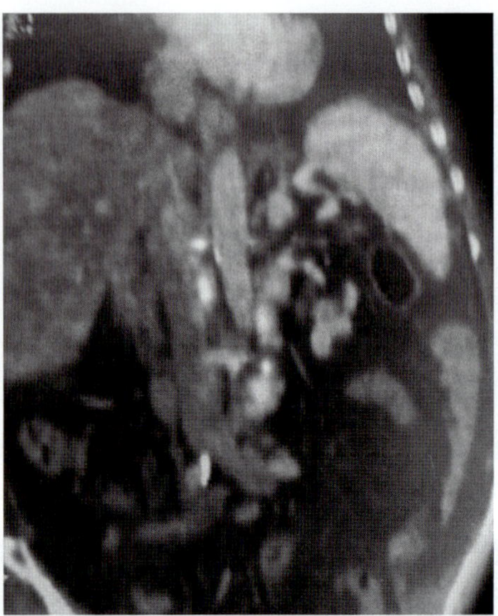

Fig. 16.12: PET scan showing pathological abdominal nodes

compound which is taken up in large quantities by areas having increased metabolic activity. The isotope accumulates in these areas and give a bright signal which is picked up by a receiver and displayed as an image.

When combined with CT or MRI, it is called PET-CT or PET-MRI (Fig. 16.12).

The CT and MRI give the anatomical location and the PET demonstrates foci of increased metabolic activity in these anatomic areas. Thus the lesion showing high signal on PET is accurately located anatomically as well.

Strength: PET detects metabolic uptake, whereas CT scan or MRI demonstrates structural changes. Metabolic uptake tells us the state of the disease in terms of disease activity. This helps identifying sites for biopsy, response to treatment, deciding if the disease is slowly progressive or otherwise, benign or malignant nature of the disease.

Weakness: Costly procedure. Uses radiation.

INTERVENTIONAL RADIOLOGY

Fluoroscopy with image intensifiers, ultrasound and CT scans have enabled accurate localization of disease processes inside the body. This has opened up a whole new field called interventional radiology.

Interventional radiology involves a wide variety of procedures. These include:

- Percutaneous catheterization and embolization in the treatment of tumours to reduce tumour size and vascularity prior to operation in difficult cases.
- Percutaneous transluminal dilatation and arterial stenosis for the treatment of localized stenosis in the arteries.
- Needle biopsy under imaging control for lung tumours and abdominal masses.
- Transhepatic catheterization of the bile ducts for draining in obstructive jaundice.
- Needle puncture and drainage of cysts in the kidneys or abscesses using ultrasound or CT.
- Pleural taps.
- Catheter drainage of pleural fluid.
- Performance of vascular studies.

The procedures are safe, quick and cheaper than surgery, do not need general anaesthesia, can be performed as outpatient procedures, but are dependent on experts to do them.

Points to Remember

- X-rays have shorter wavelength which gives them the power of penetration into different materials.
- X-rays are potentially dangerous. Adequate protective measures must be taken against repeated exposures to X-rays especially during early pregnancy.
- For viewing the lungs posteroanterior view (PA view) is taken
- Viscera are visualised by contrast radiography or by ultrasound.
- Ultrasound is a relatively safe imaging procedure during pregnancy.
- Magnetic resonance imaging is best used to visualize brain and spinal cord.
- Positron emission tomography detects functional changes at an early stage.

Multiple Choice Questions

1. **What kind of waves are X-rays?**
   a. Sound wave
   b. Electric
   c. Electromagnetic
   d. Magnetic
2. **X-rays were discovered in 1895 by:**
   a. Brain S. Worthington
   b. Howard Sochurek
   c. Wilhelm Konrad Roentgen
   d. William Harvey
3. **X-rays have the following properties *except*:**
   a. X-rays bound back toward the source
   b. X-rays cause metallic salt to fluoresce
   c. X-rays show penetrating power
   d. When they strike a photosensitive film, the film gets photosensitized
4. **Which of the properties of X-rays is used for therapeutic purpose?**
   a. Photographic effect
   b. Biological effect
   c. Penetrating power
   d. Fluorescent effect
5. **Which term is not used to describe an X-ray image?**
   a. Skiagram
   b. Roentgenogram
   c. Radiograph
   d. Sonograph
6. **Which one will produce most radiopaque shadow on X-ray film?**
   a. Enamel of tooth
   b. Muscle
   c. Bone
   d. Gas
7. **Radiography is based on:**
   a. Obstruction of X-ray by all tissue
   b. Differential absorption of X-ray by different tissue
   c. Equal absorption of X-ray by different tissue
   d. None of the above
8. **The chest X-rays are mostly taken on:**
   a. AP view
   b. Oblique view
   c. Lateral view
   d. PA view
9. **Which is the intravenous radiopaque contrast media?**
   a. Air
   b. Carbon dioxide
   c. Oxygen
   d. Iodine compounds

10. Which of the following provides images similar to transverse sections of the body part?

a. CT scan
b. Skiagram
c. Sonography
d. All of the above

11. Sound waves used for ultrasound are:

a. Within the range of human hearing
b. Above the range of human hearing
c. Below the range of human hearing
d. All of the above

12. Which scanning procedure is safe in obstetric practice?

a. X-ray
b. CT scan
c. Sonography
d. MRI

13. Which of the following technique does not show bones?

a. CT scan
b. Sonography
c. MRI
d. None of the above

14. Which one is the most effective method for examining the spinal cord?

a. CT scan
b. MRI
c. Contrast radiography
d. Sonography

15. Which procedure is used for detecting fallopian tube blockage?

a. KUB
b. Salpingography
c. Intravenous pyelogram
d. Barium enema

16. Carotid angiography is indicated in:

a. Skull fracture
b. Hydrocephalus
c. Chronic sinusitis
d. Anterior cerebral artery aneurysm

17. Which salt is used for Ba meal?

a. $BaSO_4$
b. $BaCl_2$
c. $BaCO_3$
d. BaI_2

18. What is the difference between CT scan and MRI?

a. CT scan uses sound waves
b. CT scan uses X-rays
c. MRI used sound waves
d. MRI uses X-rays
e. MRI uses magnetic fields

19. How does PET scan differ from CT scan and MR?
   a. It is used for scanning metastases
   b. It shows metabolic activity
   c. It is made of sound waves
   d. It is emitted from radioisotopes

20. Interventional radiology is:
   a. Use of radiology to OPD therapeutic and diagnostic procedures
   b. Use of radiology for biopsies
   c. Can be done under ultrasound, CT and fluoroscopy
   d. All of the above

21. X-rays are harmful if used unnecessarily:
   a. True
   b. False
   c. Harmful especially for children and pregnant women
   d. Harmful if given in high doses and repeatedly

Answers

1. c	**2.** c	**3.** a	**4.** c	**5.** d	**6.** a	**7.** b	**8.** d
9. d	**10.** a	**11.** b	**12.** c	**13.** b	**14.** b	**15.** b	**16.** d
17. a	**18.** b, e	**19.** b	**20.** d	**21.** c			

Chapter 17

Genetics

Genetic engineers don't make new genes, they rearrange existing ones.
—Thomas E Lovejoy

Genetics is the study of heredity, a process by which children inherit certain characteristics (traits) from their parents.

Heredity is controlled by genes and environmental factors. Various environmental factors may cause anomalies in chromosomes, e.g. mother's age over 40 years, viral diseases or exposure to radiation during pregnancy. One needs to compare the stages of mitosis (Fig. 17.1) and meiosis (Fig. 17.2) of the cell before the study of the genes. The comparison is shown in Table 17.1.

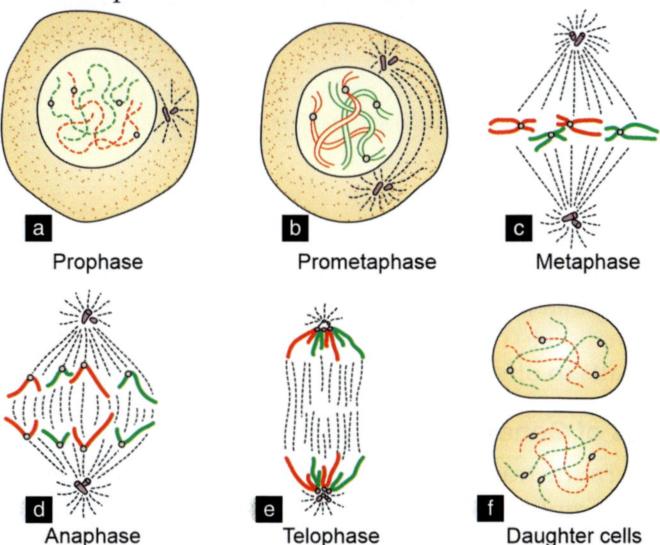

Fig. 17.1a to f: Stages of mitosis

Table 17.1: Comparison of mitosis and meiosis

	Mitosis	*Meiosis*
Prophase	• Homologous chromosomes remain separate • No formation of chiasmata • No crossing over	• Homologous chromosomes pair up. • Chiasmata form • Crossing over may occur.
Metaphase	• Pairs of chromatids line up on the equator of the spindle	• Pairs of chromosomes line up on the equator.
Anaphase	• Centromeres divide • Chromatids separate • Separating chromatids identical	• Centromeres do not divide. • Whole chromosomes separate
Telophase	• Same number of chromosomes present in daughter cells as parent cells • Both homologous chromosomes present in daughter cells if diploid	• Separating chromosomes and their chromatids may not be identical due to crossing over • Half the number of chromosomes present in daughter cells
Occurrence	• May occur in haploid, diploid or polyploid cells • Occurs during the formation of somatic (body) cells and some spores • Also occurs during the formation of gametes in plants	• Only one of each pair of homologous chromosomes present in daughter cells • Only occurs in diploid or polyploid cells • Occurs during formation of gametes or spores

THE GENES

Gene, the functional unit of DNA, is the basic unit of heredity in a living organism. All living things depend on genes. Genes hold the information to build and maintain an organism's cells and pass genetic traits to offspring.

Properties of Genes

- To determine traits, e.g. colour of skin, intelligence, height, etc.
- Undergo replication
- May undergo mutation
- Homeobox genes are groups of regulatory genes that control the expression of other genes involved in the normal development,

growth and differentiation. Teratogens like retinoic acid can activate these genes to cause abnormal gene expression (Fig. 17.2).

Functions of Genes

- Maintain the genetic specificity of an individual
- Play key role in transmission of traits from the parents to the offspring.
- Synthesise various proteins and enzymes of the cell.

Sites of Genes

Each gene occupies a specific locus on the chromosome. Both chromosomes of a given pair contain similar genes. The genes occupying the same locus on the homologous chromosomes are called alleles.

In females, the two sex chromosomes (XX) are identical in length, hence these are homologous.

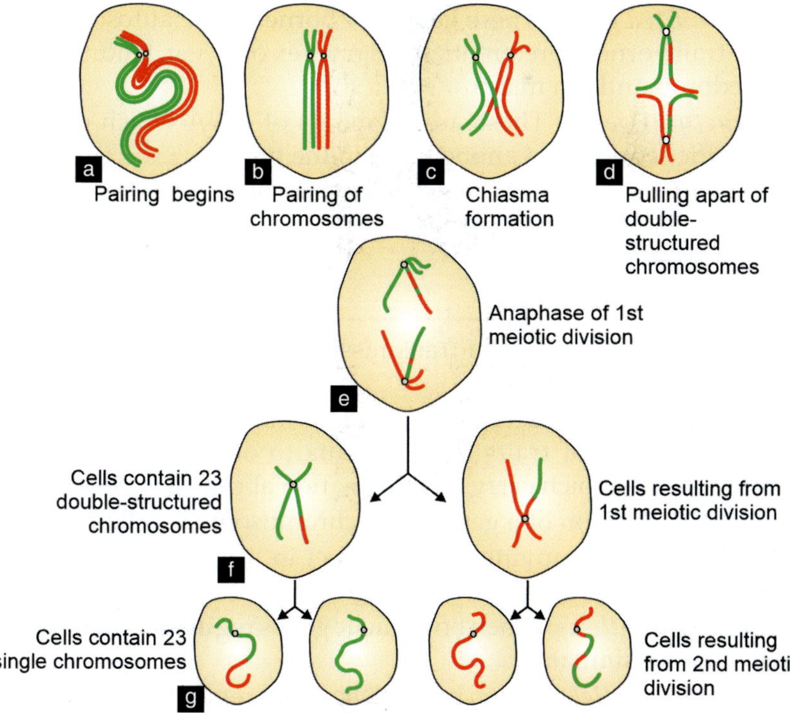

Fig. 17.2a to g: Stages of meiosis

In males, the two sex chromosomes (XY) are unequal in length. There are no alleles on the Y chromosome, for most of the loci are on the X chromosome.

Types of Genes

According to Mendelian Pattern of Inheritance

- *Dominant gene:* An allele which is always expressed in both the homozygous and the heterozygous combination.
- *Recessive gene:* When an allele is expressed only in the homozygous state, it is known as recessive gene.
- *Carrier gene:* In the heterozygous state, the recessive gene acts as a carrier gene which is not expressed in the individual but may be expressed in the subsequent generations.
- *Co-dominant gene:* When both the allelic genes are dominant but of two different types, both traits may have concurrent expression, e.g. blood group AB.
- *Sex-linked genes:* The genes located on X or Y chromosomes are sex-linked genes.
- *Sex-limited genes:* These genes are borne by the autosomes, but the trait borne is preferentially in one sex only, e.g. baldness seen predominantly in males.
- *Structural genes:* These are segments of DNA which code for specific sequence of amino acids in the protein.
- *Regulatory genes:* These are segments of DNA which control functions of structural genes.

SOME IMPORTANT TERMS

Inheritance: it is process of transmission of characters/traits from generation to generation.

Reproduction: It is essential requisite for inheritance to take place. The inheritance of traits from parents to offspring takes place through genes which carry all information about all types of traits.

Locus: The position of a gene in the chromosome is called locus.

Alleles: Genes occupying identical loci in a pair of homologous chromosomes.

Homozygous alleles: When both allelic genes regulating a particular character are similar.

Heterozygous alleles: when both allelic genes regulating a particular character are dissimilar.

Multiple alleles: When in a population, more than two different alleles exist at a given locus of a chromosome.

Mutation: It is a phenomenon which results in alteration in base pair in DNA. Under abnormal conditions, adenine may pair with cytosine or guanine, instead of thymine. This forms the basis of mutation. Some mutations involve changes in whole set of chromosomes like aneuploidy, polyploidy.

Modes of Inheritance (Mendel's Laws of Inheritance)

1. ***Law of uniformity:*** The crossing over between two homozygotes of different types results in offspring that are identical and heterozygotic. The inherited characters do not blend.
2. ***Law of segregation:*** Segregation of alleles occurs during the process of gamete formation (meiosis) and randomly united at fertilization.
3. ***Law of independent assortment:*** This law states that the traits are transmitted to the offspring independently of one another.

THE CHROMOSOMES

Structure of Chromosomes

1. All chromosomes consist of two parallel identical filaments called chromatids joined together at a narrowed constriction called centromere (Fig. 17.3).
2. As per the position of centromere, chromosomes are grouped in 3 types in humans (Table 17.2).

Groups of Chromosomes

The chromosomes are arranged in descending order of length. The first pair is the longest and the 22nd pair is the shortest. Sex chromosomes are grouped separately. The chromosomes are

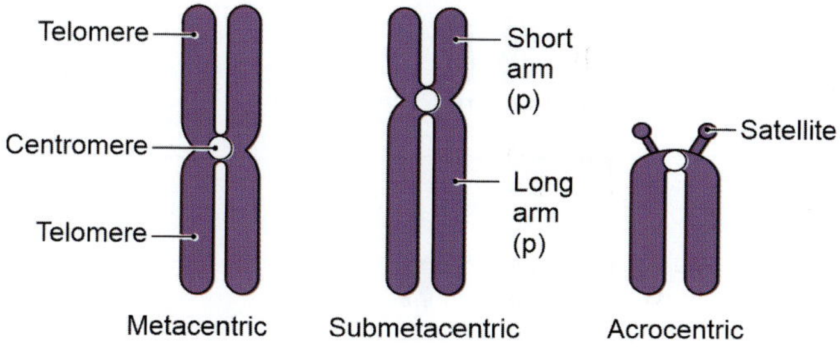

Fig. 17.3: Types of chromosomes

divided into 7 groups. They are denoted as A to G (Fig. 17.4 and Table 17.3).

Each cell contains fixed number of chromosomes which is characteristic of that species or organism. In somatic cell (body cell) of human, the number is 46, which is diploid number. In gametes, i.e. ovum and sperm it is 23, called haploid number. During fertilization, union of two haploid cells restores diploid number of chromosomes.

Table 17.2: Types of chromosomes

Type	*Position of centromere in chromosome*
Metacentric	Middle
Subcentric	Near one end
Acrocentric	Between midpoint and end of the chromosome

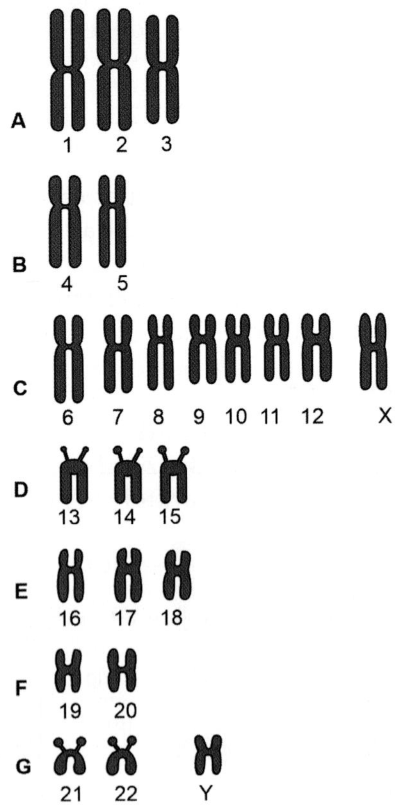

Fig. 17.4: Groups of chromosomes

Table 17.3: Groups of chromosomes		
Group	*Chromosome number*	*Feature*
A	1 to 3	Large, metacentric
B	4 and 5	Large, submetacentric
C	6 to 12 and X	Medium sized, submetacentric and X chromosome
D	13 to 15	Medium sized, acrocentric with satellite
E	16 to 18	Short subcentric
F	19 and 20	Short metacentric
G	21, 22 and Y	Very short, acrocentric, and Y chromosome

Classification of Chromosomes

According to functions:

a. Autosomes: 22 pairs in humans
b. A pair of sex chromosomes which decides the sex of the individual:
   i. In male—XY
   ii. In female—XX

According to the position of the centromere (*Denver's classification*): Shown in Table 17.4.

Clinical significance: Mapping of chromosomes according to the length of their arm and position of the centromere is called karyotyping.

Chemistry of Chromosomes

Human chromosome chiefly contains DNA and only a little RNA. The genetic material is deoxyribose nucleic acid (DNA).

Functions of DNA are to store the genetic information and to transfer the genetic information.

Table 17.4: Position of the centromere				
No.	*Particulars*	*Metacentric*	*Submetacentric*	*Acrocentric*
1	Centromere	Centrally	Subcentrally	Near one end (Fig. 11.1)
2	Arms	Equal shortest	p arm (short) q arm (long)	p arm as satellite q arm longest

Transfer of genetic information is:

1. From DNA to DNA for DNA synthesis
2. From DNA to RNA for protein synthesis

RNA is present in nucleus and in the cytoplasm. There are three types of RNA:

i. *messenger RNA:* m-RNA
ii. *transfer RNA:* t-RNA
iii. *ribosomal RNA:* r-RNA

Messenger RNA acts as an intermediate agent between DNA of the nucleus and amino acids of the cytoplasm. It plays an important role in synthesis of proteins from the pools of amino acids present in the cytoplasm.

Barr Body (Sex Chromatin)

Barr body is an inactivated X chromosome attached to nuclear membrane. It was discovered by Barr and Bertram in 1949 in the neuron of female cats. It is attached to nuclear membrane and is planoconvex in shape and darkly stained. It is also known as sex chromatin (Fig. 17.5).

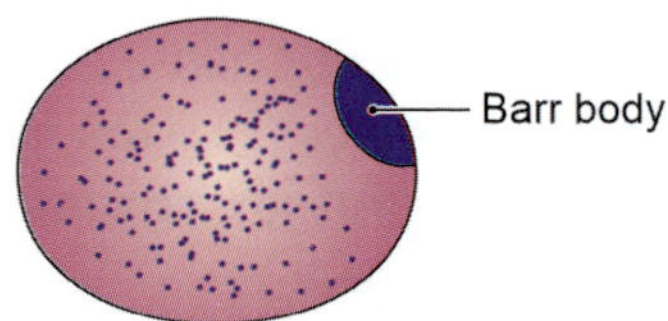

Fig. 17.5: Nucleus of a female cell showing Barr body

In female (XX): There are two X chromosomes. One of them is inactivated within 2 weeks of conception. The inactivated X chromosome becomes the Barr body. Normally, a single Barr body is present and only one X is functional. This is called Lyon's hypothesis.

In male (XY): Since there is only one X chromosome, there is no Barr body. Y chromosome is smaller and is for determination of male sex.

Sex chromatin can be stained by scraping from cheek mucosa.

Mature polymorphonuclear leucocytes in females have a drumstick like body. It is present in 6% females (Fig. 17.6).

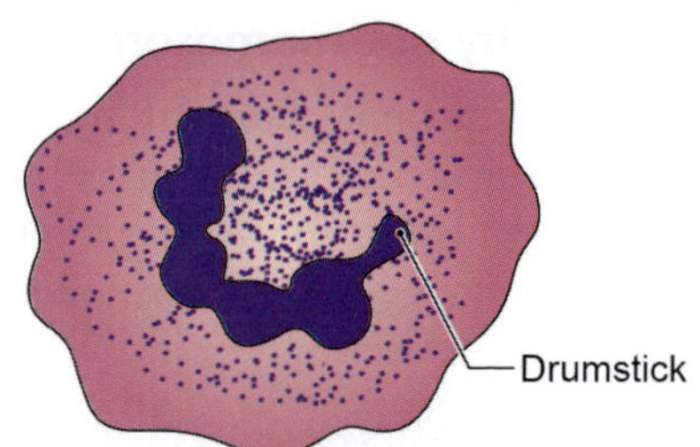

Fig. 17.6: A mature neutrophil from female showing drumstick like body

Clinical significance: It is helpful in determination of sex in case of ambiguity and also in diagnosis of various syndromes like Turner's, Klinefelter's (Table 17.5).

Table 17.5: Number of Barr bodies in different syndromes		
Name of chromosome	*Number of Barr bodies*	*Syndrome/normal*
XX	One	Normal female
XXX	Two	Triple XXX
XO	No Barr body	Turner's syndrome
XY	No Barr body	Normal male
XXY	One	Klinefelter's syndrome

Karyotyping

Introduction: Identification of chromosomes according to the length of arms including the position of centromere is called karyotyping.

Procedure: It is done by the culture of lymphocytes. The cells are grown in culture media containing phytohaemagglutinin (PHA). The cell division is arrested in metaphase by adding colchicine. The spreads of the chromosomes are counted and photographed under the microscope. The images of each chromosome are cut out and arranged in pairs according to the classification. This procedure is called karyotyping. One needs to note:

i. Total length of chromosomes
ii. Position of centromere.
iii. Relative length of two arms.
iv. Banding pattern.

The chromosomes are arranged according to their length in a descending order. Identical chromosomes are paired in karyotyping. The chromosomes paired are numbered 1 to 22 in descending order of length, i.e. pair number 1 is long, pair number 22 is short. They are grouped into 7 groups. They are noted as A to G. The chromosomes are placed separately.

Karyotyping helps to:

i. Identify pattern of abnormal chromosome.
ii. Determine the sex.

Individual chromosomes can be recognized with quinacrine banding (Q-banding) and Giemsa banding (G-banding). These methods have helped in mapping specific genes on the chromosomes (Fig. 17.7).

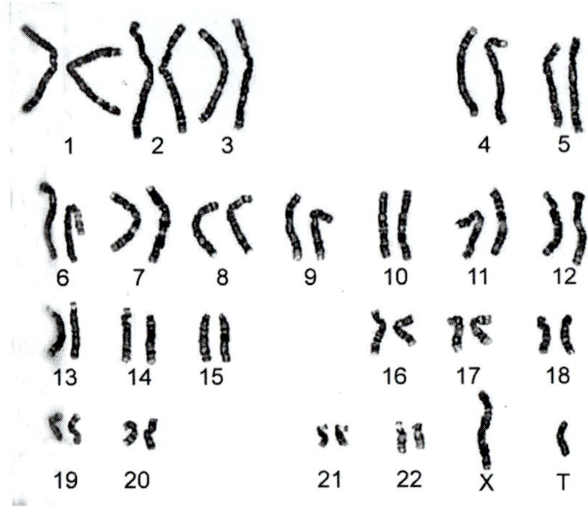

Fig. 17.7: Giemsa banding of the chromosomes

MITOCHONDRIAL DNA

A human cell has genetic material contained in the cell nucleus (the nuclear genome) and in the mitochondria (the mitochondrial genome). In human beings, the nuclear genome is divided into 23 pairs of linear DNA molecules called chromosomes. The mitochondrial genome is circular DNA molecule distinct from the nuclear DNA. Although the mitochondrial DNA is very small compared to nuclear chromosomes, it codes for 13 proteins involved in mitochondrial energy production as well as specific tRNAs.

Mitochondrial Inheritance

- The body receives its entire mitochondrial DNA only from the mother, because during fertilization mitochondria of sperm do not pass into the ovum.
- The diseases which occur due to mutation in the mitochondrial DNA are inherited entirely through mother.

The diseases are

- ***Leber's hereditary optic neuropathy (LHON):*** A condition characterized by sudden onset of blindness in adults
- ***Pearson marrow-pancreas syndrome (PMPS):*** It is a condition characterized by a loss of bone marrow cells during childhood. It is fatal.

There are symbols used in pedigree chart. Figure 17.8 shows these symbols.

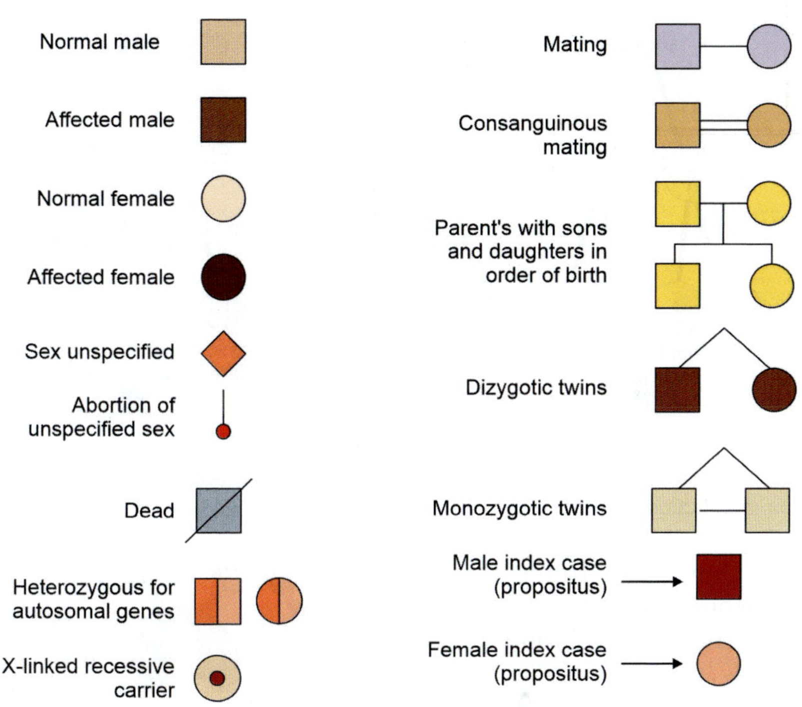

Fig. 17.8: Symbols used in pedigree charting

CHROMOSOMAL ABERRATIONS

It is the change in the structural components of the chromosome. The deletion or an addition of a segment from other chromosome results in structural aberration. The change in number results in numerical aberration. The number may be 45 or 47. Aberrations are seen in elderly primigravida or mother suffering from viral infections during pregnancy or those exposed to radiation during pregnancy.

Various chromosomal aberrations are classified:

Disease due to Autosomal Numerical Chromosomal Aberration

Down's Syndrome/Trisomy 21

- It is the most common congenital anomaly due to numerical aberration of chromosomes. This syndrome was described by Dr. Down in 1866. There is aneuploidy. In aneuploidy the chromosomes may be 2n+1, 2n–1, i.e. 47 or 45. Fertilisation with disomic gamete will result in 47 chromosomes (Fig. 17.9).

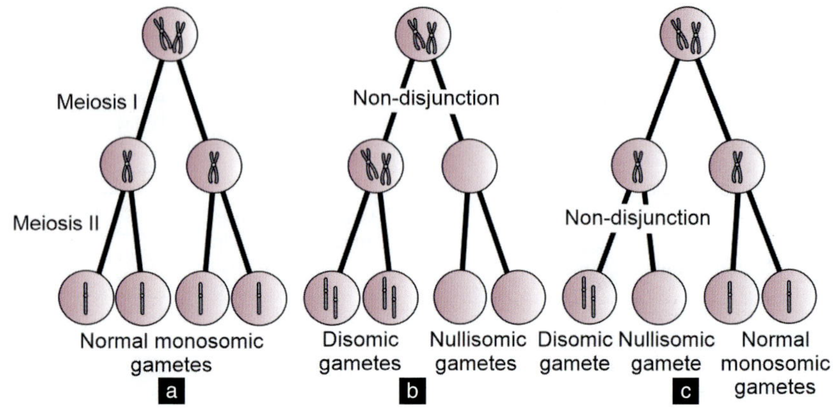

Fig. 17.9: (a) Normal meiosis showing segregation of a single pair of chromosomes, (b) gametes at non-disjunction in meiosis I, (c) gametes at non-disjunction in meiosis II

- In Down's syndrome there is trisomy of chromosome 21. The number of chromosomes is 47, i.e. 47XX or 47 XY. Sex may be male or female. It is seen to occur as one in 700 newborns (Fig. 17.10).

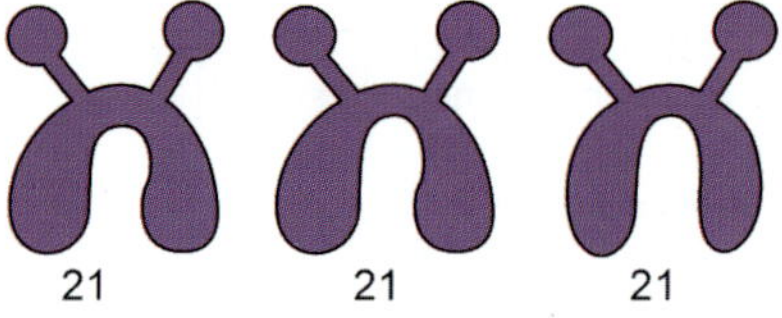

Fig. 17.10: Down syndrome

This condition is commonly seen in elderly primigravida or mother suffering from viral infection during pregnancy. In elderly primigravida the reason is the ageing of the ovum. The sperms are formed fresh every time, so ageing factor does not apply for the sperms.

Clinical Features

- Mental retardation
- Palpebral fissure is slanting upwards at lateral end
- Tongue protrudes out of the mouth
- Palate is narrow so the oral cavity cannot accommodate the tongue
- Nasal bridge is flat
- Epicanthic fold is present on the eyes
- Short broad hands have simian crease.

Edward Syndrome, Trisomy 18

Patau Syndrome, Trisomy 13

In both these syndromes, infants die within 1st month.

Disease due to Autosomal Structural Chromosomal Aberration

Autosomal structural chromosomal aberration may be due to translocations, deletions, duplications, ring chromosomes. Most of these result from unequal exchange between homologous repeated sequences on the same or different chromosomes. One syndrome due to deletion of part of an arm is described below.

Cri du chat Syndrome

This is due to deletion of a part of 'p' arm of chromosome 5 (Fig. 17.11). The following symptoms are seen:

- Septal defects in heart
- "Cat like cry" due to underdevelopment of larynx.
- Severe mental retardation.

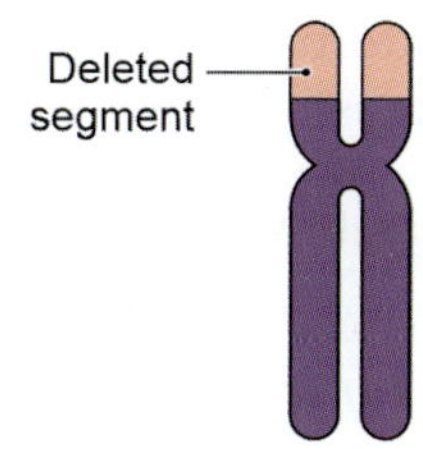

Fig. 17.11: Cri du chat syndrome

Diseases due to Numerical Aberration of Sex Chromosomes

Turner's Syndrome (45X)

This syndrome was discovered by Mr. Turner in 1938. It occurs once in 5000 births (Fig. 17.12).

Chromosomes are only 45X. One chromosome is missing, so no Barr body is seen though the individual is a female.

The patient is of short height with webbed neck. The breasts and genitalia are underdeveloped with wide carrying angle at the elbow.

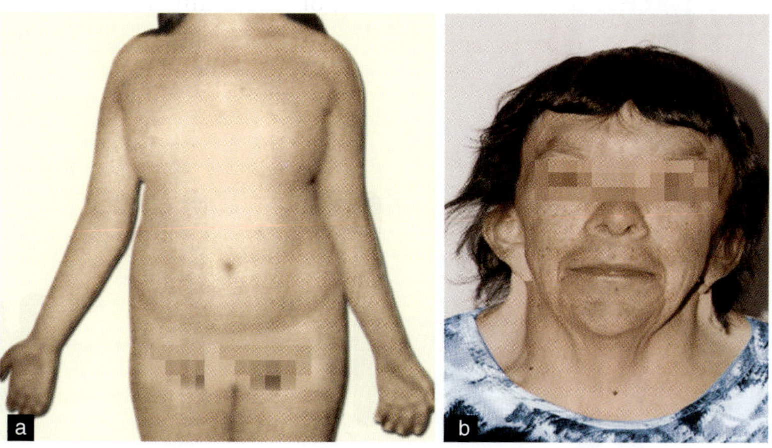

Fig. 17.12: Turner's syndrome showing (a) wide carrying angle, and (b) webbing of the neck

Klinefelter's Syndrome (47 XXY)

The Klinefelter's syndrome was described in cases of tall males in 1942.

Its incidence is 1 in 1000 male newborns (Figs 17.13 and 17.14).

The genotype is 47 XXY.

The individual is male with an extra X chromosome. Since there are two X chromosomes, Barr body is present.

External genitalia including testes are underdeveloped. In contrast, breasts are well developed.

Single Gene Inherited Diseases

Autosomal Dominant Inheritance

Characters: Commonest mating normal with heterozygote.

1. Parents show the trait.
2. There is horizontal and vertical transmission (50% affected at every conception).
3. Trait appears in each generation.
4. Normal (unaffected) individual does not carry the gene and does not transmit the trait.
5. No sex predilection.
6. Both the chromosomes carry the trait. Mating is heterozygous.

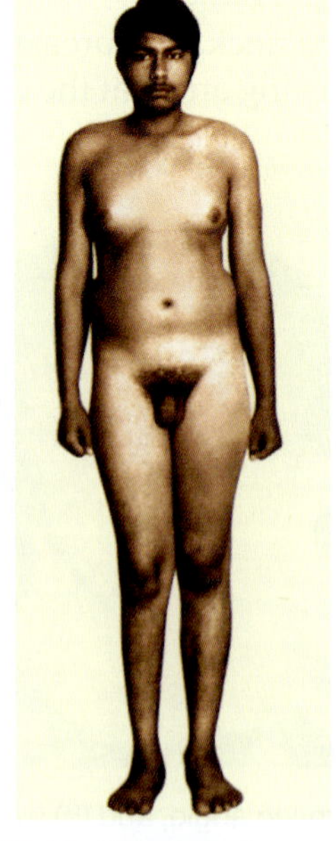

Fig. 17.13: Klinefelter's syndrome

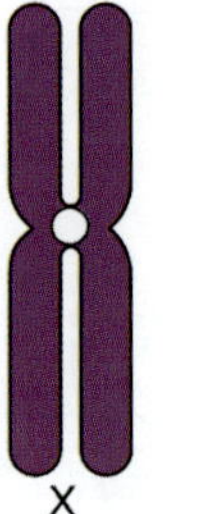

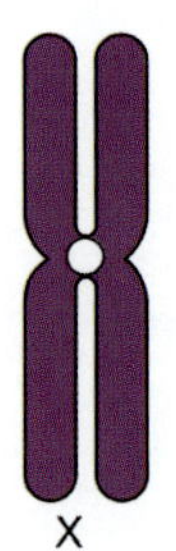

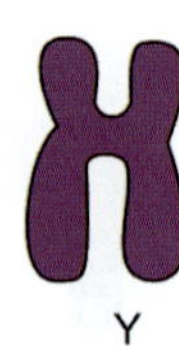

Fig. 17.14: Chromosomal pattern in Klinefelter's syndrome

The disease is inherited by both male and female in each generation. Examples are seen in brachydactyly, syndactyly, achondroplasia, Huntington's chorea.

Pedigree chart is shown in Fig. 17.15.

Autosomal Recessive Inheritance

This condition is common in homozygous mating, 25% are affected in every conception.

Carriers are present and look normal. Parents are from consanguineous marriage. Traits are seen only in the siblings and not parents. Examples are albinism and deaf mutism.

Pedigree chart is shown in Fig. 17.16.

X-linked Dominant Condition

The X-linked dominant trait is seen in homozygous and heterozygous females. It is also seen in male having a gene under

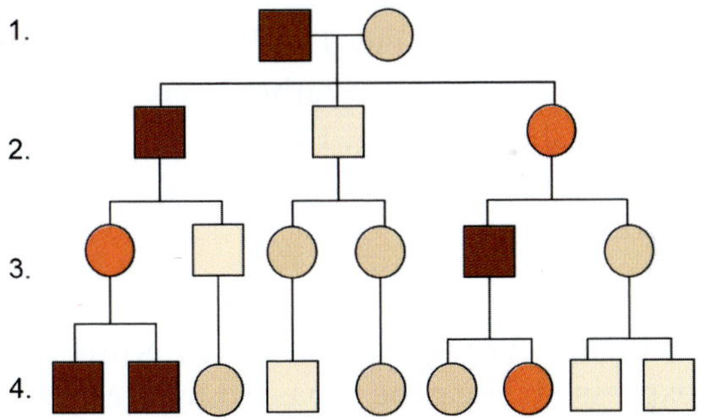

Fig. 17.15: Pedigree chart of autosomal dominant inheritance

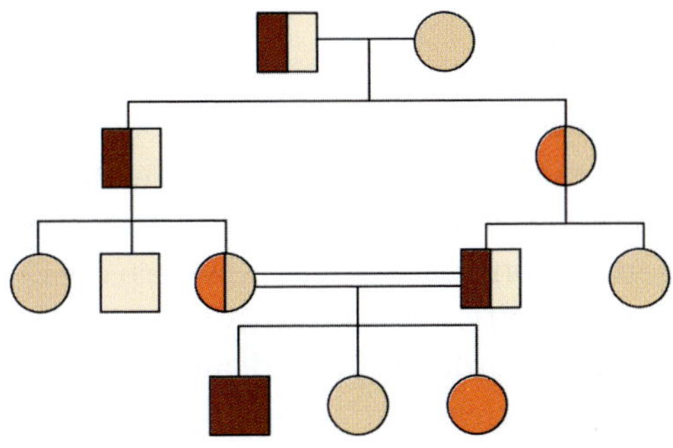

Fig. 17.16: Pedigree chart of autosomal recessive inheritance

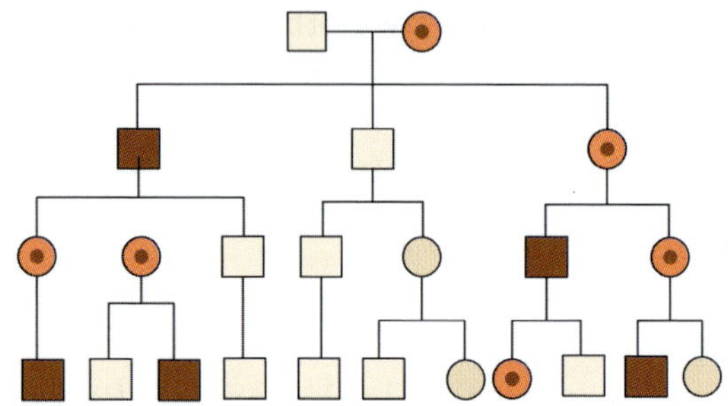

Fig. 17.17: Pedigree chart of X-linked recessive traits

question on his single X chromosome. Common in females, ratio of female: male is 2:1.

Example is seen in vitamin D resistant rickets.

X-linked Recessive Traits

The females are always the carriers and do not show the symptoms.

The females are rarely affected

Pedigree chart is shown in Fig. 17.17.

Disease is not transferred from father to son.

Pedigree chart is shown in Fig. 17.17.

Examples are hemophilia, colour blindness and Duchenne muscular dystrophy.

Y-linked Conditions

Male has only single Y chromosome. The gene is unpaired. If present, it should be expressed. The gene is passed from affected male to his sons but none to his daughters as she does not get Y chromosome.

Example is hypertrichosis, i.e. growth of hair on the outer rim of the pinna of the auricle.

PRENATAL DIAGNOSIS

Genetic abnormalities in a conceptus can result in the following:

1. Spontaneous miscarriages: First trimester losses, mostly associated with chromosomal abnormalities.
2. Gross congenital abnormalities in newborn are 2–3%. This leads to perinatal morbidity and mortality.
3. Abnormalities in childhood and adult life, e.g. blindness, deafness, malignancies.

Prenatal diagnosis helps the doctors in early detection and appropriate management in high-risk cases.

Indications of Prenatal Diagnosis

1. Advance maternal age at conception.
2. Previous history of a genetically abnormal child or a child with gross congenital anomaly.

In addition, routine assessment of normal growth of conceptus and to screen for the various congenital malformations, prenatal diagnosis with special tests is indicated in high risk pregnancies which include:

Maternal risk factors

- Advanced maternal age (>35 years)
- Family history of previous child with neural tube defects
- Previous gestation with chromosomal abnormalities
- One or both parents carrier of X-linked or autosomal traits
- A child born with an unbalanced translocation
- History of recurrent miscarriages

Prenatal risk factors

- Oligohydramnios,
- Polyhydramnios,
- Decreased fetal activity,
- Severe intrauterine growth retardation,
- Presence of soft tissue markers of chromosomal anomaly on routine ultrasonography

METHODS OF DIAGNOSIS

I. Pre-implantation Genetic Diagnosis (PGD)

Following techniques are used whenever indicated:

- Polar body biopsy,
- Blastomere biopsy (from 6 to 8 cell stage) and
- Trophectoderm biopsy.

II. Prenatal Diagnostic Techniques

1. ***Ultrasonography:*** It is a non-invasive technique used for routine antenatal check up to assess fetal growth as well as to detect structural abnormalities whenever indicated.

   Assessment of fetal growth is done by serial ultrasonography for following parameters:

   - Fetal age and growth is assessed by crown rump length (CRL) during 5th to 10th week of gestation.

- Other parameters which help in assessment of fetal growth are biparietal diameter (BPD) of the skull, femur length and abdominal circumference.

Congenital malformations that can be determined by ultrasonography include the:

- Neural tube defects (anencephaly and spina bifida),
- Abdominal wall defects such as omphalocele and gastroschisis,
- Heart defects, and
- Facial defects including cleft lip and cleft palate.

Soft tissue markers for chromosomal anomalies: When observed on ultrasonography, fetal karyotyping is indicated for confirmation.

Blood Flow Velocity

Blood flow velocity is measured in the Doppler ultrasonography to detect the vascular resistance secondary to fetal hypoplasia and IUGR.

2. ***Maternal serum screening tests*** recommended to search for biochemical markers of fetal status are:
   i. *Serum fetoprotein levels*
      - Elevated in twinning, neural tube defects, intestinal atresia, and fetal demise
      - Lowered in trisomies and aneuploidy

   ii. *Human chorionic gonadotropins* (*HCG*) levels are also lowered in trisomies and aneuploidy.

   iii. *Circulating fetal cells in maternal blood for* molecular DNA genetic analysis.
3. ***Amniocentesis:*** In this technique about 20–30 ml of amniotic fluid is withdrawn with the help of a needle inserted into the amniotic cavity transabdominally under ultrasound guidance. It is indicated to perform the following tests:
   - *Biochemical analysis* for fetoprotein and acetylcholine esterase.
   - *Karyotyping* (cystogenetics) from the fetal cells present in the fluid.
   - *Molecular genetic* DNA diagnosis genome detection, etc. by using various tests including polymerase chain reaction (PCR).
   - *Fetal maturity assessment* from the levels of creatinine and lecithin.
4. ***Cordocentesis***, i.e. percutaneous umbilical cord blood sampling is used for:

- *Fetal blood disorders* such as anaemia, hemoglobinopathies, thrombocytopenia.
- *Response to infection* by IgM antibody levels in fetal blood.
- *Rapid karyotyping* and *molecular* DNA genetic diagnosis.

5. ***Fetal tissue biopsies*** indicated in certain specific conditions are as follows:
   - *Chorionic villus sampling* (CVS) involves transabdominally needle aspiration of about 5 to 30 mg of villus tissue from the placenta. The material obtained is used for karyotyping, molecular DNA genetic analysis and enzyme analysis.
   - *Fetal skin biopsy* is indicated with history of hereditary skin disorders.
   - *Fetal liver biopsy* may sometimes be required for enzyme assay.

III. Postnatal Tests to Detect Congenital Malformations

1. Clinical evaluation at birth. Gross anomaly can be seen on routine clinical examination of newborn. Look specifically for:
   - Imperforate anus, and
   - Tracheoesophageal fistula
2. Imaging techniques like ultrasonography, MRI, radiography, etc. can be employed in a newborn if indicated to detect:
   - Anomalies of gastrointestinal tract like oesophageal or duodenal atresia, extent of imperforate anus,
   - Cardiac abnormalities,
   - Intracranial abnormalities and
   - Gross skeletal abnormalities.

FETAL THERAPY

Modern prenatal diagnostic techniques have made it possible to diagnose and treat some fatal diseases. Following modes of therapy are in vogue for fetal diseases:

1. ***Medical therapy to mother*** for prevention as well as treatment of certain fetal disorders being used are:
   - *Administration of folic acid* before and during pregnancy has markedly reduced the incidence of neural tube defects.
   - *Administration of steroids to mother* to accelerate fetal lung maturation and decrease the incidence of respiratory distress syndrome during the risk of premature delivery

- *Medical treatment* of fetal infections, cardiac arrhythmias, compromised thyroid functions, anaemias, can be done successfully.

2. ***Fetal transfusion*** through umbilical cord vein (ultrasound guided cordocentesis) is recommended in cases of fetal anaemia produced by maternal antibodies or other causes.
3. ***Fetal surgery*** in most advanced ultramodern centers is possible for following conditions with guarded risk to mother and fetus:
   - Obstructive urinary diseases to prevent renal damage,
   - Congenital diaphragmatic hernia,
   - Cystic lesions in the lungs,
   - Neural tube defects (spina bifida).
4. ***Stem cell transplantation and gene therapy*** before 18 weeks still under research includes:
   - *Transplantation of hematopoietic stem cells* for treatment of immunodeficiency and hematologic disorders.
   - *Gene therapy* for inherited metabolic disorders such as Tay-Sachs disease and cystic fibrosis.

Note. Tissue or cell transplantation is possible before 18 weeks of gestation, as before this time fetus does not develop any immunocompetence.

MOLECULAR REGULATION OF DEVELOPMENT

A cell contains 23000 genes approximately. These genes are able to make 100000 proteins. The control of development is described below:

Several processes which control differentiation and development include:

- Cell differentiation
- Regulated cell migration
- Induction
- Apoptosis

Cell Differentiation

Totipotent cells are present only in the zygote during first few days before the embryo develops. Each such cell is capable of forming a normal embryo.

Pluripotent cells are present in the blastocyst. They are capable of forming a variety of cell types.

Multipotent cells are present as some undifferentiated stem cells in adult organs and act as source of new cells. These can be cultured to form entirely different tissues than in their organ of origin.

Regulated Migration of Cells

Most events in the embryogenesis involve the migration of cells. Following factors play role in cell migration:

- Connective tissue fibres help to guide the cells
- Chemical signals induce migration
- Hyaluronic acid, creates a favourable environment for cell migration.

Induction

Induction is the interaction between two separate histological tissues or primordial in the embryo that result in morphological differentiation. One tissue usually induces the other. The signals travel from one cell to another by any of the following methods:

- Diffusion of signaling molecules from one cell to other.
- Extracellular matrix mediated signaling.
- Direct cellular contact between the two embryonic tissues.

Growth factors: The signaling molecules.

Growth factors are a group of more than 50 naturally occurring proteins that bind to specific cell receptors to stimulate cell division, differentiation and tissue proliferation. Some common growth factors can be grouped as follows:

1. ***Fibroblast growth factors (FGFs).*** These are particularly important for:
   - Angiogenesis,
   - Axon growth,
   - Mesoderm differentiation (limb development (FDFs—2, 4 and 8).
2. ***WNT proteins.*** There are about 15 WNT proteins. These are particularly important for:
   - Regulating limb patterning,
   - Regulating mid-brain development, and
   - Regulating some aspects of somites and urogenital differentiation.
3. ***Hedgehog proteins.*** There are three hedgehog protein genes: Desert, Indian and sonic hedgehog.

Sonic hedgehog is particularly important for:

- Limb patterning,
- Neural tube induction and patterning,
- Somite differentiation, and
- Gut regionalization.

4. ***Transforming growth factor* β *(TGF-*β*) super family***
   The TGF-β super family has over 30 members.
   - TGF-β *members* are particularly important for extracellular matrix formation and epithelial branching that occurs in the development of lungs, kidneys and salivary glands.
   - *Bone morphogenic proteins* (MBPs) belonging to this family induce bone formation and is involved in regulating cell division, cell death (apoptosis), and cell migration among other functions.
5. ***Epidermal growth factor (EGF)*** is concerned with growth and proliferation of cells of ectodermal and mesodermal origin.
6. ***Nerve growth factors (NGFs)*** stimulate the growth of sensory and sympathetic neurons.
7. ***Insulin-like growth factors (IGF)***
   - IGF-1 acts as a factor for bone growth, and
   - IGF-2 is a fetal growth factor.

Morphogens, e.g. retinoid acid, neurotransmitters and products of Wnt genes are reported to activate homeobox genes.

Growth factor receptors

Growth factor receptors are present in the cell membrane. Two types of growth factor receptors known are:

1. ***Transmembrane receptors*** are present within the cell membrane and protein in nature. They bind to the signaling molecules on the outer side of the membrane and initiate tyrosine kinase activity on the inner side of membrane.
2. ***Notch receptors:*** These play important role in the induction process during embryonic development. These are involved in *juxtacrine signaling* in which a protein on one cell surface interacts with a receptor on adjacent cell surface. Juxtacrine signaling is involved in:
   - Neuronal differentiation,
   - Blood vessel specification, and
   - Somite segmentation.

Apoptosis

Apoptosis, refers to programmed cell death.

Some roles played by apoptosis in development of the following structures are:

- Disappearance of a large number of tissues and structures during development is an obvious function of apoptosis. Fingers and toes are formed by the elimination of tissue between them.
- The lumens of vessels, ducts, hollow organs, other spaces in the body are formed via apoptosis.
- In nervous system a large number of neurons are lost by apoptosis to allow for the proper connections and functions of the remaining cells.

Molecular Control of Development

Most of the information about genetic control of development has come from studies in other organisms, especially Drosophila fruit flies.

Genes controlling development: Three hierarchial groups of genes controlling development have been identified in Drosophila. These include:

- Maternal effect genes,
- Segmentation genes, and
- Homeotic genes

1. ***Maternal effect genes.*** These genes begin producing their proteins within the oocyte before fertilization. With fertilization, mRNA from a specific gene is translated into its corresponding protein. This defines the craniocaudal and dorsoventral axes.
2. ***Segmentation genes*** of the Hox gene family are responsible for defining the segments. Segmentation is expressed throughout the embryo in the formation of:
   - Cranial and spinal nerves,
   - Vertebral column and ribs,
   - Early muscle development, and
   - Pattern of blood vessel formation

   Segmentation of the embryonic head is more obvious than anywhere else in the embryo, with neuromeres in the hindbrain, somites and somitomeres, and the pharyngeal arches of mesoderm.
3. ***Homeotic genes.*** These genes are activated by the segmentation genes to determine the fate of segments.

Homeobox gene clusters: Homeobox (HOX) genes are a group of genes which represent the genes controlling development in Drosophilia. In human they exist as four copies: HOX-A, HOX-B, HOX-C and HOX-D.

Paralogus group is formed by genes with the same number, but belonging to different clusters, for examples, HOX-A4, HOX-B4, HOX-C4 and HOX-D4 form a paralogus group of genes.

Cranial-to-caudal patterning of the derivatives of all three germ layers is determined by the HOX genes.

Paired-box (pax) genes, eight in number have been identified in humans. They encode DNA-binding proteins, which act as transcription control factor, and play an important role in the development across the animal kingdom.

Timing, amount and sequencing of the signalling molecules results in proper development.

Points to Remember

- Genetics is the study of heredity, a process by which children inherit certain characteristics (traits) from their parents.
- Each cell contains fixed number of chromosomes which is characteristic of that species/organism.
- Inactivated X chromosome forms Barr body. The inactivation occurs within 2 weeks of conception. Females do "so much" with one X chromosome only.
- Y chromosome of males is smaller and is for determination of male sex. Hairy pinna is the only condition associated with Y chromosome.
- Down's syndrome/trisomy 21 is a disease due to autosomal numerical chromosomal aberration.
- Cri du chat syndrome is a disease due to autosomal structural chromosal aberration.
- Turner's syndrome and Klinefelter's syndrome are diseases due to numerical aberration of sex chromosomes.
- Single gene inherited diseases may be:
  i. Brachydactyly/syndactyly due to autosomal dominant inheritance.
  ii. Albinism and deaf mutism due to autosomal recessive inheritance.

iii. Vitamin D resistant rickets due to X-linked dominant condition.
iv. Haemophilia due to X-linked recessive traits.

- Prenatal diagnosis is possible in some clinical cases.
- Genetic counselling is advisable in some cases.
- Genetic therapy is possible in selected cases.

Multiple Choice Questions

1. The number of chromosomes after a mitotic division is:
a. Halved
b. Same number
c. Doubled
d. Tripled

2. The number of chromosomes after a meiotic division is:
a. Doubled
b. Tripled
c. Halved
d. None of the above

3. Mendel's laws of inheritance are:
a. Law of uniformity
b. Law of segregation
c. Law of independent assortment
d. All of the above

4. Turner's syndrome patient has following number of Barr body:
a. One
b. Two
c. None
d. Three

5. Ultrasonography can detect following congenital malformations:
a. Neural tube defects
b. Heart defects
c. Facial defects
d. All of the above

Answers

1. b 2. c 3. d 4. c 5. a

Chapter 18

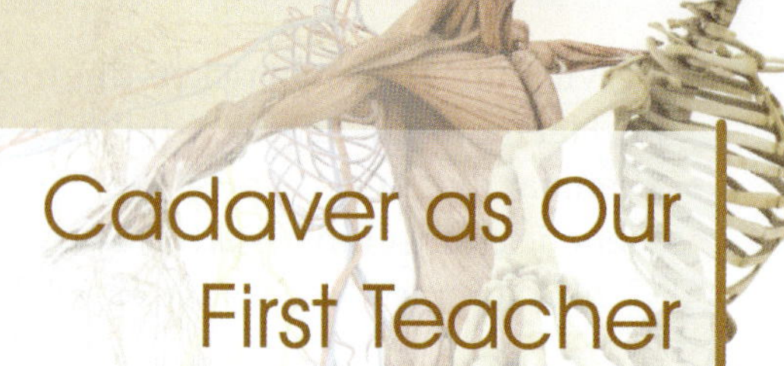

Cadaver as Our First Teacher

Doctors are always learning from cadavers. —***Krishna Garg***

Cadaver as a First Teacher

Once a senior secondary school student with biology gets admission in a medical college, he/she is renamed a medical student, who is mentally prepared to study for about 10 years before becoming a specialized doctor. During the first professional period a medical student needs to study anatomy, physiology and biochemistry.

From time immemorial, anatomy has been viewed as a complex and challenging subject to be learnt from embalmed human cadaver who is slowly and steadily being dissected. As one does dissection in a group, one is incorporating a great skill including the teamwork and patience. So, globally it is acclaimed that the cadaver is the 'First Teacher'.

How to Obtain a Cadaver

Cadaver is a dead human body used in scientific or medical research.

Earlier and even at present, unclaimed dead bodies usually belonging to poor strata are taken by the police. Police personnel inform the medical college (anatomy department) to collect the body. Even if postmortem has been done, the body is taken by the anatomy department for the dissection of the limbs. For the last decade or so many persons make a 'Will' to donate their bodies. To promote this scheme, many anatomy departments give it as a news item in the local newspapers. The department puts the photograph of the voluntary donor outside the Dissection Hall.

Preservation of the Cadavers

The dead body starts putrifying and decaying within a few hours after death depending on the weather. To prevent this, bodies are embalmed with formalin mixture. Procedure of embalming takes a few hours to complete.

Embalming is also done if a dead body or cadaver is to be transported to a distant place in the country or abroad. Even if a VIPs body is to be kept for public viewing before the last rites, the body has to be embalmed. Embalming can be done as: (i) Arterial embalming, (ii) cavity embalming, (iii) hypodermic embalming and (iv) surface embalming.

Embalming fluid—the fluid is prepared by thoroughly mixing up 5 litres of water, 3 litres of formalin (40%), 2 litres of spirit, 1 litre of glycerine, sodium chloride, etc.

The cadaver is put in a supine position on a table. It is shaved and cleaned.

Procedure for arterial embalming: A 6 cm long vertical incision is given in the upper medial side of thigh. After reflecting skin and fasciae, femoral sheath is incised to visualise the femoral artery. The prepared embalming fluid is put in the embalming machine which is connected to a cannula.

A small nick is given in the femoral artery and cannula introduced so that its tip points towards the head end and 8.5 litres of fluid is pumped under 20 pounds pressure. Then the direction of cannula is reversed and rest of the fluid is pumped in. Lastly, the skin and fasciae are stitched.

Cavity embalming: The internal fluids inside the body cavities are replaced with embalming chemicals with the use of an aspirator and trochar.

Hypodermic embalming: Injection of embalming fluid into tissues with the help of a syringe and needle. It is done in an area where arterial fluid has not reached.

Surface embalming: Preserves areas on skin damaged by accidents or skin donations.

Embalming and Ethics

The decision for embalming is taken by close relatives usually when there is a 'Will' to the same effect. This trend is 'catching up' and some people are 'making a Will' to donate their body for education or research to the department of anatomy. Earlier and even now many bodies are the 'unclaimed ones'.

Care of the cadaver: The cadaver has to be handled with care and respect. Only the part being dissected is kept open and exposed, rest is to be covered by a sheet. After dissection the dissecting part must also be covered, palms and soles are wrapped till their dissection is reached. Over the weekend or a holiday the cadaver or the body is put in a formalin tank to be taken out after the weekend. There is always an irritating smell of formalin causing watering of the eyes but it gets over within 30–40 minutes. Detached limbs are to be wrapped up by a bandage to prevent drying. If fungus is seen on a part, it must be removed by using dilute carbolic acid. "You care for the cadaver, he or she takes care of your learning anatomy".

So, a cadaver, a dead human body is showing his internal features to help you learn anatomy and cadaver is the first teacher. The students of University of Taiwan are told about the family of the cadaver. They visit the family to pay their respects as their deceased family member is assisting them to become a doctor for treating the patients.

Many institutions start their anatomy dissection classes with a prayer to thank Almighty for giving them a body to learn. At a college in Mumbai, the cadaveric oath is administered to first year medical undergraduates who pledge to honour the dignity and integrity of the human remains that they are about to work on. Anatomical memorial services are held in Mayo Medical College, Rochester, USA, to enable students to reflect on the life of the departed souls who facilitated their education. The cadaver, in addition to teaching anatomy, also teaches to work in a team. Even after many years of dissection one remembers colleagues of your dissection table and the happy hours spent together. We must all remember that the cadaver was one of us and deserve great respect. Cadaver not only teaches gross anatomy but also surface anatomy and embryology from dissection of the fetuses.

Disposal of the cadaver: The remains of the cadaver are buried in the burial ground attached to the department of anatomy.

The cadaver continues to be a teacher in Forensic Medicine. Here the cause of death has to be established by postmortem so that guilty persons may be punished.

Computers potential for teaching anatomy: In 1988, the Visible Human Project of US National Library of Medicine began. Now anatomy is being integrated with radiographs. CT, MRI, sectional anatomy scans to provide a 3D view of anatomy. The alternatives to dissection are computer programmes, videos, etc. being developed with the help of computers. This method is as dynamic as a cinema. Table 18.1 shows comparison of human cadaveric dissection to alternative to dissection.

Table 18.1: Comparison of human cadaveric dissection to alternative to dissection

Human cadaveric dissection	*Alternative to dissection/artificial cadaver synthetic corpse*
Preservation required	No preservation required
More staff required for maintenance	Less staff required for maintenance
Trained staff can manage	Highly trained staff can manage to teach
Scalpels, etc. required	Scalpels, etc. not required
Cannot be used repeatedly	Can be used repeatedly
Actual feel of a nerve, artery is there	Actual feel of nerve, artery, muscle is not there

Ideal method is dissection with added technology.

Dress code for the students: The students must wear an apron or overall, a cap, gloves to protect from any injury, etc.

DISSECTION INSTRUMENTS

Large instruments like hammer, saw, chisel, etc. are provided in the department. Every medical student must have the following instruments in his/her dissection box.

Scalpel: The scalpel is used for giving incisions. It should have a detachable blade of 3–4 cm. Scalpel blade should be sharp and scalpel handle need to be metallic. Care must be taken not to injure oneself.

Forceps: Forceps are used to hold the part being dissected. One pair should be serrated tip forceps for lifting the nerve, artery or vein, etc. Another pair should be toothed forceps for holding the structure firmly while dissection is being done. Size of the forceps may be 7.5 to 15 cm.

Scissors: Pair of small scissors is necessary for cutting a small structure. Another pair of big scissors (15 cm) is also required at times.

Probe: The probe is useful for doing blunt dissection and for cleaning the dissecting region.

Hand lens: The hand lens is required to magnify the smaller structures for better and correct identification.

Points to Remember

- Cadaver is the first teacher for a first year medical student.
- Preservative fluid mainly contains formalin, glycerin, sodium chloride, spirit.

- Bodies can be obtained from police as unclaimed bodies, or of persons who make a 'will' to donate their bodies for education and research.
- Cadaver or any of its body parts must be looked after with care and respect.
- Medical students can act as volunteers for promoting body donation.

Multiple Choice Questions

1. **Embalming is done for:**
   a. Dissection during 1st year
   b. For postmortems
   c. For autopsy
   d. For study during 2nd–4th years
2. **Which procedures can be used for embalming?**
   a. Arterial embalming
   b. Cavity embalming
   c. Hypodermic embalming
   d. All of the above
3. **Which methods are more popular for learning anatomy?**
   a. Human cadaveric dissection
   b. Artificial cadaveric dissection
   c. No dissection
   d. Cadaveric dissection with technology
4. **Which dissection procedure is very easy?**
   a. Human cadaveric dissection
   b. Artificial cadaveric dissection
   c. Cadaveric dissection with technology
   d. All of the above
5. **Use of embalmed cadaver lies:**
   a. In doing routine dissection
   b. In workshops for specialised clinical procedures
   c. During MD examinations
   d. All of the above

Answers

1. a **2.** d **3.** d **4.** b **5.** d

Anatomical Terms and Historical Names

A	Anglo-Saxon	Du	Dutch	G	Greek	L	Latin
Ar	Arabic	E	English	Gr	German	S	Sanskrit
C	Chinese	F	French	It	Italian		

	Term	Meaning
	Afferent	coming towards
	Anus	ring
(G)	Artery	blood vessel
(L)	Articulation	joint
(G)	Arytenoid	like a pitcher
(G)	Ascites	bag-like (fluid collection)
	Astrocyte	star-shaped
	Atavism	a remote ancestor (epiphysis)
	Atelectasis	incomplete expansion
	Atheroma	tumour
	Atlas	carry earth on head—1st cervical vertebra
	Atresia	no hole
(L)	Atrium	central open part
(G)	Atrophy	ill-nourished
(L)	Auditory	related to hearing
	Auerbach (German anatomist)	Auerbach's plexus of autonomic nerves between longitudinal and circular coats of gastrointestinal tract
(L)	Auricle	diminutive of ear
	Auscultation	to hear with attention
	Autonomic	self-controller
(G)	Autopsy	self-seeing
(L)	Avulsion	to tear away
(L)	Axilla	armpit
(L)	Axis	carry (pillar)—2nd cervical vertebra
(G)	Azygous	unpaired—azygous vein in thorax
(F)	Ballotment	tossing
	Basilic	medial vein of arm
	Basophilic	basic stain of nucleus
(L)	Bile	fluid

	Biliverdin	green bile
	Bilirubin	red bile
(G)	Bio	life
	Birth	bearing of offspring
(A)	Bladder	watery swelling
(G)	Blepharitis	eyelid inflammation
(L)	Bolus	mass
(A)	Bone	bar
(F)	Boss	a hump
(G)	Botany	grass
	Bowman (English surgeon)	Bowman's capsule, Bowman's memb, Bowman's muscle of ciliary body
(L)	Brachium	arm
(G)	Brady	slow
(G)	Brain	upper part of head
(G)	Branchia	gills of fishes—branchial arches
(A)	Breast	bursting forth
(A)	Breech	lower part of trunk and thigh
(G)	Bregma	forepart of head
	Brown-Séquard (British neurologist)	Brown-Séquard syndrome—hemisection of spinal cord
	Broca (French surgeon)	Broca's area—speech centre
(G)	Bronchus	windpipe
(G)	Bronchiole	terminal air tube
(F)	Bruise	to break
	Brunner (Swiss anatomist)	Brunner's duodenal glands
(L)	Bucia	cheek
(L)	Buccinator	trumpeter
(E)	Buffer	cushion to soften blow
(L)	Bulb	as onion
(L)	Bulbar	medulla oblongata
(L)	Bulbocavernosus or	
(L)	Bulbospongiosus	accelerator of urine
(L)	Bulla	bubble
(It)	Bunion	swelling
(G)	Burdach (Greek anatomist)	posterior column of spinal cord
	Bursa	a purse
(E)	Buttock	end (prominence posterior to hip)
(L)	Cadaver	a dead body
(L)	Caecum	blind
	Cesarean section (Julius Caesar was born)	cutting uterus for taking out a baby
(F)	Caisson	box
	Cajal (Spanish histologist)	Cajal stain
(L)	Calamine	red

(L)	Calculus	little stone
(L)	Calvaria	vault of cranium
(L)	Calcaneus	bone of foot
(L)	Calcar	spur (calcarine sulcus)
(L)	Calcar femorale	strong plate of bone in front of lesser trochanter supporting neck of femur (spur-shaped)
(L)	Calcarine fissure	spur-shaped
	Calcination	to make bone
	Calyx	covering of bud/shell
	Calveria	vault
	Camper (Dutch anatomist)	superficial fascia of anterior abdominal wall
(L)	Canal	channel or furrow
	Canal of Arnold	for lesser petrosal nerve
	Canal of Schlemm	at cornea-scleral junction
(L)	Cancellous	lattice work
(L)	Cancer	crab-like
(L)	Canine	related to dog (teeth)
	Cannula	hollow, tubular instrument
(L)	Capillary	like hair of head (caput), fine tube
	Capsule	a small box
(L)	Caput	head
	Capitulum	in humerus (lateral part of lower end)
	Caput Medusae	(head of witch) seen because of dilatation of veins at umbilicus due to cirrhosis of liver
(L)	Carbohydrate	made of carbon, hydrogen and water
	Caput succedaneum	swelling produced on presenting part of fetal head during labour
(G)	Cardia	heart
(L)	Caries	decay of bone and teeth
(L)	Carina	structure with a projecting central ridge
(L)	Caro	flesh
(G)	Carotid	to throttle (blood vessel)
	Carotid tubercle	anterior tubercle of 6th cervical vertebra
(L)	Carpus	wrist
(L)	Cartilage	gristle
(L)	Castrate	to cut off
(G)	Catarrh	to flow down
	Catgut	from intestine of sheep
(L)	Cauda	tail
	Caudate	caudate nucleus, caudate lobe (tail-shaped)
(E)	Caul	cap (fetal membrane with fluid)
(G)	Causalgia	burning pain
(L)	Cavernous	full of compartments
(L)	Cell	small room
	Cement	binding
	Centrifuge	fleeing away from centre
(G)	Centrosome	body centre
(G)	Cephalic	to head (cephalic vein)

(L)	Cera	wax
(L)	Cerebellum	little brain
(L)	Cerebrum	brain
(L)	Cerumen	ear wax
(L)	Cervix	neck, e.g. cervix of uterus, cervical rib
(G)	Chancre	venereal disease
	Chemotaxis	reaction of living cells to chemical agents
	Chest	box
(G)	Chiasma	crossing over
(G)	Chitin	coat
(G)	Chole	bile
(G)	Cholesterin	solid bile
(G)	Chord	a cord of string, e.g. chorda tympani nerve
	Chordata	animals with notochord
(G)	Chorea	dancing (disease of basal ganglia)
(G)	Chorion	skin
(G)	Chromosome	coloured bodies
(G)	Chyme	juice
	Cilium	eyelid
(L)	Cingulum	girdle
(L)	Circle of Haller	venous circle in areola of female breast
(L)	Circular sinus	sinus around pituitary
	Circle of Willis	arterial circle at base of brain
(L)	Circulation	motion in circle
(L)	Circum	around, e.g. circumflex artery
	Cirrhosis	to turn reddish yellow
	Cisterna	reservoir (at base of brain)
(L)	Claustrum	barrier
	Clavicle	diminutive of key
	Cledio	closes the thorax, clavipectoral fascia
(G)	Climacteric	step of a stair (menopause)
	Clinic	at the bed side
	Clinoid	surround pituitary fossa like four posts of bed
(G)	Clitoris	tender (female external genitalia)
(L)	Clivus	slope of a hill—part of cranial fossae
(L)	Cloaca	drain or sewer (dilated part of hindgut)
(G)	Clonus	confused motion
(L)	Coagulation	to curdle
(L)	Coarctation	to press together (coarctation of aorta)
(G)	Coccyx	cuckoo (coccyx resembles bill of a cuckoo)—lowest part of vertebral column
(L)	Cochlea	snail (internal ear)
(G)	Coelenterate	hollow (internal)
(G)	Coeliac	belly (coeliac axis artery for stomach)
(G)	Coelome	hollow
	Cohnheim (scientist)	Cohnheim's areas in skeletal muscle
	Colic	pain in intestine
(G)	Collagen	glue producing substance
	Colloidion	glue-like
	Colon	large intestine

	Colostrum	first milk secreted by breasts
	Colpotomy	cutting through vagina
(L)	Commissure	join together
(L)	Complement	I fill up
(L)	Concha	shell (in lateral wall of nose)
(L)	Concussion	a shaking
(G)	Condyle	knob formed by knuckle of any joint
(L)	Conjugate	yoked together
(L)	Conjunctiva	mucus membrane of eye
(L)	Conus	cone
(G)	Coracoid	a crow-like process of scapula
(L)	Corneum	most superficial layer of epithelium of skin
(G)	Corona	crown, e.g. corona radiata and coronal suture corona glandis (coronary arteries, coronary sulcus)
(L)	Corpus	body, e.g. corpus callosum, corpus luteum
(L)	Corpuscle	a little body, pacinian corpuscle, thymic corpuscle
(L)	Corrugator	wrinkler
(L)	Cortex	outer bark (grey matter)
(L)	Cortex	rind (outer layer)
(L)	Costa	rib
(A)	Cough	violent expulsion
	Cowper	Cowper's gland near upper end of male urethra
(S)	Coxa	hip
	Cramp	to contract
(L)	Cranium	skull
(G)	Creatine	(flesh) a non-protein nitrogenous substance from flesh
(G)	Cremaster	a suspender (of testis)
	Crepitus	a little noise
(L)	Creta	a chalk ($CaCO_3$)
(F)	Cretin	congenital myxoedema
(L)	Cribriform	sieve-like, e.g. cribiform fascia of thigh
(G)	Cricoid	ring, e.g. cricoid cartilage
(L)	Crista	crest
	Crista galli	cockscomb
(L)	Crus	shin bone or leg
(L)	Crural	leg
(L)	Cruciate	cross-like
(L)	Crypt	underground vault (hidden)
(G)	Crystal	clear ice
(L)	Cubitus	elbow
(G)	Cuboid	cube-like
(L)	Culture	growth
(L)	Cuneiform	wedge-shaped
	Cupola	dome-shaped
(L)	Curriculum	a course of study
(L)	Cusp	point of a spear (cusp of valve)
(L)	Cutis	skin
(F)	Cuvier (anatomist)	ducts of Cuvier

(G)	Cyclops	one-eyed giant
(L)	Cyst	bladder, cystic duct
	Cytoplasm	spread outside the nucleus
(G)	Dacryocyte	tear-drop
(G)	Dactylitis	finger inflammation
	Dale (English physician)	histamine discovered by Dale
(E)	Dandruff	skin scabs
(S)	Dartos	leather
	Darwin tubercle	projection in upper part of ear
(L)	Decalcify	process which extracts Ca++
(L)	Deci	one tenth
(L)	Deciduous	falling off
	Decompression	decreased pressure
(L)	Decubitus	lying down
(L)	Decussate	intersection of two lines
(L)	Defecate	to evacuate the bowels
(L)	Degenerate	structural impairment of a tissue
(L)	Deglutition	action of swallowing
	Deiters (German anatomist)	Deiters cells in internal ear
(G)	Deltoid	triangular in shape, deltoid muscle, deltoid ligament
(L)	Dementia	to be mad
(F)	Demilune	half moon, demilune of Giannuzzi
(G)	Dendron	tree, dendrites of neuron
	Denonvilliers (French surgeon)	fascia between rectum and prostate is Denonvilliers' fascia
(L)	Dens	tooth-like dens of 2nd vertebra/axis
(L)	Dentate	tooth-like, dentate ligament of pia mater, dentate gyrus of brain
(Gr)	Dermis	skin
	Descemet (French surgeon)	Descemet's membrane of cornea
(L)	Desquamate	to scale off
(L)	Detrusor	to thrust away, detrusor muscle of urinary bladder
(L)	Dexter	right
(G)	Diagnosis	through knowledge
(G)	Dialysis	to loose from one another
(G)	Diapedesis	leading through
(G)	Diaphragm	a partition
(G)	Diaphysis	growing through
(G)	Diarrhoea	flowing through
(G)	Diarthrosis	joint
(G)	Diastole	a pause
(G)	Diathermy	very hot
(G)	Dichotomous	cut in half
(G)	Didelphys	double uterus
(G)	Diencephalon	between brain
(G)	Diet	a way of living

(G)	Digastric	double belly
(L)	Digestion	to dissolve
(L)	Digit	finger
(G)	Diphtheria	leather-like membrane
(G)	Diploë	double layers (diploë of some of the skull bones)
(F)	Disease	not well
(L)	Dislocation	pulled out of place
(L)	Dissect	cut apart
(G)	Diuresis	increased urination
(L)	Diverticulum	a small cul-de-sac
(L)	Doctor	a teacher and a healer
(G)	Dolichocephalic	long head
(L)	Dorsum	back
(It)	Douche	to pour
	Douglas (Scottish anatomist)	pouch of Douglas (rectouterine pouch)
(L)	Duct	to conduct
(L)	Duodenum	width of 12 fingers
	Dupuytren (French surgeon)	Dupuytren's contracture
(L)	Duramater	hard mother
(G)	Dys (prefix)	bad, e.g. dysentery, dyspepsia, dysmenorrhoea
(G)	Ectoderm	outside skin
(G)	Ectopia	displacement (out of place)
(G)	Ectropion	to turn from
(G)	Eczema	anything thrown out by heat
	Edinger (German anatomist)	Edinger-Westphal nuclei of III N
	Effector	to effect
(L)	Efferent	going away
(L)	Element	a rudiment
(G)	Elephantiasis	elephant-like legs
(G)	Embed	holding in place
(G)	Embolus	a plug
(G)	Embryo	something that grows in another's body
(G)	Emesis	vomiting
(L)	Emissary	escape channels (emissary veins connecting intracranial sinuses with extracranial veins)
(L)	Empirical	experienced, not scientific
(L)	Emulsion	milk-like mixture
(F)	Enamel	coating on metal
(F)	Enarthrosis	ball and socket joint
(G)	Encephalon	brain plus head
(G)	Endarteritis	blockage within arteries
(G)	Endemic	native
(G)	Endo (prefix)	within, e.g. endocrine, endolymph, endomet-rium, endothelium
(G)	Enema	to inject
(L)	Ensiform	sword-like, xiphoid process

(G)	Enteric	gut
(G)	Enuresis	urine passed
(G)	Enzyme	which causes fermentation
(G)	Eosin	pink
(G)	Ependyma	wrap
(G)	Epicondyle	upon a knob
(G)	Epicranius	upon head
(G)	Epicritic	fine touch
(G)	Epidermis	upon dermis
(G)	Epididymis	upon testis
(G)	Epigastrium	upon belly
(G)	Epiglottis	upon tongue
(G)	Epihyal	part of 2nd arch
(G)	Epilepsy	a seizure
(G)	Epinephrine	hormone
(G)	Epiploic	omental
(G)	Episiotomy	cutting the pudendum (perineum)
(G)	Epispadius	upon a tear
(G)	Epistaxis	to trickle
(G)	Epithelium	upon nipple
(G)	Epoophoron	upon egg-bearing
	Erb (German neurologist)	Erb's palsy (C 5, 6)
(L)	Erector	to stand up
(G)	Erotic	love
(L)	Eructation	throwing upwards
(G)	Ethmoid	sieve-like
(G)	Etiology	giving the cause
(G)	Etymology	true analysis of a word
(G)	Euthanasia	painless death
(L)	Eustachius (Italian anatomist)	eustachian valve
(L)	Evolution	to unroll
(G)	Exacerbation	to irritate
(L)	Exogenous	on the outside
(L)	Experiment	an active test
(L)	Extension	stretch out
(L)	Exteroceptor	outward receptor
(L)	Exude	to sweat out
(L)	Facet	a little face
(L)	Facial	related to face
	Falciform/Falx	sickle-shaped
	Fallopius (Italian anatomist)	fallopian tube
(L)	Fascia	a bandage
(L)	Fasciculus	a passage
(L)	Febris	fever
(L)	Femur	thigh
(L)	Fenestra	window

(L)	Ferment	warm
(L)	Fetus	offspring
(L)	Fibula	needle of brooch (bone)
(L)	Filament	small thread
(L)	Filaria	a thread
(L)	Fimbria	a fringe/border
(L)	Fissure	cleft
(L)	Fistula	a pipe
(L)	Flagellum	a whip
(L)	Flatus	to blow
(L)	Flavine	yellow
(L)	Flex	to bend
(L)	Flocculus	a tuft of wool
(L)	Folium	leaf
(L)	Follicle	a bag
	Fontana (Italian anatomist)	spaces of Fontana
(L)	Fontanelle	small fountain
(L)	Foramen	hole
(L)	Forensic	pertaining to law, courts—Forensic medicine
(L)	Fornix	an arch
(L)	Fossa	ditch
(L)	Fourchette	little fork
(L)	Fovea	a small pit
(L)	Frenulum	bridle, e.g. Franulum of tongue, of clitoris, of penis
(L)	Frontal	forehead
(L)	Fundus	larger part
(L)	Fundiform	sling-shaped
(L)	Funiculus	cord
(L)	Fusiform	spindle-shaped
(E)	Gag	to suffocate
	Galea	helmet, galea aponeurotica
	Galen (Roman physician)	vein of Galen (great cerebral vein)
(A)	Gall	bile
(G)	Gamete	a married person
(G)	Ganglion	a knot
(L)	Gastric	belly
(G)	Gastrocnemius	calf of leg
(G)	Gastrula	belly
(G)	Gene	unit of heredity
	Genetics	study of natural development of race
(L)	Genial	chin
(L)	Genu	bend, knee (genu of corpus callosum)
(G)	Genus	family
(G)	Geriatrics	study and treatment of old persons
(L)	Gustatory	sense of taste
(L)	Gyrus	convolution
(L)	Haeme	blood
	Haematoxylin	stain

(L)	Hallux	big toe
(A)	Hamstring	a little hook
	Hartman (German anatomist)	gall bladder cyst near cystic duct
(L)	Haustrum	bucket-shaped haustration of large intestine
	Havers (English physician)	haversian gland—pad of fat in joints
	Heister (German anatomist)	Heister's valve (in gall bladder)
(G)	Helicotrema	an opening between two scala of cochlea
(G)	Helix	a coil
	Helmholtz (German physician)	Helmholtz theory of color vision
	Henle (German anatomist)	Henle's loop, Henle's layer in hair follicle
	Hensen (German physician)	Hensen's node
(G)	Hepar	liver
(G)	Hermaphrodite	both sexes
(L)	Hernia	rupture
(G)	Herpes	to spread
(G)	Hetero	different
	Hilton (English surgeon)	Hilton's line
(L)	Hilum	depression
(G)	Hippocampus	sea horse
	Hirschsprung (Danish physician)	Hirschsprung's disease (congenital megacolon)
(G)	Histamine	tissue amine
(G)	Histo	anything woven
(G)	Histology	study of woven structures/tissues
(L)	Homo	a man
(G)	Hormone	to set in motion
	Horner (Swiss ophthalmologist)	Horner's syndrome
	Hunter (Scottish surgeon)	Hunter's canal (adductor canal)
(G)	Hyaline	glass-like; hyaline cartilage
(G)	Hybrid	of double origin
(F)	Hydatid	a drop of water
(G)	Hydrocele	water + hernia
(G)	Hygiene	healthy
(G)	Hymen	membrane
(G)	Hyoid	U-shaped
(G)	Hyper	in excess of
	Hypnosis	state of being asleep
(G)	Hypoblast	endoderm
(G)	Hypodermic	under the skin

(G)	Hypothesis	placing under
(G)	Hyster	uterus
(G)	Icterus	a yellow bird (jaundice)
(G)	Idiopathic	'unknown'
(G)	Idiosyncrasy (allergy)	individual peculiarity
(G)	Ileum	twisted gut
(L)	Ilium	hip bone
(L)	Immunity	exemption or protection
(L)	Incise	to cut into
(L)	Incubation	to sit or brood
(L)	Incus	an anvil (ear ossicle)
(L)	Index	a pointer
(8)	Indigo	blue dye
(L)	Inducium	a tunic
	I. griesum	a grey tunic
(L)	Infant	not speaking
(L)	Infarct	necrotic
(L)	Infection	a bending inward
(L)	Inflame	to set aflame
(L)	Infra	below
(L)	Inguinal	the groin—inguinal canal
(G)	Inion	below occiput
(L)	Injection	putting in
(L)	Innominate	unnamed
(L)	Inoculate	to ingraft
(L)	Inquest	inquire
(L)	Insanity	unsound mind
(L)	Insemination	seed
(L)	In situ	manner of lying in local position
(L)	Instrument	to equip
(L)	Insufflation	to blow into
(L)	Insula	island
(L)	Internuncial	inter-messenger
(L)	Intestine	internal
(L)	Intoxication	to smear with poison
(L)	Intra	inside
	Intrinsic	special to the thing itself
(L)	Intussusception	within receive
(L)	Invagination	enclose in a sheath
(L)	Involution	to roll up
(G)	Iodine	violet
(G)	Iris	coloured membrane of eye
(G)	Ischaemia	lack of blood supply
(G)	Ischium	bone (part of hip bone)
(G)	Isotonic	equal tension
(G)	Isotope	equal place
(L)	Isthmus	narrow, isthmus of fallopian tube
(L)	Iter	a passage (iter cerebri)
(F)	Jaundice	yellowness

(L)	Jejunum	empty or fasting
(L)	Joint	to join
(L)	Jugular	the throat
	Jugam	yoke
(G)	Karyo	a nut (nucleus)
	Keith (English anatomist)	Keith's SA node
(G)	Keratin	horn-in hairy layer of skin
(G)	Kilo	one thousand
	Klumpke (French neurologist)	Klumpke's paralysis
	Kupffer (Greek anatomist)	Kupffer cell (sinusoids of liver)
	Kymograph	a wave writer
(G)	Kyphosis	hump on back
(L)	Labrum	lip
	Labial	pertaining to lips
(L)	Labour	work
(L)	Lac	milk
(G)	Labyrinth	maze
(L)	Lacrimal	tear
(L)	Lacunae	hollow
(G)	Lambda	inverted Y-shaped suture
(L)	Lamina	a thin plate
(L)	Lancet	a slender spear
	Langerhans (German anatomist)	islet of Langerhans (pancreas)
(L)	Lanugo	first soft hair of beard
(L)	Larva	ghost
(G)	Larynx	upper part of wind pipe
(L)	Latent	to lie hidden
(L)	Laxative	loosening
(Gr)	Lemniscus	bandage
(Gr)	Leprosy	scaly disease
(Gr)	Leptomeninx	tender membrane (pia and arachnoid)
(L)	Lethal	death
(Gr)	Lethargy	forgetful
(Gr)	Leuc	white, leucocyte, leucoplakia, leucorrhoea
(L)	Levator	one who lifts
(L)	Libido	desire, lustre
(G)	Lieberkuhn (German scientist)	crypts of Lieberkuhn (intestine)
	Lienal	spleen
	Ligament	to bind, e.g. deltoid ligament, falciform ligament, etc.
(L)	Limbus	a border
(L)	Limen	edge or threshold—L. insulae
(L)	Linea	a line
(L)	Lingual	the tongue
(S)	Lipoma	fat

(Gr)	Lithos	a stone
(L)	Locus	a place
(G)	Lordosis	increased anterior curvature of lumbar spine
	Louis (French physician)	Louis's angle of sternum (sternal angle)
	Lower (English physician)	projection in the right atrial wall between the two caval openings
(L)	Ludwig (German surgeon)	Ludwig's angina
(L)	Lumbar	loin
	Lumbrical	a worm (a muscle)
(L)	Lumen	light passage
(L)	Lunar	the moon
	Lutein (German anatomist)	yellow pigment of corpora lutea
(L)	Lymph	clear water
(Gr)	Macro	big
	Macroscopic	big to see
(L)	Macula	a small patch (macula lutea, macula densa)
	Magendie (French doctor)	Foramen of Magendie
(G)	Malacia	softness
(F)	Malady	illness
(L)	Malar	cheek bone
	Malaria	bad air
(L)	Malignant	ill-disposed
(L)	Malleus	hammer—ear ossicle
(L)	Malleolus	a little hammer
	Mallory (Irish anatomist)	Mallory's stain
	Malpighi (Italian anatomist) Founder of Histology	Malpighian corpuscle, Malpighian layer in skin
(L)	Mamma	the breast
(L)	Mandible	lower jaw
(Gr)	Mania	madness
(L)	Manubrium	a handle (manubrium sterni)
(Gr)	Marasmus	waste away
	Marchi (Irish anatomist)	Marchi's staining for nerve fibres
	Marginal	artery border, along large intestine
(L)	Marrow	medulla
	Marshall (English surgeon)	Marshall's vein—oblique vein of left atrium
(Gr)	Masseter	the chewer
(Gr)	Mast	to feed
(Gr)	Mastos	breast
(L)	Mastication	to chew
(L)	Matrix	mould

(L)	Mature	to ripe—maturation
	Maxilla	cheek
	McBurney (American surgeon)	McBurney point for appendicectomy
(L)	Meatus	canal
	Meckel (German anatomist)	Meckel's cave for 5th nerve ganglion, Meckel's cartilage
	Meatus	canal
(L)	Median	central
(L)	Mediastinum	middle space
(L)	Medicine	the art of healing
(L)	Medulla	marrow
	Medusa (Greek goddess)	caput medusa
(L)	Mega	big
	Meibom (German anatomist)	meibomian glands
(L)	Meiosis	lessening
	Meissner	Meissner's plexus in submucous coat of GIT
(L)	Melan	black
	Melanin	black pigment
(G)	Meninges	a membrane
	Meningocoele	membrane + hernia
(G)	Meniscus	crescent (medial and lateral menisci in knee joint)
(G)	Men (prefix)	month, e.g. menopause, menorrhagia, menstruation, menarche
(Gr)	Merkel	corpuscle sensory nerve ending
(Gr)	Mesencephalon	mid-brain
(Gr)	Mesenchyme	middle infusion or juice
(Gr)	Mesentery	middle intestine
	Mesoderm	middle skin
(G)	Mesonephros	middle kidney
(G)	Mesothelium	middle nipple
(G)	Metacarpus	from wrist
(G)	Metamorphosis	changed form
(G)	Metanephros	after kidney
(G)	Metastasis	removal from one place
(G)	Metencephalon	after brain
(G)	Metopic	frontal, space between eyes—metopic suture
(G)	Metre	unit of length
	Meynert (Austrian physician)	Dorsal tegmental decussation
(G)	Microbe	small life
(G)	Microcyte	small cell
(G)	Microglia	small glue (cells)
(G)	Micrometer	small measure
(G)	Microscope	small eye-view
(G)	Microtome	small cutting
(G)	Mitochondria	the thread grain

(G)	Mitosis	thread
(L)	Mitral	kind of cap
(G)	Mneomonic	relating to memory
(L)	Molar	milestone—a tooth
(E)	Mole	spot
	Monro (English scientist)	foramen of Monro—interventricular foramen of brain
	Montgomery (Irish obstetrician)	Montgomery's tubercles in the nipple
(L)	Morbid	ill
	Morgagni (Italian anatomist)	appendix of testis
(F)	Morgue	mortuary
	Morison (English surgeon)	Morison's pouch (hepatorenal pouch)
	Moron	dull
(G)	Morphology	shape/discourse
(L)	Morula	mulberry
(L)	Mucus	thin watery fluid, mucosa
	Muller (German anatomist)	Müller's muscle in eye (circular), mullerian duct
(L)	Multiparous	more than once pregnant
(L)	Murmur	a humming sound
(L)	Muscle	a little mouse; myology
(G)	Museum	temple of muses
(L)	Mutation	to change
(L)	Mydriatic	unnatural dilatation of pupil
(G)	Myopia	close to eyes
(G)	Myxoma	mucus + tumor
	Naboth (German anatomist)	Nabothian glands
(L)	Naevus	birth mark
	Nagek (German obstetrician)	Nagek pelvis (obliquely contracted pelvis)
(E)	Nape	external depression, knob
	Narcolepsy	numbness
(L)	Nares	nostril, nasal
(G)	Nausea	sickness
(A)	Navel	umbilicus
(L)	Navicular	boat-shaped
(G)	Necrosis	a dead body
(G)	Neo	new
	Neolithic	new stone
	Neoplasm	new form
(G)	Nephr	kidney
	Nephropexy	kidney + fastening
(L)	Nerve	string, nerve root
(G)	Neuralgia	pain in nerves
(G)	N. crest	on either side of neural tube

(G)	Neurasthenia	nerve weakness
(G)	Neurilemma	nerve covering
(G)	Neurobiotaxis	nerve + life + arrangement of nerves in living
(L)	Neutrophil	neuter (not fond of any color)
	Nipple	beak
	Nissl (German neurologist)	Nissl granules in neurons
(L)	Nodus	knot
(L)	Nomenclature	a list of names
(G)	Nostalgia	home coming + pain
(G)	Notochord	back + a string
(Ar)	Nucha	spinal cord
(Du)	Nuck	canal of Nuck
(L)	Nucleus	nut
(L)	Nullipara	none + bring forth, not yet pregnant
(L)	Nurse	to nourish
(G)	Nyctalopia	night blindness
(G)	Nystagmus	nodding
(Gr)	Obelian	a pointed pillar portion of sagittal suture between 2 parietal bones
(L)	Obstetrix	midwife
	Obstetrics	surgery, dealing with pregnancy, labour
	Obturator	a stopper of
	Occiput	back of head
	Occult	hidden
	Oculus	eye
	Oddi (Irish physician)	sphincter of Oddi
(G)	Odontoid	tooth-like
(G)	Oesophagus	gullet
(L)	Oestrus	madness or frenzy
(G)	Olecranon	point of elbow
(L)	Olfaction	to smell
(G)	Oligo	few
(G)	Omohyoid	shoulder + hyoid bone
(G)	Omphalos	omphalocoele (umbilicus)
(G)	Oopheron	ovary
(L)	Operation	to work
(L)	Operculum	lip
(Gr)	Ophth	eye
(Gr)	Optics	belonging to sight, optic chiasma; optic disc
(L)	Oral	of mouth
(L)	Orbicularis	circular
(G)	Orchitis	testicle inflammations
(L)	Organ	any part of the body with a special function
(Gr)	Osmosis	push
(L)	Ossicle	small bone
(Gr)	Otic	ear, otic ganglion
(L)	Ovary	egg receptacle

(G)	Oxyntic	to make sour
	Pacchioni (Italian anatomist)	arachnoid granulations
(Gr)	Pachymeninx	thick membrane
	Pacini (Italian anatomist)	pacinian corpuscle
(G)	Paediatrics	child + healing
	Paget (English surgeon)	Paget's disease
(G)	Palaco	old
(L)	Pallid	pale
(L)	Pallium	clock or mantle
(L)	Palpate	to touch
(L)	Palpebra	eyelid
	Palsy	paralysis
(L)	Pampiniform	tendril
(G)	Panacea	all healing
(G)	Pan	sweet bread
(G)	Pandemic	all people
(L)	Panniculus	a piece of cloth, a layer of membrane, panniculus carnosus
(L)	Paraffin	little affinity
	Paradidymus	beside + twin-like
(Gr)	Paralysis	weakening
	Parametrium	beside the uterus
	Paraphimosis	constriction of the prepuce behind the glans penis
	Paraplegia	paralysis of lower limbs
	Parenchyma	functional
	Parietal	a wall
	Paronychia	beside nail
	Para	beside
	Passavant (German surgeon)	Passavant's ridge
(L)	Patella	a small dish (sesamoid bone)
(L)	Pecten	a comb
(L)	Pectoral	belonging to breast
(L)	Pedicle	a little foot
	Peduncle	a foot
	Pellagra	skin attack
(L)	Pelvis	a basin
(L)	Penis	tail
(L)	Percussion	beating
(L)	Perforator	to bore through
(G)	Peri	around
(G)	Perilymph	clear watery fluid all around
(G)	Perineum	swim around penis
(G)	Periosteum	around bone
(G)	Periphery	circumference
	Peristalsis	contracting around
	Peritoneum	serous membrance lining abdomen

(G)	Peroneus	anything pointed for piercing
(L)	pes-a foot	hippocampus (foot-like)
(L)	pessary	an oval body (plug)
	Petit (French surgeon)	Petit's triangle
(L)	Petrous	stony, rock, petrous temporal bone
	Peyer (Swiss anatomist)	Peyer's patch (ileum)
(G)	Phagocytosis	eat + cell + osis (fullness), i.e., eating cells
(G)	Phalanx	closely knit row
(G)	Pharynx	musculo membranous sac behind the mouth
(L)	Philtrum	a love charm
(Gr)	Phimosis	stopping up (in relation to prepuce of penis)
(Gr)	Phonation	sound or voice
(Gr)	Physiotherapy	nature + treatment
(L)	Pia mater	soft mother
(L)	Pineal	pine cone
(L)	Pinna	ear
(L)	Piriform	pear-shaped
(L)	Pisiform	pea-shaped
(L)	Pituitary	mucus secretion
(L)	Placenta	flat cake
	Planes	flat
	Plantar	sole of foot
(Gr)	Platysma	flat
(Gr)	Pleo	more
(Gr)	Plethora	fullness
(Gr)	Pleura	serous membrane enfolding lung
(L)	Plexus	woven
(L)	Plica	to fold
(L)	Plumbus	lead
(L)	Pneumo	gas
(Gr)	Podagra	foot
(Gr)	Podalic	foot
(L)	Polarity	relating to pole
(Gr)	Polio	grey matter + inflammation
(L)	Pollex	thumb (strong)
(Gr)	Poly	many
(L)	Pons	bridge
(L)	Popliteus	ham
(L)	Porta	gate
(L)	Post	behind
	Poupart (French anatomist)	Poupart's ligament (inguinal ligament)
(L)	Pregnant	with child
(L)	Prepuce	foreskin
(Gr)	Presbyopia	old age hypermetropia
(Gr)	Proposis	elephant's trunk
(L)	Process	advance

(L)	Procidentia	parts that fall out of place
(Gr)	Prodo	anus
(Gr)	Prodromal	in advance
(L)	Progesterone	before to bear
(Gr)	Prognosis	to know beforehand
	Prolapse	falling
	Proliferate	create or reproduce in quick succession
(L)	Promontory	prominence
(L)	Pronator	to bend forward
(Gr)	Pronephros	before kidney
(Gr)	Prophylaxis	to keep guard (the prevention of a disease)
(L)	Proprioceptive	one's own, to take
(Gr)	Prosencephalon	forward + brain
(Gr)	Prostate	before + stand
(Gr)	Prosthetic	in addtion
(Gr)	Protamine	first + amine
(Gr)	Protein	comprised of amino acid
(Gr)	Protocol	first glue
(Gr)	Protopathic	first + suffering
(L)	Pruritis	itching
(Gr)	Psoas	loin
	Psyche	breath
(Gr)	Pterion	wing
(Gr)	Pterygoid	wing-like
(Gr)	Ptoma	a corpse
(Gr)	Ptosis	falling
(Gr)	Ptyalin	saliva
(L)	Pubis	puberty
(L)	Pud	to be ashamed (pudendal)
(L)	Puerperal	after delivery
(E)	Puke	to vomit
(L)	Pul (prefix)	lung
(L)	Puke	beating
(L)	Pulvinar	cushion, pillow
(L)	Punctum	point
(L)	Putamen	cutting
(Gr)	Pyelo	basin
(Gr)	Pylorus	gatekeeper
(Gr)	Pyramid	swelling
(Gr)	Pyrexia	fever
(L)	Quadri	four
	Quadratus	square
	Quadriceps/quadri	geminus four heads/two twins
(G)	Quartz	rock crystal
(L)	Rabies	rage/madness
(L)	Racemose	cluster of grapes (glands)
(Gr)	Rachitis	spine
(L)	Radical	roots
(L)	Radium	radioactive element

(L)	Radius	small bone of forearm
(L)	Ramus	branch
	Ranvier (French histologist)	node of Ranvier
(Gr)	Raphe	suture
(L)	Rash	eruption of skin
	Rathke (German anatomist)	Rathke's pouch
(L)	Receptor	to receive
(L)	Rectum	upright (misnomer)
(L)	Recurrent	running back
(L)	Refraction	broken (bend)
	Reid (Scottish anatomist)	Reid's base (from lower margin of orbit through centre of external auditory meatus)
	Reil (Greek physiologist)	island of Reil-Insula
	Reissner (Greek anatomist)	Reissner's fibres running through the length of brainstem and spinal cord
	Remarc (German neurologist)	Remarc fibre/non-medullated nerve fibre
(L)	Resection	cut off
(L)	Resin	to flow
(L)	Restiform body	rope-shape (inferior cerebellar peduncle)
(L)	Rete	a net, rete mirabile—a wonderful network, rete testis—tubular network
(L)	Reticulum	a little net
(L)	Retinaculum	to hold back
(L)	Retort	twisted back
(L)	Retro (prefix)	behind, retroverted, retroflexed uterus, retro-pharyngeal space
	Retzius (Swedish scientist)	space of Retzius
(Gr)	Rheumatism	a liability
(Gr)	Rhinencephalon	nose + brain
(Gr)	Rhinoplasty	nose moulding
(Gr)	Rhomboid	rhombus-like
(Gr)	Rhonchus	snoring
(L)	Rigor	rigidity
(L)	Rima	slit, rima glottidis
(L)	Risus	to laugh, risus sardonicus
	Robertson (Scottish ophthalmologist)	Argyll Robertson pupil (pupil sign)
	Robin (German histologist)	perivascular/space in brain
	Rolando (Italian anatomist)	fissure of Rolando
	Rosenmuller (German anatomist)	fossa of Rosenmuller (lateral pharyngeal recess)

	Term	Meaning
(L)	Rostrum	beak of a bird
(L)	Rebella	red
	Ruffini (Italian anatomist)	nerve endings of skin
(L)	Rugat	wrinkled
(L)	Saccharin	sugar
(L)	Sacrum	holy
(L)	Sagittal	arrow
(Gr)	Salpina	trumpet
	Santorini (Italian anatomist)	Santorini's cartilage, Santorini's duct accessory duct of pancreas
(Gr)	Saphenous	clear, easily seen saphenous vein
(Gr)	Sarco	flesh, sarcolemma
(L)	Sartorius	tailor
(L)	Scala	stairway (scala tympani, scala vestibuli)
(Gr)	Scalenus	irregular
(L)	Scalpel	knife
(Gr)	Scaphoid	boat-shaped
(L)	Scapula	shoulder blades
	Scarpa (Italian anatomist)	Scarpa's fascia, (deeper membranous layer of superficial fascia) Scarpa's ganglia 8th nerve ganglia
(Gr)	Schizophrenia	split mind
	Schlemm (German anatomist)	Schlemm's canal at corneo-scleral junction
	Schwann (German anatomist)	cell of Schwann
(L)	Sciatica	pain in loins
(L)	Scirrhus	hard
(Gr)	Sclera	hard
(Gr)	Scoliosis	curvature (lateral)
(L)	Scrotum	skin or hide
(L)	Sebum	grease
(L)	Segmentation	to cut
(L)	Sella turcica	Turkish saddle
(L)	Semen	that which is sown
(L)	Semi	half
(L)	Septum	a dividing wall
(L)	Serratus	like saw
(Gr)	Sesamoid	seed-like (patella)
	Sharpey (English anatomist)	Sharpey's fibres in compact bone
	Sibson	Sibson's fascia
(Gr)	Sigmoid	sigma-like
	Sims position	lithotomy position
(L)	Sinus	anything hollowed out
(Gr)	Skeleton	dried up
(L)	Soleus	sole
(Gr)	Soma	body

(L)	Soporific	deep sleep
(L)	Spatula	flat wooden instrument
(Gr)	Sperm	seed
	Sphenoid	butterfly shaped
(Gr)	Sphincter	bind/tight
(L)	Spine	thorn
(Gr)	Splanchnic	relating to bowels
(Gr)	Splenius	bandage
(Gr)	Spondylitis	vertebra inflammation
(Gr)	Spondylolisthesis	vertebra + sliding
(L)	Squama	scale of fish
(L)	Stapes	stirrup (ear ossicle)
(Gr)	Stasis	standing
(Gr)	Stenosis	narrowing
	Stensen (Danish anatomist)	Stensen's duct, parotid gland duct
(Gr)	Stethoscope	instrument of listening the auscultatory sounds
(L)	Stimulus	to prick
(Gr)	Stoma	mouth
(Gr)	Stomach	mouth bed
(Gr)	Strabismus	squinting
(L)	Stratum	covering
(L)	Stria	furrow
(L)	Stricture	contraction
(L)	Strider	harsh
(Gr)	Stroma	bed
(Gr)	Styloid	pointed
(L)	Sub	under
(L)	Subclavian	under clavicle
(L)	Substantia	essence
(L)	Sudor	sweat
(L)	Sulcus	furrow
(L)	Super	over, above
(L)	Supination	bent backwards
(L)	Sural	calf of leg
(Gr)	Surgeon	hand + work (operator)
(L)	Sustentaculum	support (sustentacular tali)
(L)	Stitch	sewing together
	Sylvius (German anatomist)	Sylvius' fissure, lateral fissure of the brain
(Gr)	Symbiosis	living with
(Gr)	Symphysis	natural union
(Gr)	Syndrome	running together
(G)	Synovia	along with + egg
(L)	Syringe	like a pipe (tube)
(Gr)	Syringomyelia	pipe + marrow
(Gr)	Systole	contraction
(L)	Tabes	wasting away

(Gr)	Taenia	rope-like structure, taenia thalami, taenia coli, hookworms
(L)	Talipes	weak on feet
(L)	Talus	ankle bone
(L)	Tapetum	carpet
(Gr)	Tarsus	Crate—bones of posterior part of foot
(L)	Tectum	to cover
(Gr)	Telangiectesis	end vessel dilatation
(L)	Tellurium	earth
(L)	Temple (temporal)	temple region
(L)	Tendon	to stretch out
	Tenon (German surgeon)	Tenon's capsule (back of eyeball)
(L)	Tensor	stretch out
(L)	Tentorium	tent
(L)	Teres	round
(L)	Testicle	testis (singular)
(Gr)	Tetanus	stretch, tetany
(Gr)	Thalamus	inner chamber
(Gr)	Thallium	young
	Thebesius (German physician)	Thebesian valve, valve of coronary sinus
(Gr)	Thenar	the part of the hand with which one strikes
(Gr)	Theory	speculation
(Gr)	Therapy	care
(Gr)	Thrombus	rump
(L)	Thymus	leaf used for worship
(Gr)	Thyroid	shield (oblong)
(L)	Tibia	shin bone (flute)
Gr)	Tissue	woven
(Gr)	Tone	which can be stretched
(A)	Tooth	an organ of mastication
(Gr)	Topography	a place + description
(L)	Torticollis	twisted
(L)	Torus	bulging place
(Gr)	Tourniquet	instrument for turning
(Gr)	Toxin	poison
(L)	Trabeculae	a little beam
(Gr)	Trachea	wind pipe
(L)	Tract	pathway
(Gr)	Tragus	ear
(L)	Transfusion	pouring out
	Trapezium	table
(Gr)	Trauma	wound
	Treitz (Austrian physician)	lig of Treitz at duodeno-jejunal flexure
(Gr)	Trema	hole
(L)	Tremor	shaking
	Trendelenburg (German surgeon)	Trendelenburg's position, Trendelenburg's sign and Trendelenburg's test

	Term	Meaning
	Trephine	a saw for cutting out circular piece of bone especially skull
	Treves (English surgeon)	bloodless fold of Treves
(L)	Triceps	having three heads
(Gr)	Trichiasis	hair (trichionis)
(Gr)	Tricuspid	three cusps
(L)	Trigeminal	three + twin-like (3 divisions)
(Gr)	Trigone	triangle
(L)	Triquetral	having 3 corners
(Gr)	Trocar	3 quarters
(Gr)	Trochanter	bony process
(L)	Trochlea	pulley
(Gr)	Trophic	nourishment (trophoblast)
(Gr)	Tropism	burning
(L)	Tube	a trumpet
(L)	Tumour	swelling
(L)	Turbinate	spinning top
(L)	Tympanum	kettle drum
	Typhoid	fever typhus like
	Tyson (English anatomist)	Tyson's glands, sebaceous glands on inner side of prepuce
(L)	Ulcer	sore
(L)	Ulna	elbow
(L)	Umbilicus	naval
	Umbo	tympanic membrane
(L)	Unciform	hook-shaped
(L)	Undulant	fever, wave
(Gr)	Urachus	urinary canal of foetus
(Gr)	Uranium	heaven
(Gr)	Ureter	urinary duct
(Gr)	Urethra	to make water
(Gr)	Urobilin	urine + bile
(L)	Urticaria	to burn
(L)	Uterus	womb
	Utricle	a little uterus
(L)	Uvea	grape
(L)	uvula	a little grape
(L)	Vaccine	lymph from cowpox vesicle
(L)	Vagina	sheath
(L)	Vagus	vagabond (wanderer)
(L)	Valency	capacity
	Valentine (German physician)	discovered nucleolus and sex cords of ovary
	Valentine (German anatomist)	Valentine bodies in nervous tissue
(L)	Valgus	bow-legged
	Valsalva (Italian anatomist)	Valsalva sinuses-aortic sinuses

(L)	Valve	leaf of folding door
(L)	Varix (varicose)	dilated veins
	Varolius (Italian anatomist)	pons varolii
(L)	Varus	grown inwards, knock knee—genu varus
(L)	Vas	vessel
(L)	Vastus	large
	Vater (German anatomist)	ampulla of Vater
(L)	Vector	one that bears
(L)	Velum	curtain
(L)	Venereal	belonging to Venus (goddess of love)
(L)	Venter	belly, ventricle
(L)	Vermis	worm
(L)	Vertebra	turning place or joint
(L)	Vertigo	to turn around
	Vesalius (Belgian anatomist)	Father of anatomy
(L)	Vesica	bladder
(L)	Vestibule	enclosed space
(L)	Vestigeal	remnant of something formerly present
(L)	Veterinary	cattle doctor
	Vidius (Italian physician)	vidian nerve, nerve of pterygoid canal
(L)	Villus	tuft of hair
	Virchow (German pathologist)	Virchow-Robin space
(L)	Virus	poison
(L)	Viscus/viscera	vital organ/plural
(L)	Vision	act of seeing
(L)	Vital	to life
(L)	Vitamin	life + amine
(L)	Vitelline	yolk of egg
(L)	Vocal cords	uttering of voice
(L)	Volar	palm of hand
	Volkmann (German physician)	Volkmann's canal
(L)	Voluntary	willing
(L)	Volvulus	to roll
(L)	Vomer	thin plate of bone between nostrils
(L)	Vulva	to roll, to turn around
	Waldeyer (German anatomist)	Waldeyer's ring at oropharyngeal isthmus
	Waller (English physician)	Wallerian nerve degeneration
	Westphal (German neurologist)	Westphal nucleus (part of oculomotor complex)
	Wharton (English anatomist)	Wharton's duct (Submand. duct), Wharton's jelly

	Whisky	water of life
	Whitlow	painful swelling in finger
(E)	Whooping cough	to call/shout
	Widal (French physician)	Widal reaction
	Willis (English anatomist)	circle of Willis
	Winslow (Danish anatomist)	foramen of Winslow
	Wirsung (German anatomist)	pancreatic duct
	Wistar (American anatomist)	pyramids (in kidneys)
	Wolff (German anatomist)	Wolfian or mesonephric
	Wright (American anatomist)	Wright's stain
(Gr)	Xanthine	yellow
	Xeroderma	dry or parched
(Gr)	Xiphoid	sword-like
	Xylol	wood + oil
	Yellow fever	an infectious viral fever
	Young (English physician)	Young's rule
	Zenker (German histologist)	Zenker's solution
	Zinn (German anatomist)	annulus of Zinn (origin of rectus)
(L)	Zona	zone
(Gr)	Zoology	animal + treatise
	Zuckerkandl (Austrian anatomist)	Zuckerkandl's gyrus, subcallosal gyrus
	Zygoma	like a yoke
	Zymogen	ferment producer, zymogen granules in serous acini

Compiled by Dr Krishna Garg

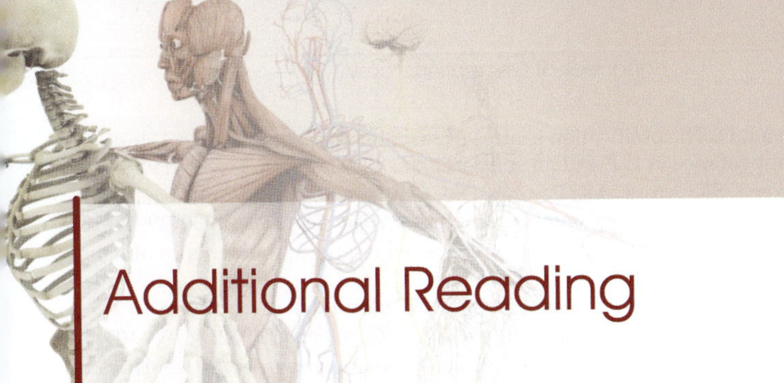

Additional Reading

CHAPTER 1

Field, EJ; Harrison, RJ. Anatomical Terms, their Origin and Derivation, 2nd edn. Heffer, Cambridge, 1957.

Major, RH. A History of Medicine, 2 volumes. Thomas, Springfield, 1954.

Singer, C. A Short History of Anatomy from the Greeks to Harvey. Dover, New York, 1957.

Singh, S. Cadaveric supply for anatomical dissections, a historical review. Indian J. History Med. 1973; 18: 35–39.

Singh, S. Grave-robbers all. Science Reporter, 1972; 9: 492–493.

Singh, S. Susruta, pioneer in human dissections. Souvenir, Anat. Soc. India, 1974; 31–32.

Singh, S. The Illustrious Hunters and the Anatomy Museums. Indian Med. Gaz., 1972; 12: 62–66.

CHAPTER 2

Athawale, MC. Estimation of height from lengths of forearm bones: A study of one hundred Maharashtrian male adults of ages between twenty-five and thirty years. *Am. J. Phys. Anthropol*, 1963; 21: 105–112.

Bajaj, ID; Bhardwaj, OP; Bhardwaj, S. Appearance and fusion of important ossification centres: A study of Delhi population. *Indian J. Med. Res.* 1967; 55: 1064–1067.

Charnalia, VM. Anthropological study of the foot and its relationship to stature in different castes and tribes of Pondicherry State. *J. Anat. Soc. India* 1961; 10: 26–30.

Chhatrapati, DN; Misra, BD. Position of the nutrient foramen on the shafts of human long bones. *J. Anat. Soc. India* 1967; 16: 1–10

Choudhry, R, Raheja, S; Gaur, H; Choudhry, S; Anand, C. Mastoid canals in adult human skulls. *J Anat.* 188: 217–210; 1996.

Das Gupta, SM; Prasad, V; Singh, S. A roentgenologic study of epiphysial union around elbow, wrist and knee joints and the pelvis in boys and girls of Uttar Pradesh. *J. Indian Med. Assoc.* 1974; 62: 10–12.

Garg, K; Bahl, I; Mathur, R; Verma, RK. Bilateral asymmetry in surface area of carpal bones in children. *J. Anat. Soc. Ind.* 1985; 34: 167–172.

Garg, K; Kulshrestha, V; Bahl, I; Mathur, R; Mittal SK; Verma, R. Asymmetry in surface area of capitate and hamate bones in normal and malnourished children. *J. Anat. Soc. Ind.* 1988; 37: 73–74.

Gupta, A; Garg, K; Mathur, R; Mittal, SK. Asymmetry in surface area of bony epiphysis of knee in normal and malnourished children. *Ind. Paed.* No. 10: 1988; 999–1000.

Halim, A. Siddiqui MS. Sexing of atlas. *Indian J. Phys. Anthropol. Hum. Genet.*, 1976; 2: 129–135.

Hasan, M; Narayan, D. Radiological study of the postnatal ossification of the upper end of humerus in UP. Indians. *J. Anat. Soc. India*, 1964; 13: 70–75.

Hasan, M; Narayan, D. The ossification centres of carpal bones: A radiological study of the times of appearance in U.P. Indian subjects. *Indian J. Med. Res.*, 1963; 51: 917–920.

Jeyasingh, P; Saxena, SK; Arora, AK; Pandey, DN. Gupta, CD. A study of correlations between some neonatal and placental parameters. *J. Anat. Soc. India*, 1980; 29: 14–18.

Jit, I. Observations on prenatal ossification with special reference to the bones of hand and foot. *J. Anat. Soc. India* 1957; 6: 12–23.

Jit, I. The house of skeletons case. *J. Anat. Soc. India* 1979; 28: 106–116.

Jit, I. Times of ossification in India (editorial). *Bull. PGI* (*Chandigarh*) 1972; 6: 100–103.

Jit, I; Gandhi, OP. The value of preauricular sulcus in sexing bony pelvis. *J. Anat. Soc. India* 1966; 15: 104–107.

Jit, I; Jhingan, V; Kulkarni, M. Sexing of human sternum. *Am. J. Phys. Anthropol.* 1980; 53: 217–224.

Kate, BR. Nutrient foramina in human long bones. *J. Anat. Soc. India* 1971; 20: 139–144.

Kate, BR. The angle of the femoral neck in Indians. *East. Anthropologist* 1967; 20: 54–60.

Kate, BR; Majumdar, RD. Stature estimation from femur and humerus by regression and autometry. *Acta Anat.* 1976; 94: 311–320.

Kolte, PM; Bansal, PC. Determination of regression formulae for recons-truction of stature from the long bones of upper limb in Maharashtrians of Marathwada region. *J. Anat. Soc. India* 1974; 23: 6–11.

Krogman, WM. *The Human Skeleton in Forensic Medicine*. Thomas, Springfield, Ill, 1962.

Longia, GS; Ajmani, ML; Saxena, SK; Thomas, RJ. Study of diaphysial nutrient foramina in the human long bones. *Acta Anat.* 1980; 107: 399–406.

Maniar, BM; Seervai, MH; Kapur, PL. A study of ossification centres in the hand and wrist of Indian children. *Indian Pediatr.* 1974; II: 203–211.

Modi, NJ. *Modi's Textbook of Medical Jurisprudence and Toxicology* 1977; 20th edn, pp. 27–38 and 80–88, Tripathi, Bombay.

Mysorekar, VR. Diaphysia nutrient foramina in human long bones. *J. Anat.* 1967; 101: 813–822.

Mysorekar, VR; Nandedkar, AN. Diaphysial nutrient foramina in human phalanges. *J. Anat.* 1979; 128: 315–322.

Mysorekar, VR; Nandedkar, AN; Sarma, TCSR. Estimation of stature from parts of humerus and radius. *Medicine. Science and Law* (*Lond.*)

Mysorekar, VR; Verma, PK; Nandedkar, AN. Sarma, TCSR. Estimation of stature from parts of bones, lower end of femur and upper end of radius. *Medicine Science and Law* (*Lond.*) 1980; 20: 283–286.

Narayan, D; Bajaj, JD. Ages of epiphysial union in long bones of inferior extremity in UP subjects. *Indian J. Med. Res.* 1957; 45: 645–649.

Patake, SM; Mysorekar, VR. Diaphysial nutrient foramina in human metacarpals and metatarsals. *J. Anat.* 1977; 124: 299–304.

Pillai, MJS. The study of epiphysial union for determining the age of South Indians. *Indian J. Med. Res.* 1936; 23; 1015–1017.

Prakash, S; Chopra, SRK; Jit, I. Ossification of the human patella. *J. Anat. Soc. India* 1979; 28: 78–83.

Qamra, SR; Jit, I; Deodhar, SD. A mode for reconstructing height from foot measurements in an adult population of north-west India. *Indian J. Med. Res.* 1980; 71; 77–83.

Raheja S, choudhry R, Kakar S, Tuli A. Lateral supracondylar crest of humerus. An unusual presentation JIMSA 14(3): 166–167 (2001).

Raju, BP; Singh, S. Sexual dimorphism in hip bone. *Indian J. Med. Res.* 1979; 69; 849–855.

Raju, PB; Singh, S. Sexual dimorphism in scapula. *J. Indian Acad. Forens. Sci.* 1978; 17: 23–34.

Raju, PB; Singh, S; Padmanabhan, R. Sex determination and sacrum. *J. Anat. Soc. India* 1981; 30: 13–15.

Saxena, SK; Jeyasingh, P; Gupta, AK; Gupta, CD. Estimation of stature from measurement of head length. *J. Anat. Soc. India* 1981; 30: 78–79.

Saxena, SK; Maewal, S; Pandey, DN; Gupta, CD. A study of correlationships between CR length and neonatal and placental parameters. *J. Anat. Soc. India* 1981; 30: 67–69.

Siddiqui, MAH; Shah, MA. Estimation of stature from long bones of Punjabees. *Indian J. Med. Res.* 1944; 32: 105–108.

Singh S; Potturi, BR. Greater sciatic notch in sex determination. *J. Anat.* 1978; 127: 619–624.

Singh, B; Sohal, HS. Estimation of stature from the length of clavicle in Punjabees, a preliminary report. *Indian J. Med. Res.* 1952; 40: 67–71.

Singh, I. The architecture of cancellous bone. *J. Anat.* 1978; 127: 305–310.

Singh, S; Gangrade, KC. The sexing of adult clavicles. Demarking points for Varanasi zone. *J. Anat. Soc. India* 1968; 17: 89–100.

Singh, S; Raju, PB. Identification of sex from the hip bone, demarking points. *J. Anat. Soc. India* 1977; 26: 111–117.

Singh, S; Singh, G; Singh, SP. Identification of sex from the ulna. *Indian J. Med. Res.* 1974; 62: 731–735.

Tandon, BK. A study of the vascular foramina at the two ends of ulna. *J. Anat. Soc. India* 1964; 13: 24–27.

Tuli, A; Choudhry, R; Choudhry, S; Raheja, S; Agarwal, S. Variation in shape of the lingula in the adult human mandible. *J. Anat.* 2000; 197: 313–317.

Ujwal, ZS. Nutrient canal of long bones. *Univ. Rajasthan Studies* 1964; 6: 39–43.

Vare, AM; Bansal, PC. Estimation of crown–rump length from diaphysial lengths of foetal long bones. *J. Anat. Soc. India* 1977; 26: 91–93.

CHAPTER 3

Barnett, CH; Davies, DV; MacConail, MA. *Synovial Joints: Their Structure and Mechanics.* Longmans, London, 1961.

Freeman, MAR. *Adult Articular Cartilag*. Pitman Medical, London, 1973.

Gardner, ED. The innervation of the knee joint. Anat. Rec. 1948; 101: 109–131; The innervation of the shoulder joint. *Anat. Rec.* 1948; 102: 1–18, 1948.

Hilton, *J. Rest and Pain*, Ed. by W.H.A. Jacobson, reprinted from the last London edition, P.W. Garfield, Cincinnati 1891.

Kapandji, IA. *The Physiology of the Joints*. Livingstone, London 1970.

Kellgren, JH; Sarnual, EP. Sensitivity and innervation of the articular capsule. *J. Bone Jt. Surg*. 1950; 32b: 84–92.

MacConail, MA. The function of intra-articular fibrocartilages, with special reference to the knee and inferior radioulnar joints. *J. Anat.* 1932; 66: 210–227.

MacConail, MA; Basmajian, JV. Muscles and Movements. Krieger Publishing Company, New York 1977.

Steindler, *A. Kinesiology of the Human Body*. Thomas, Springfield, Ill 1955.

CHAPTER 4

Gauthier, GF, Schaeffer, SF. Ultrastructural and cytochemical manifestations of protein synthesis in the peripheral sarcoplasm of denervated and newborn skeletal muscle fibres. *J. Cell Sci.* 1974; 143: 113–137.

Jain, P; Tuli, A; Raheja, S; Agarwal, S. Morphological description of variations in the origin of Long Head of Biceps Brachii. An evolution and embryological interpretation. International medical journal. Manuscript No. GS 6109224 Nov. 12, 2012.

Jaya, Y. A brief exposition of AVA, histologically and radiologically. *Proc. Acad. Med. Sc., Hyderabad,* 1957; 1: 15–21.

Jaya, Y. Quantitative anatomy of the capillaries in the rat muscles. *J. Anat. Soc. India* 1962; 11: 32–34.

Kakar, S; Raheja, S; Dinesh, K. Bilateral accessory extensor digitorum muscle in hand. A case repart JIMSA 17(4): 235–236 (2004).

Kate, BR. The cartilage modification of the periosteum. *J. Anat. Soc. India* 1971; 20: 28–32.

MacConail, MA; Basmajian, JV. *Muscles and Movements*. Krieger Publishing Company, New York 1977.

Sadasivan, G; Hanmant Rao, G. Arteriovenous anastomosis in skeletal muscle. *J. Anat. Soc. India* 1964; 13: 90–95.

CHAPTER 5

Bennett, HS; Luft, JS; Hampton, JC. Morphological classification of vertebrate blood capillaries. *Am. J. Physiol.*, 1957; 196: 381–390.

Clark, ER. Arteriovenous anastomosis. *Physiol. Rev.*, 1938; 18: 229–247.

Grant, RT; Payling Wright, H. Anatomical basis for non-nutritive circulation is skeletal muscle exemplified by blood vessels of rat biceps femoris tendon. *J. Anat.*, 1970; 106: 125–134.

Rhodin, JAG. The diaphragm of capillary endothelial fenestrations. *J. Ullrastruct. Res.*, 1962; 6: 171–185.

Rhodin, JAG. Ultrastructure of mammalian arterioles and precapillary sphincters. *J. Ultrastruct. Res.*, 1967; 18: 181–223.

Rhodin, JAG. Ultrastructure of mammalian venous capillaries, venules and small collecting veins. *J. Ultrastruct. Res.*, 1968; 25: 452–500.

Simionescu, N; Simionescu, M; Palade, GE. Permeability of muscle capillaries to small hemepeptides. Evidence for the existence of patent transendothelial channels. *J. Cell Biol.*, 1975; 64: 586–607.

Zweifach, BW. The microcirculation of the blood. *Scient. Am.*, 1959; 200: 54–60.

CHAPTER 6

Allen, L. Lymphatics and lymphoid tissue. *A. Rev. Physiol.*, 1967; 29: 197–12.4.

Boggon, RP; Palfrey, AJ. The microscopic anatomy of human lymphatic trunks. *J. Anat.*, 1973; 114: 389–405.

Jamieson, JK; Dobson, JF. On the injection of lymphatics by Prussian blue. *J. Anat.*, 1910; 45: 7–10; *Lancet*, 1: 1061–1066, 1907; *Proc. R. Soc. Med.*, 2: 149–174, 1908; *Lancet*, 1: 493–495, 1910; *Br. J. Surg.*, 8: 80–87, 1920.

Kinmonth, JB. Some general aspects of the investigation and surgery of the lymphatic system. *J. Cardiovasc. Surg.*, 1964; 5: 680–682.

Nopajaroonskri, C; Luk, SC; Simon, GT. Ultrastructure of the normal lymph node. *Am. J. Path.*, 1971; 65: 1–24.

Roitt, IM. *Essential Immunology*, 3rd edn. Blackwell, Oxford, 1977.

Shridhar. Roentgenographic visualization of human lymphatics, *J. Anat. Soc. India*, 1964; 13: 15–17.

Steinman, RM; Lustig, DS; Cohn, ZA. Identification of a novel cell type in peripheral lymphoid organs of mice. II. Functional properties *in vitro*. *J. Exp. Med.*, 1974; 139: 380–397.

William, PL; Warwick, *R. Gray's Anatomy*, 36th edn. Churchill Livingstone, London, 1980.

CHAPTER 7

Garg, K; Kaul, M; Bahl, I. Textbook of Neuroanatomy with Clinical orientation 6th edn. CBS Publishers & Distributors, New Delhi (2015).

Glees, P; Hasan, *M. Lipofuscin in Neuronal Aging and Diseases*. Georg Thieme Verlag, Stuttgart, 1976.

Glees, P; Hasan, M; Tischner, K. Trans-synaptic atrophy in the lateral geniculate body of the monkeys. *J. Physiol.* (*Lond.*) 1966; 188: 17–19.

Gregson, NA. The chemistry of myelin. In: *The Peripheral Nerve* (London, D.N., Ed.). Chapman & Hall, London, 1975.

Grey, EG. Morphology of synapses. *J. Anat.*, 1959; 93: 420–423, *J. Anat.*, 1961; 95: 345–356, *Prog. Brain Res.*, 1969; 31: 141–155, In: *Essays on the Nervous System* (Bellairs, R. and Gray, E.G., Eds). Clarendon Press, Oxford, 1974.

Hasan, M, Glees, P. Electron microscopic study of the changes in fibrous astrocytes of the lateral geniculate body of blinded monkeys. *J. Anat. Soc. India*, 1974; 23: 1–4.

Hasan, M; Shipstone, AC; Bajpai, VK. Scanning electron microscopy of ventricular ependyma. *Bull. Electron Microscopic Soc. India*, 1978; 2: 1–2.

Jacob, M; Weddell, G. Neural intersegmental connections in the spinal roots and ganglion region of the rat. *J. Comp. Neurol.*, 1975; 161: 115–123.

Jacobs, S; Jacob, M. Intersegmental anastomoses between adjacent dorsal roots of spinal cord in the human. *Neurol. India*, 1971; 19: 51–54.

Linge, EA, et al. Identification of glial cells in the brain of young rats. *J. Comp. Neurol.*, 1973; 146: 43–72.

Palay, SL. Chan Palay, V. General morphology of neurons and neuroglia. In: *Handbook of Physiology* (Kandel, ER, Ed.), Vol. 1, Part 2. Physiological Society, Bethesda, 1977.

Shepherd, GM. *The Synaptic Organization of the Brain*. Oxford University Press, New York, 1974.

CHAPTER 8

Cummins, H; Midlo, C. Finger Prints, Palms and Soles: *An Introduction to Dermatoglyphics*. Dover, New York, 1961.

Montagna, W; Lobitz, WC. *The Epidermis*. Academic Press, New York, 1964.

Montagna, W; Parakkal, PF. *The Structure and Function of Skin*, 3rd edn. Academic Press, New York, 1974.

Sinclair, *D. Cutaneous Sensation*. Oxford University Press, London, 1967.

Zelickson, AS. *Ultrastructure of Normal and Abnormal Skin*. Kimpton, London, 1967.

Zelickson, AS. Ultrastructure of the human epidemis. In: *Modern Trends in Dermatology* (Borrie, P., Ed.), volume 4, Butterworth, London, 1971.

CHAPTER 9

Garg, K; Rath G, Chandra M. *A Textbook of Histology*. CBS Publishers & Distributors, New Delhi, 2023 6th ed.

Mitra, NL. *A Short Textbook of Histology*. Scientific Book Agency, Calcutta, 1979.

Ramachandran, GN. *Treatise on Collagen*. Academic Press, New York, 1967.

Serafini-Fracassini, A; Smith, JW. *The Structure and Biochemistry of Cartilage*. Churchill-Livingstone, Edinburgh, London, 1974.

Wagner, BM; Smith, DE. *The Connective Tissue*, Williams & Wilkins, Baltimore, 1967.

CHAPTER 10

Chandrupatla M, Krishnaiah. The study of bronchial tree. *International Journal of Pharma and Biological Sciences* 2011;2:166–72.

Hush A. Asthma research: The real action is in children. *Paediatr Respair Rev* 2005;6:101–10.

CHAPTER 11

Datta D, Tripathi A, Anand C, Singh AP, Jain S, Khare S. Common Hepatic Artery Variations: A cadaveric Study. *Intl J Med Res Prof* 2017;3(3):155–58.

Jackson JE. Vascular anatomy of the gastrointestinal tract. In: Butler P, Mitchell AWM, 1999.

Kakar S, Raheja S, Anand C, Gupta SR. *Reevaluation of the blood supply of sigmoid colon.* IJCP 1994;4(9):26–30.

CHAPTER 12

Allam AF. Pneumatization of the temporal bone: Ann Otol Rhino Laryngol 1969;78:49–64.

Anderson SD. The Intratympanic muscles. In: Hinchcliffe R (ed). *Scientific Foundations of Otolaryngology*. London: Heinemann; 1976; pp. 257–80.

O'Rahilly R. The timing and sequence of events in the development of the human eye and ear during the embryonic period proper. *Anat Embryol Berl* 1983;168:87–99.

Tabinda Hasan, Satyam Khare, Shilpi Jain, Puneet Gupta, Sanjay Sharma. Retinal Vasculature—an imaging based morphological study. *Journal of the Anatomical Society of India*, 2013;62:146–56.

Netter FH. *Atlas of Human Anatomy*. Los Angels: Icon Learning Systems, 1997.

Whillis J. Movements of tongue in swallowing. *Journal of Anatomy*, 1996;80:115–16.

CHAPTER 13

Mohebati A, Shaha AR. Anatomy of thyroid and parathyroid glands and neurovascular relations. *Clin Anat* 2012;25:19–31.

Rhoton AL. *Cranial Anatomy and Surgical Approaches*. Baltimore: Lippincortt Whilliams & Wilkins 2007.

CHAPTER 14

Braithwaite JL. The arterial supply of the male urinary bladder. *Br J Urol* 1952;24:64–71.

Oelrich TM. The striated urogenital sphincter muscle in the female. *Anat Rec* 1983;205:223.

Oelrich TM. The urethral sphinceter muscle in the male. *Am I Anat* 1980;158:229–46.

CHAPTER 15

Dietz HP. Lanzarone V. Levator trauma after vaginal delivery. *Obstet Gynecol* 2005;106:707–12.

Shoja MM, Sharma A, Mirzaya N, et al. Neuroanatomy of the female abdominopelvic region: A review with application to pelvic pain syndromes. *Clin Anat* 2013;26:66–76.

Garg K, Rath G, Chandra M. Histology of prostate. In: *Textbook of Histology* 6th ed. 2023.

Shenoy KR, Shenoy AN. Vasectomy. In: *Clinical Methods in Surgery*, CBSPD, 2019;520.

CHAPTER 16

Griffiths, HJ; Sarno, RC. *Contemporary Radiography. An Introduction to Imaging*. Saunders, Philadelphia, 1979.

Halim, A. *Surface and Radiological Anatomy*, 3rd edn. CBS, New Delhi, 2011.

CHAPTER 17

BD Chaurasia's Human Anatomy for Dental Students 5th ed: Ch.43.

CHAPTER 18

AETCOM Manual (2021) NA John–Editor

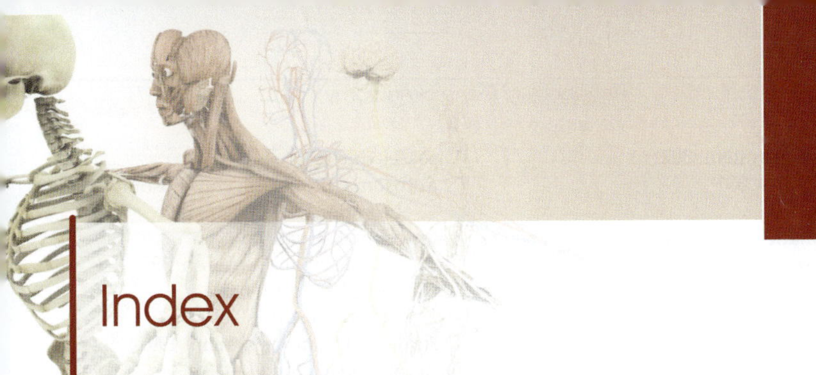

Index